Environmental Gerontology

Environmental gerontology – the research on aging and environment – evolved during the late 1960s, when the domain became a relevant topic due to societal concerns with the problems of housing for elderly people. The field proliferated during the 1970s and 1980s, and remains viable and active today on an international scale. However, in recent times, the viability of the field and its future has been brought into question.

In this volume, international experts across diverse areas reflect on the current progress of their respective disciplines, illustrating research-grounded benefits emerging from their work, and suggesting new agenda that can guide progress in the future. The contributors address a wide range of issues, including: evaluation of existing paradigms and new theories that might advance both research and training; issues and applications in methods, measures, and empirically-generated research agenda; innovative approaches to environmental transformations in home, community, and long-term care settings; and understudied populations and issues in environmental gerontology.

This book was originally published as a special issue of the *Journal of Housing for the Elderly*.

Rick J. Scheidt is a Professor of Lifespan Human Development at Kansas State University, USA. His research focuses on the ecology of aging in small rural towns. He has served on numerous editorial boards and is a Fellow of the Gerontological Society of America, the American Psychological Society, and the Association for Psychological Science.

Benyamin Schwarz is a Professor in the Department of Architectural Studies at the University of Missouri, USA. He has designed numerous facilities for the elderly in Israel and in the United States. His research addresses issues of long-term care settings and fundamentals of Environmental Gerontology. He has been the Editor of the *Journal of Housing for the Elderly* since 2000.

Environmental Gerontology
What Now?

Edited by
Rick J. Scheidt and Benyamin Schwarz

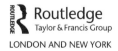 Routledge
Taylor & Francis Group

LONDON AND NEW YORK

First published 2013
by Routledge
2 Park Square, Milton Park, Abingdon, Oxfordshire OX14 4RN

Simultaneously published in the USA and Canada
by Routledge
711 Third Avenue, New York, NY 10017

First issued in paperback 2015

Routledge is an imprint of the Taylor & Francis Group, an informa business

British Library Cataloguing in Publication Data
A catalogue record for this book is available from the British Library

ISBN13: 978-1-138-94449-7 (pbk)
ISBN13: 978-0-415-62616-3 (hbk)

Typeset in Garamond
by Taylor & Francis Books

Publisher's Note
The publisher would like to make readers aware that the chapters in this book may be referred to as articles as they are identical to the articles published in the special issue. The publisher accepts responsibility for any inconsistencies that may have arisen in the course of preparing this volume for print.

Contents

CONTENTS

Citation Information

The chapters in this book were originally published in the *Journal of Housing for the Elderly*, volume 26, issues 1-3 (2012). When citing this material, please use the original page numbering for each article, as follows:

Chapter 1
First Words
Benyamin Schwarz and Rick J. Scheidt
Journal of Housing for the Elderly, volume 26, issues 1-3 (2012) pp. 1-3

Chapter 2
Environmental Gerontology: What Now?
Benyamin Schwarz
Journal of Housing for the Elderly, volume 26, issues 1-3 (2012) pp. 4-19

Chapter 3
The Quest for a New Paradigm: A Need to Rewire the Way We Think
Leon A. Pastalan
Journal of Housing for the Elderly, volume 26, issues 1-3 (2012) pp. 20-25

Chapter 4
Out of Their Residential Comfort and Mastery Zones: Toward a More Relevant Environmental Gerontology
Stephen M. Golant
Journal of Housing for the Elderly, volume 26, issues 1-3 (2012) pp. 26-43

Chapter 5
Environmental Gerontology for the Future: Community-Based Living for the Third Age
Lyn Geboy, Keith Diaz Moore and Erin Kate Smith
Journal of Housing for the Elderly, volume 26, issues 1-3 (2012) pp. 44-61

Chapter 6
Implementation of Research-Based Strategies to Foster Person–Environment Fit in Housing Environments: Challenges and Experiences during 20 Years
Susanne Iwarsson
Journal of Housing for the Elderly, volume 26, issues 1-3 (2012) pp. 62-71

Notes on Contributors

Addie M. Abushousheh, Executive Director, Association of Households International, Manhattan, Kansas, USA.

Matthew Bressette, Fall Prevention Center of Excellence, Andrus Gerontology Center, University of Southern California, Los Angeles, California, USA.

Kate Clark, MPA, Planner, Philadelphia Corporation for Aging, Philadelphia, Pennsylvania, USA.

Stefani Danes, Principal, Perkins Eastman Architects, Pittsburgh, Pennsylvania, USA.

Patrick J. Doyle, PhD Candidate, Center for Aging Studies, Department of Sociology & Anthropology, University of Maryland, Baltimore County Baltimore, Maryland, USA.

J. Kevin Eckert, PhD, Center for Aging Studies, Department of Sociology & Anthropology, University of Maryland, Baltimore County Baltimore, Maryland, USA.

Ann Christine Frankowski, PhD, Center for Aging Studies, Department of Sociology & Anthropology, University of Maryland, Baltimore County Baltimore, Maryland, USA.

Lyn Geboy, PhD, Independent Research and Planning Advisor, Milwaukee, Wisconsin, USA.

Allen Glicksman, PhD, Director of Research and Evaluation, Philadelphia Corporation for Aging, Philadelphia, Pennsylvania, USA.

Stephen M. Golant, PhD, Department of Geography, University of Florida, Gainesville, Florida, USA.

Regina Hrybyk, MA, Center for Aging Studies, Department of Sociology & Anthropology, University of Maryland, Baltimore County Baltimore, Maryland, USA.

Susanne Iwarsson, PhD, Faculty of Medicine, Lund University, Sweden.

Roman Kaspar, PhD, Department of Interdisciplinary Ageing Research, Faculty of Educational Sciences, Goethe University Frankfurt, Germany.

Migette L. Kaup, PhD, College of Human Ecology & K-State Center on Aging, Kansas State University, Manhattan, Kansas, USA.

Lynn Keimig, PhD Candidate, Center for Aging Studies, Department of Sociology & Anthropology, University of Maryland, Baltimore County Baltimore, Maryland, USA.

Morton Kleban, PhD, Director of Psychometrics, Abramson Center for Jewish Life, North Wales, Pennsylvania, USA.

Sonne Lemke, PhD, Research Psychologist in the Center for Health Care Evaluation, VA Palo Alto Health Care System, California, USA.

James Lubben, D.S.W, M.P.H, Boston College, Graduate School of Social Work, Chestnut Hill, Massachusetts, USA.

Keith Diaz Moore, PhD, School of Architecture Design and Planning, University of Kansas, Lawrence, Kansas, USA.

Mary Nemec, MSW, Center for Aging Studies, Department of Sociology & Anthropology, University of Maryland, Baltimore County Baltimore, Maryland, USA.

Anna Quyen Do Nguyen, OTD, Fall Prevention Center of Excellence, Andrus Gerontology Center, University of Southern California, Los Angeles, California, USA.

Carolyn Norris-Baker, PhD, Professor Emerita Kansas State University, Manhattan, Kansas, USA.

Julie A. Norstrand, PhD Candidate, School of Social Work, Boston College, Chestnut Hill, Massachusetts, USA.

Frank Oswald, PhD, Department of Interdisciplinary Ageing Research, Faculty of Educational Sciences, Goethe University Frankfurt, Germany.

Leon A. Pastalan, PhD, Professor Emeritus Taubman College of Architecture and Urban Planning, the University of Michigan, Ann Arbor, Michigan, USA.

Amanda D. Peeples, PhD Candidate, Center for Aging Studies, Department of Sociology & Anthropology, University of Maryland, Baltimore County Baltimore, Maryland, USA.

Mark Proffitt, PhD Candidate, Institute on Aging and Environment, School of Architecture and Urban Planning, University of Wisconsin, Milwaukee, Wisconsin, USA.

Jon Pynoos, PhD, Fall Prevention Center of Excellence, Andrus Gerontology Center, University of Southern California, Los Angeles, California, USA.

Erin Roth, MA, Center for Aging Studies, Department of Sociology & Anthropology, University of Maryland, Baltimore County Baltimore, Maryland, USA.

Robert L. Rubinstein, PhD, Center for Aging Studies, Department of Sociology & Anthropology, University of Maryland, Baltimore County Baltimore, Maryland, USA.

Rick Scheidt, PhD, School of Family Studies and Human Services, Kansas State University, Manhattan, Kansas, USA.

Benyamin Schwarz, PhD, Department of Architectural Studies, University of Missouri, Columbia, Missouri, USA.

Erin Kate Smith, PhD Candidate, Gerontology Center, University of Kansas, Lawrence, Kansas, USA.

Bernard A. Steinman, PhD, Senior Research Associate, Institute for Community Inclusion, University of Massachusetts, Boston, Massachusetts, USA.

Ruth Brent Tofle, PhD, Department of Architectural Studies, University of Missouri, Columbia, Missouri, USA.

First Words

BENYAMIN SCHWARZ and RICK J. SCHEIDT

Place makes a difference. This statement is highlighted in the *Handbook of Theories of Aging* (Gans, Putney, Bengtson, & Silverstein, 2009), whose editors write in the concluding article: "There appears to be a consensus across disciplines in gerontology that understanding the environment and the individual's place within it is crucial for understanding the aging process" (p. 732). The authors go on to state that "despite recognition of the importance of integrating personal and environmental factors in aging research ... prior to today there have been few attempts to develop aging theory by integrating comparable concepts of individual and environment across disciplines" (p. 732). This is a surprising statement for anyone who is immersed in the field of environmental gerontology because research on aging and environment has existed as a significant line of inquiry within the wide array of gerontological research since the late 1960s.

Gerontologists have recognized that although the inherent genetic and biological program drives the aging process of each organism, aging is equally dependent on the soicophysical environment in which the individual resides. Researchers have acknowledged the role of place in the aging process and the manner in which it affects aging as it unfolds and manifests itself in different contexts. Contrary to the above statement, various theories have been suggested since the inception of the field to address the complex interaction of elderly people with the environment on a range of scales from private homes to neighborhoods and complete cities (Scheidt & Windley, 1998; Wahl, 2001). However, "the in-depth understanding of person–environment processes and outcomes has so far not been achieved by one major theory; rather, a multitude of conceptual approaches that augment and build on each other in a pluralistic manner infuse the field" (Wahl & Gitlin, 2007, p. 497).

Environmental gerontology strives to understand the continually changing interrelations between aging people and their sociophysical environment and how these relationships shape the human aging progression. The underlying assumption of the field is that as people age and their competencies decline, they become particularly vulnerable to features of their environments. As a result, place makes a difference in connection with individuals' sociocultural background, somatic and psychic health, and cognitive and physical, functional abilities. Studies of aging and the environment stress ordinary contexts of aging individuals, highlighting the notion that these everyday milieus deserve attention and rigorous research. Given the focus of the field on modification and optimization, researchers in environmental gerontology endeavor to contribute to the improvement of quality of life of elderly people.

Through involvement in modification and the design of housing and public places, practitioners in the field strive for enhancing the well-being of older adults as they age. The field focuses on attributes of person–environment relationships, such as accessibility, privacy, independence, autonomy, and personal control, among elders within various contexts across a continuum of conditions, from high competence to chronic frailty. Environmental gerontology was founded and continues to be nurtured by a diversity of scholarly inputs and interdisciplinary approaches. Many disciplines, such as psychology, sociology, social work, nursing, architecture, interior design, urban planning, social geography, occupational therapy, health and social policy, contribute to the field. Consequently, the disciplines coincide with other research and practice fields in gerontology, such as housing, institutional care, and technology. Although the grounding in a specific disciplinary orientation is generally considered a necessity for scientific research, studying complex phenomena such as the environment and aging calls for an interdisciplinary approach and cross-fertilization of different theoretical perspectives and knowledge bases.

The title "Environmental Gerontology: What Now?" reflects the intention of this special issue. It seeks to explore the current state of the field and to discuss alternative prescriptions for sustaining the vibrant future of studies in aging and the environment. This special issue consists of 16 articles written by 35 nationally and internationally recognized experts who responded to a "Call for Papers" to discuss current and future agendas from their diverse perspectives. Although they do not represent the entire field, their work and leadership have brought the field, to a significant extent, to its present point. We accommodated the wishes of the authors to respond in their own fashion. Some offer thoughtful overviews, some offer new conceptual and methodological approaches, and others illustrate how their specific current work contributes to the needs within the field of environmental gerontology. Their efforts create a rather natural taxonomy, reflecting the current status of studies in the field and future directions these disciplines may take.

1. Paradigms, theories, and context: Stock-taking and new ground
2. Methods and measures: Issues and applications
3. Transforming environments: Home and community contexts
4. Transforming environments: Care-based settings
5. Into the light: Populations and topics deserving more attention

Although each of the contributions has a "stand alone" quality, at the conclusion of the special issue we extract both specific and broader agendas for future research and practice. This diverse triangulation offers *points of light*, so to speak, that may aid our navigation toward *true North*—the goal of improving the quality of life of older individuals by conducting, translating, and applying good science within the ecology of aging.

REFERENCES

Gans, D., Putney, N. M., Bengtson, V. L., & Silverstein, M. (2009). The future of theories of aging. In V. L. Bengtson, M. Silverstein, N. M. Putney, & D. Gans (Eds.), *Handbook of theories of aging* (2nd ed., pp. 723–737). New York, NY: Springer.

Scheidt, R. J., & Windley, P. G. (Eds.). (1998). *Environment and aging theory*. Westport, CT: Greenwood Press.

Wahl, H.-W. (2001). Environmental influences on aging and behavior. In J. E. Birren & K. W. Schaie (Eds.), *Handbook of the psychology of aging* (5th ed., pp. 215–237). San Diego, CA: Academic Press.

Wahl, H.-W., & Gitlin, L. N. (2007). Environmental gerontology. In J. E. Birren (Ed.), *Encyclopedia of gerontology* (2nd ed., vol. 1, pp. 494–502). Amsterdam, The Netherlands: Elsevier.

PART I: PARADIGMS, THEORIES, AND CONTEXT: STOCK-TAKING AND NEW GROUND

Environmental Gerontology: What Now?

BENYAMIN SCHWARZ

Department of Architectural Studies, University of Missouri, Columbia, Missouri, USA

*During the past two decades, environmental gerontology has not flourished as scholars in the field once anticipated. This article considers reasons for this claim, focusing specifically on the place of theory and, more broadly, on the undergirding functions of paradigms for the field. It is argued that progress in this diverse field has slowed in recent years due the decline of useful theoretical research on practice, the limited applicability of current research in the field, and a positivist approach that focuses on predictive, context-*independent *processes while ignoring the physical environment is an essential contextual element in the aging process. Moreover, it is argued that claims that adoption of a natural or "hard" science paradigm will reinvigorate research in environmental gerontology are misguided. Rather, the case is made that environmental gerontology is not a "normal" science (judged against Kuhnian criteria) but appears currently to be in a pre-paradigmatic stage. Debates within the social-behavioral sciences about their "real science" status directly affect environmental gerontology, particularly with regard to context-dependent and independent findings. Consistent with an interpretive perspective, it is argued that because environmental gerontology ultimately solution-driven, it must focus on practical activity and practical knowledge generated from context-bound, every-day practices. This requires holistic methodologies such case studies, precedents, and exemplars necessarily and directly tied to their actual local contexts.*

Since its inception approximately half a century ago, environmental gerontology has aspired to understand, explain, and optimize the interaction between older adults and their environment. Environmental gerontology is concerned with varieties of housing arrangements for the elderly; the nature and effect of home modifications; the range of facilities for institutional care; the role of neighborhoods and community settings; and rural and urban socio-physical contexts (Wahl, 2001; Wahl & Weisman, 2003). Currently, the field consists of a loose confederation of disciplines (e.g., psychologists, sociologists, social workers, allied health professionals, architects, interior designers, community planners, and social policy makers). Investigators in these fields are interested in understanding the ongoing changes in the encounters between older individuals and their social and physical environment (Scheidt & Windley, 2006). As a result of this pluralism within environmental gerontology, the theoretical approaches and the varied research agenda "address very different levels of analysis regarding both place type and scale of social aggregation (from home to neighborhood, to city, and to rural region as well as individual, to group, to organization) and very different processes (such as perceptual, cognitive, and affective" (Wahl & Weisman, 2003, p. 617). Multiplicity of perspectives also confronts empirical research in the field and its application, which extends from information for social policy decisions to planning and to guidelines for the continuum of accommodations for older adults.

In the early 1960s, environmental gerontology was propelled by the mission to improve the lives of the increasing elderly populations, as well as the increasing demand for applied research (Lawton, 1980; Lawton, 1990). At that time, new federal programs for purposely designed housing for older people, and age-segregated public housing was being developed in the United States. Prior to this era, most elderly people and their families were ignored and largely existed as a neglected part of American society. Medicare and Medicaid were still being deliberated in Congress at the time, and when this Social Security Act Amendment finally passed in 1965, it radically transformed the delivery of medical care for American older adults. When the new law was implemented, there were virtually no specialized housing for the elderly and no long-term care services. The majority of the nation's nursing homes were unable to meet Medicare standards for extended-care facilities, and some homes were even having difficulties meeting Medicaid's loose, interim skilled nursing home regulations (Schwarz, 2003). Thus, both the socio-political conditions and the needs of elderly people were in alignment for the development of the new field of environmental gerontology.

The need for the type of research that the newly launched environmental gerontology endeavored was going to undertake was fueled by the incentives created and by the needs in housing and services of an escalating population of older people and the timeliness of the Social Security Act Amendment. The results of this research would provide new knowledge for planners, architects, and administrators, who were eager to know more about environmental attributes and features associated with better outcomes for aging populations. During the 1970s and the early 1980s, Congressional committees, the Department of Housing and Urban Development, the Administration on Aging, the Farmers Home Administration, and the White House were genuinely interested in studies about environment and aging. These agencies and many other organizations funded research, facilitated the dissemination of research findings, and influenced the national policy in congregate housing, design standards for housing, and the design of institutions such as nursing homes (Lawton, 1990). This awareness and attention generated the theory-driven research for creating and improving the settings for older adults. In the initial stages of the field's evolution, the core was driven by applied research, which paved the way to theory development. However, over the years, the orientation of the field has shifted toward more theoretical research with an emphasis on the positivist approach. The field began to focus on predictive, context-independent theories despite its own recognition that the physical environment is an essential contextual element in the aging process.

However, environmental gerontology has not flourished as scholars in this field anticipated. In their effort to explain the widespread dissatisfaction about the state of empirical research in the field, Parmelee and Lawton (1990) noted:

> Several factors may be responsible for the lull in empirical research during the past decades. One possible explanation is the relative standstill in federally assisted housing program development since 1980. Similar factors are the relatively small trickle of new nursing home construction and the slowing of community development funds, both of which spurred the research in the 1970s. Another trend that resulted at least partly from diminished federal funds was the somewhat belated interest of the policy and housing services professions in older persons living in ordinary communities. (p. 464)

Concerns over the sluggish state of the field center on the place of theory in environmental gerontology and its relevance for the applied fields, research funding and its influence on knowledge development, and the shift in public construction priorities for programs and services pertaining to elderly people and their environment (Kendig, 2003). The decline in the effect of theoretical research on practice and the enhancement of the elderly's quality of life, as well as the limited applicability of current research in the field, is reflected in the preferences of funding agencies and policymakers who have been looking for more applications of existing studies rather than new theoretical endeavors.

The aims of this article are to call attention to the challenges confronting environmental gerontology and to chart some directions that may make the field meaningful again. I argue that the nature of today's environmental gerontology requires that we look for alternative, more effective direction based on the philosophy of pragmatism and centered around the method of the systematic case study. My intention is not to abolish other philosophical points of view or methodologies in environmental gerontology, but rather to suggest a way to recover environmental gerontology from its current irrelevant position by adopting the conceptually promising perspective of pragmatism.

IS ENVIRONMENTAL GERONTOLOGY A SCIENCE?

Because of the exceptional status of science in western societies and the claim that scientific methodological procedures are the only certain mode of knowing, practitioners in environmental gerontology, as in other human sciences, are commonly asked by governments, institutions, and agencies "to limit their activities to those that have been scientifically validated through experimentation to produce desired effects" (Polkinghorne, 2004, p. 174). Clearly, science developed an amazing ability to articulate and control important features within specific fields of human experience. However, it is also clear that not everything can be achieved by such means. This is obviously apparent when scientific research is translated to fields of practice. For example, although scientific research is a unique mode of inquiry that can inform and guide architectural practice in housing for the elderly, designers typically do not base their design on theoretical scientific findings. Furthermore, scientists and designers work within irreconcilable paradigms of inquiry. Efforts to reconcile them or search for commonalities might not serve either profession. Scientific research with the theories it produces is grounded in past observations and bases its predictions on the assumption that the patterns found in the past will persist in the future. This kind of knowledge is of less relevance for designers who are intent on changing the world in ways not predictable from natural scientific research (Krippendorff, 2006). Designers use empirical knowledge of so-called practice that they accumulate from experience. Clearly, this kind of knowledge is subjective—that is, mostly unverifiable and volatile.

What we call science today is a reasonably distinctive set of claims that have particular characteristic features. Science attempts to understand the empirical world in a search for order. "More specifically, science looks for unbroken, blind, natural regularities (*laws*). Things in the world do not happen in just any old way. They follow set paths, and science tries to capture this fact. Bodies of science, therefore, known variously as 'theories' or 'paradigms' or 'sets of models,' are collections of laws" (Ruse, 1998, p. 39).

The most significant activities in science involve the use of laws to effect explanations. Scientists attempt to show why things are the way they are and how they follow from these laws. A scientific explanation hinges on law and must demonstrate that what is being explained had to occur. In addition, scientific law indicates what is going to happen; in other words, it can predict what will occur under certain conditions. Linked to explanation and prediction is the notion of testability. Any scientific theory needs to be tested against the real world. It can prove to have some empirical support and be confirmed or it can be refuted if the facts speak against it. A scientific theory can be falsified. Thus, science is tentative. Eventually, a scientist must be ready to reject his or her theory. Scientists are not expected to discard their theories as soon as a rival contender surfaces, but they need to be able to change their minds in the face of empirical evidence that falsify their theory. Modern science is distinguished by its capacity to organize, based on mathematical models, concrete information about observable phenomena under general laws. One aim of science is describing the real world and telling us what the world is like. It is also common to think that science tells us why certain things happen and that it seeks to explain and describe.

However, science is only one way to look at, interpret, and develop knowledge about the world. Scientific theories are premised on the idea "that knowledge can be value free, that it can explain the actual workings of the empirical world, and that it can be revised by a better theory as a result of careful observations of empirical events" (Turner, 1991, p. 3). Most scientific theories are essentially deductive theories. They start with definitions of general concepts and suggest several logically ordered propositions about the relationships among concepts. The concepts are linked to empirical phenomena from which hypotheses are derived and then tested against empirical observations (Turner, 1991). These theories are perceived, particularly by governmental funding agencies, as useful tools for predicting and manipulating the environment. As a result, theories of this nature are considered critical for the design of programs devised to ameliorate problems associated with aging (Bentson et al., 2005).

Much of the lament about the lack of progress in environmental gerontology takes its evidence from an awkward comparison with the natural sciences. Just like gerontology, environmental gerontology has always endeavored to become a science (Achenbaum, 1995). Academics who aspire to make the field into a science tend to assure themselves that to advance its research program, the discipline should emulate the hard sciences and concentrate on testing and rejecting hypotheses. Critics of this tendency nicknamed it physics envy (Achenbaum, 1991). The underlying philosophical justification for a scientific approach to environmental gerontology is naturalism, which can be defined in different ways "but in social sciences it is usually taken to mean that human beings belong to an objective natural order and that the social world is continuous with, or arise from, the physical world" (Williams, 2000, p. 49). Therefore, the assumption is that the methodological approach of natural sciences can be applied to the study of the social world.

IS ENVIRONMENTAL GERONTOLOGY A PARADIGMATIC SCIENCE?

According to Kuhn (1962/1970), normal science is characterized by a scientific work that is well organized and occurs within the framework provided by a paradigm. By Kuhn's (1962/1970) account, a mature science always has a paradigm. In the narrow sense, a paradigm is an exemplar, an influential presentation of scientific theory. In the broader sense, a paradigm represents an entire constellation of beliefs, values, techniques, and methods shared by the members of a scientific field. When the activities in a discipline amount to normal (real) science, various puzzles are solved in a manner of the exemplary work and scientists agree on how to approach problems and how to assess possible solutions. However, after some time, several unresolved puzzles occur, and as anomalies multiply, science in that area enters a period of crisis. At that point, a scientific revolution occurs and a new paradigm replaces the old one (Godfrey-Smith, 2003).

Clearly, environmental gerontology is not a normal science. However, some academics argue that all the field needs to become a real science is to give itself a paradigm. However, it is a naïve proposition to think that getting a paradigm is a sufficient condition to assure that a discipline will become real science. A paradigm is not a fantasy or something that can be imposed on a field of investigation. Paradigm, as Kuhn (1962/1970) suggested, cannot be forced on a discipline; it must emerge naturally (Read, 2009). The question then arises as to whether environmental gerontology has a paradigm. For example, can the Press-Competence Model (Lawton, 1982; Lawton & Nahemow, 1973) be considered as the field's paradigm?

The model is unquestionably one of the central theories in the field. The central principle of the theory has been the congruence between the abilities of the individual and the demands and resources available in the environment (Gitlin, 2003; Kahana, 1982; Lawton, 1982, 1989, 1998; Parmelee & Lawton, 1990). As humans age and their competencies decline, the demands from the environment increase, resulting in the need to compensate with environmental prosthetics to reduce the environmental press or to adapt to new conditions to avoid negative outcomes. Lawton (1989) expanded his model over time by adding the notion of proactive behaviors that people adopt to maintain the right balance between the environmental pressures and their declining competencies (Scheidt & Schwarz, 2010).

Nevertheless, despite its prominence, the General Ecological Model of Aging, as this theory is interchangeably called, does not function as a unifying element for organizing the scientific work in environmental gerontology. Regardless of its elegance, the theory cannot be used as an integrating framework, linking all of the fragmented association of disciplines that now constitute environmental gerontology. The plurality of disciplines in environmental gerontology and the growing diversity of outcomes and data make it almost impossible to find a minimal overlap in theoretical explanations or a designation of common ground in the field. However, the questions of whether a field has a paradigm or whether it makes progress are irrelevant, as Kuhn (1962/1970) noted:

> To a very great extent the term 'science' is reserved for fields that do progress in obvious ways. Nowhere does this show more clearly than in the recurrent debates about whether one or another of the contemporary social sciences is really a science ... Probably questions like the following are really being asked: Why does my field fail to move ahead in the way that, say, physics does? What changes in techniques or method or ideology would enable it to do so? These are not, however, questions that could respond to an agreement on definition. Furthermore, if precedent from the natural sciences serves, they will cease to be a source of concern not when a definition is found, but when the groups that now doubt their own status achieve consensus about their past and present accomplishments. (pp. 160–161)

In this passage, Kuhn (1962/1970) articulated the uselessness of the attempt to define a field of studies as a science. The efforts to emulate natural science's success as a gold standard for every field of inquiry simply do not work. Thus, the efforts to transform environmental gerontology into science through the prescriptive approaches for getting a paradigm, changing techniques or methods to emulate the hard sciences, are misguided. In his analysis of the concept of paradigm in sociology, Turner (1991) made the point that perhaps the concept is too strong; he suspects that "no theoretical approach is sufficiently coherent, precise, and established as to constitute paradigm of abstract concepts and laws as well as verified research findings" (p. 29). Environmental gerontology appears to be in a pre-paradigmatic stage. The field has a succession of orientations that guide theoretical activity, but these perspectives do not constitute a paradigm. Currently, no normal-science theories exist in environmental gerontology, and there is no reason to believe in any abstract, context-independent concepts that will evolve in the field in the near future, which will lead the field to an agreed on paradigm.

ENVIRONMENTAL GERONTOLOGY AND THE DEBATE IN THE SOCIAL SCIENCES

Because environmental gerontology is mostly associated with the social-behavioral sciences, the question whether it is a science is part of the larger problem of whether the social sciences constitute real sciences. This has been a continuous debate in the social sciences since the 1960s. On one side, some scholars support the naturalist approach with its scientific theories (positivist theories) that are based on a hierarchical structure of observations and concepts. On the other side, some reject naturalism and instead explore meanings in a social context, whereby situations are interpreted and meanings are constructed and shared. This non-scientific methodology for the social sciences has been called interpretivism since Weber laid the foundation for an interpretive sociology, or what has been termed the sociology of understanding (Layder, 2004; Williams, 2000). Weber's (1949) social theory holds that individuals create the social world through their own meaningful actions and interpret social reality in a subjective way. This philosophical approach is difficult to define clearly. It has no theory or distinctive paradigm. However, interpretive research assumes that the research is conducted in natural settings and offers thick descriptions in the quest to understand what people are doing in these settings and what is happening in social situations. Data analysis is predominantly qualitative, searching for meanings of behaviors and practices. Interpretive research is used widely in the social sciences and often takes the form of a case study. It includes a range of theoretical views and technical procedures, such hermeneutics, field research, social constructionism, phenomenology, symbolic interactionism, and ethnomethodology (Gubrium & Holstein, 1999). It prioritizes the interpretation of human actions and their meanings over measurement, explanation, and prediction.

These well-established perspectives assume that the standard view of science, with its search for laws and regularities, fails to understand the world of everyday life, which is fundamentally open and different from the closed systems that occur only in the science laboratory. Furthermore, social problems are stratified; they consist of complex entities on multiple levels. Moreover, because of the internal structures of individuals, an antecedent representation does not enable prediction of behavior; individuals may behave differently in the same environmental circumstances because they may be in different internal conditions. In other words, the scientific principle that links the same cause to the same effect does not work in the social world. Therefore, an explanation of one's actions or behavior is entirely individual and cannot explain the same action of others. Because the variability between actions and meaning in the social universe is so large, it does not allow causal explanation. Consequently, scholars who conduct research under these perspectives believe that the nature of the social universe excludes science as a useful mode of inquiry. They contend that human beings can change the nature of their world and constantly remake their universe. Therefore, the social sciences cannot have laws like those that characterize the natural science, and the strategy of explanation used in the natural sciences must be replaced by one of interpretive understanding.

In his book *Making Social Science Matter*, Flyvbjerg (2001) argued that the natural sciences are better equipped for testing hypotheses to unveil abstract principles and rules among variables, whereas the social sciences are more suitable for producing contextual knowledge about how to understand

and act in contextualized settings based on values and interests. Although the social sciences are well-suited to deliberate about values and interests, the natural sciences are not. The natural sciences are particularly appropriate for conducting decontextualized experiments to understand abstract and generalizable relationships, whereas the social sciences are more suitable for understanding localized, intimate human relationships and generating subjective knowledge based on values and interest. Scholars such as Pierre Bourdieu (1977) and Hubert Dreyfus (1982) contend that social science is not a normal science. As Flyvbjerg (2001) notes "[t]he study of individuals and society can never be "normal" in the Kuhnian sense because of the relationship between ideal scientific theory on the one hand and human activity on the other" (p. 38). Similarly, environmental gerontology, with its variability in developing systems that helps enable and sustain the daily functions of life for older adults, grapples with what it can and cannot be.

Discussing Dreyfus' (1982) six criteria for an ideal type of scientific theory, Flyvbjerg (2001) maintains that theory first needs to be explicit; it should be clearly laid out to be understood. Second, a theory must be universal; it should be applicable in all places and across time. Third, a theory should be abstract; it should not be based on concrete examples. Fourth, a theory should be discrete; it should be context-independent, free of human interests, traditions, or organizations. Fifth, a theory should be systematic; "that is, it must constitute a whole, in which context-independent elements (properties, factors) are related to each other by rules or laws" (Flyvbjerg, 2001, p. 39). And sixth, a theory must be complete and predictive. The last property is crucial and is obligatory for scientific theories, but it seems challenging for the social science disciplines.

Flyvbjerg's (2001) central point is that a fundamental problem exists with the attempt to establish theories about the social world by mirroring natural science theories because explaining and predicting social activities using abstract, context-independent theories is not feasible. The reason is primarily due to the centrality of context in human social life. Dreyfus (1982) stated that excluding the context from everyday problems to better follow the characteristics of natural science cause the theory to collapse. As a result, he observes:

> If Dreyfus is right he has identified a fundamental paradox for social and political sciences: a social science theory of the kind which imitates the natural sciences, that is, a theory which makes possible explanation and prediction, requires that the concrete context of everyday human activity be excluded, but this exclusion of context makes explanation and prediction impossible. (Flyvbjerg, 2001, p. 40)

Dreyfus's (1982) analysis created a significant predicament for environmental gerontology because any attempt to study older adults' interaction with the environment cannot be context-free. The context of the socio-physical environment is in the heart of the field—it is its fundamental essence. Therefore, if scientific theory is, by definition, supposed to be context-independent, theory is prohibited in a context-dependent discipline. Stated in another way, although context is essential for defining the relationship between humans and the environment, it needs to be excluded in a theory in order for theory (rules and laws) to be a theory at all. As Flyvbjerg (2001) wrote:

> It is the contradiction between scientific theories' necessary freedom from context and the actual context-dependent of people's expert decisions on what counts as relevant actions that causes predictions on the basis of "theories" about human activity to err at a specific moment; namely, at precisely the moment when action which according to the theory belongs to a distinct category of action, is no longer considered to belong to this category by the people within the group to which the theory applies. (p. 43)

The individuality of the aging process and its dynamic quality, as well as the complexity of the socio-physical environment and the constant changing interactions between the two, reduces the ability of producing cumulative and predictive theory. This contradiction between the essential properties of scientific theory and the nature of the field obviously compromise the aspirations of environmental gerontology to become a normal science.

THEORIES OF ENVIRONMENTAL GERONTOLOGY

Environmental gerontology is inundated with many variations on theoretical approaches, as well as empirical research and research application. However, no particular theoretical approach dominates the discipline (Wahl, & Weisman, 2003). Currently, the field is split between those who concur with the scientific approach to the development of knowledge and environmental gerontologists who believe that there are other, non-scientific ways to conduct research in this context-dependent field. Researchers who endorse the social constructivist and critical perspectives are concerned with the lack of attention to the subjective experience of the aging individual and his or her interaction with the environment, and question the need for additional theoretical models based on positivist logic and quantifiable measurements. They claim that the positivist approach restricts understanding of multifaceted relationships between elderly people and the environment and tends to reduce complex phenomena into graphic charts and simplified analytical schemes. The interpretivist approach to environmental gerontology prefers to describe and understand how the social reality is interpreted and then to concentrate on the subjective meaning of environment and aging. These researchers often use inductive theoretical approaches through qualitative research methods, starting with data gathering and leading through rigorous analysis to the emergence of key concepts.

Regrettably, recent theoretical developments have not had the anticipated effect on empirical research in environmental gerontology and the limited theoretical progress has not lead to new questions and new theoretical perspectives (Wahl & Weisman, 2003). This begs the question: Are scientific theories of environmental gerontology necessary? From the traditional science perspective, theories are essential. Theories help us describe and explain the observable parts of the world. Theories are crucial for useful research about aging and the environment. Lack of theories may limit the application of research findings and hinder cumulative knowledge building (Bengtson, Gans, Puney, & Silverstein, 2009).

However, from another perspective, scientific theories in environmental gerontology are not only uncalled for, but also may be impossible, as mentioned earlier in this essay. According to this view, the development of scientific explanations may be interesting and occasionally productive, but mostly it constitutes an intellectual exercise that is not only unnecessary, but also may be largely irrelevant (Bengtson, Putney, & Johnson, 2005). A third perspective, shared by many advocates, practitioners, and officers of funding agencies, tends to ignore theory altogether and instead tries to pursue solutions to the problems of aging. These practical reformers argue that there are enough theories about aging and the environment and that research should focus on application, assisting elderly people and their families overcome the problems associated with the environment. Another argument is that there are no theories of environment and aging as such—there are only theories in environmental gerontology that explain the continuing interaction between older people and the environment.

One of the crucial arguments in this article is that although scientific knowledge embodies the victory of the general (of the rule) over the particular, we need to be aware of its limitations and realize that the normal scientific ideal has not been achieved and probably cannot be achieved in environmental gerontology. I argue that context must have a more central position in environmental gerontology, and scientific theory a less central one. We need to recognize the significance of the particular and the non-rule-based approach. The certainty and neatness of science that rarely appears in life should not dominate environmental gerontology.

So what should researchers and students in the field do? What are the implications for the practical elements of our research? What kind of methods we should use for our studies of environmental gerontology?

THE FUTURE OF RESEARCH IN ENVIRONMENTAL GERONTOLOGY

The answers to these questions lay in the reevaluation of the central objectives of the field. To create better environments for older adults, the research in environmental gerontology has to lead to sensible and useful knowledge. It cannot simply follow in the footsteps of the natural sciences. Generating more theoretical models and concentrating the research efforts on basic science to guide practitioners with scientific knowledge is ineffective; their occupation requires action under far less certain conditions. However, shifting to a more context-based, social science-influenced theoretical approach can fuel the future direction of environmental gerontology as it continues to seek implementable ways to answer the needs of an increasingly evolving population.

Kurt Lewin, the practical theorist, has been credited for the maxim "There is nothing so practical as a good theory" (Marrow, 1969, p. viii). His famous field theory, which states that the behavior of an individual a function of both the person and the environment (B $=$ f [P, E]), has guided the field of environment and behavior studies and notably influenced the field of environmental gerontology (Parmelee, 1998). However, Lewin (1951) is also recognized as the forefather of action research, which attempts to bridge the gap between social research and social practice. I believe that the link between theory and practice is a central tenet of environment and aging; it stands or falls with the practicality of the research. For example, if a design theory for creating better environments for frail elderly people is not helpful for making design decisions leading to predictable outcomes, it is immaterial. Like in other "communities of practice," research in environmental gerontology hinges on the willingness of those who are supposed to benefit from it to implement the outcomes and continuously evaluate them. The definitive test of the success of any research results lies in the question of whether those results will be accepted or rejected by the social body that they are supposed to benefit. To remain relevant, researchers in environmental gerontology have to ensure that their studies do not only determine causal relationships among variables with the hope of producing theoretical results. We need to address real-world problems that matter and produce meaningful knowledge that practitioners such as policymakers, designers, and providers can use to affect elderly people, their families, and other caregivers.

Currently, research in environmental gerontology focuses on the collection of empirical observations that are used inductively to produce overarching statements about the relationships among the elderly and the environment. The features of this positivist-inspired science include requirements for completeness and precision and for observing causal relations under controlled condition to assure objectivity. However, this type of research produces theories that are too complex to be used by practitioners who must function in real time and respond to situations that are in a constant flux. At issue is the usefulness of this knowledge for practitioners in the realm of aging and the environment that includes care providers, nursing staff, social workers, and others who treat individual people (whether individually or in groups) on a daily basis. The problems are that, at the individual level, people vary in their responses to interventions and that knowledge, which takes the form of statements, rules, and general laws, may produce valid positivist explanations of social problems but fails to provide answers for the particular individual. As a result "practitioners themselves have to inter-pret human science knowledge in terms of its applicability to the particular situation in which they are engaged. Research-generated knowledge does not provide direct instruction that is certain to produce the desired results" (Polkinghorne, 2004, p. 94).

Practice is essentially an activity directed toward accomplishing a goal. Thus, in addition to seeking knowledge about the goal of a practice, in-quiry about practice is concerned with what actions need to be taken to achieve those goals. This type of knowledge is intended to be useful for practice, and it needs to be pragmatic. It is embedded in the prag-matic philosophy, which rather than focusing on a search for underlying laws and truths of the universe, makes efforts to collect, organize, and dis-tribute the practices that have produced their intended results (Polkinghorne, 2004). Following pragmatism, environmental gerontology research should contribute to solutions of real-life problems by using actual cases with all their complexity and contextual dependence. Practice means not only what one can make, but it also involves choice and prioritizing options, which in some cases are based on incomplete knowledge. As Gadamer (1996) explained:

> Science is essentially incomplete; whereas practice requires instant deci-sions. The incompleteness of all experimental science thus means that it not only raises a legitimate claim of universality by virtue of its readi-ness to process new experience, but also is not wholly able to make good this claim. Practice requires knowledge, which means that it is obligated to treat the knowledge available at the time as complete and certain. The knowledge from science, however, is not of this sort. There is thus a fundamental difference between modern science and the pre-modern aggregate of knowledge, which under the name "philosophy" comprehended all human knowledge. This difference is precisely that what we know from "science" is incomplete and therefore, can no longer be called a "doctrine." It consists of nothing other than the current state of "research." (Gadamer, 1996, p. 4)

If we want to make environmental gerontology relevant and transform it from a field of study that has been gradually morphing into a sterile academic activity performed for its own sake, environmental gerontology research should focus on practical activity and practical knowledge that are generated from actual, everyday practices. It needs to focus on case studies, precedents, and exemplars that should not be disconnected form their contexts, and it should function on the basis of practical rationality and judgment. It needs to concentrate on application by solving particular problems in local situations, and it must deal with problems as they holistically present themselves in actual situations.

REFERENCES

Achenbaum, A. W. (1991). Critical gerontology. In A. Jamieson, S. Harper, & C. Victor (Eds.), *Critical approaches to ageing and later life* (pp. 16–26). Buckingham, England: Open University Press.

Achenbaum, A. W. (1995). *Crossing frontiers: Gerontology as a science*. New York, NY: Cambridge University Press.

Bengtson, V. L., Gans, D., Puney, N. M., & Silverstein, M. (2009). Theories about age and aging. In V. L. Bengtson, M. Silverstein, N. M. Putney, & D. Gans (Eds.), *Handbook of theories of aging* (pp. 3–24). New York, NY: Springer.

Bengtson, V. L., Putney, N. M., & Johnson, M. L. (2005). The problem of theory in gerontology today. In Johnson, M. L. (Ed.), *The Cambridge handbook of age and ageing*. Cambridge, MA: Cambridge University Press.

Bourdieu, P. (1977). *Outline of a theory of practice*. Cambridge, UK: Cambridge University Press.

Dreyfus, H. (1982, October). Why studies of human capacities, modeled on ideal natural science can never achieve their goal. Paper presented at The Boston Colloquium for the Philosophy of Science, Boston, MA.

Flyvbjerg, B. (2001). *Making social science matter: Why social inquiry fails and how it can succeed again*. Cambridge, UK: Cambridge University Press.

Gadamer, H.-G. (1996). *The enigma of health: The art of healing in a scientific age*. Stanford, CA: Stanford University Press.

Gitlin, L. N. (2003). M. Powell Lawton's vision of the role of the environment in aging processes and outcomes: A glance backward to move us forward. In K. Warner Schaie, H. W. Wahl, H. Mollenkopf, & F. Oswald (Eds.), *Aging independently: Living arrangements and mobility* (pp. 62–76). New York, NY: Springer.

Godfrey-Smith, P. (2003). *Theory and reality*. Chicago, IL: The University of Chicago Press.

Gubrium, J. F., & Holstein, J. A. (1999). Constructionist perspectives on aging. In V. L. Bengtson, & K. W. Schaie (Eds.), *Handbook of theories of aging* (pp. 287–305). New York, NY: Springer.

Kahana, E. (1982). A congruence model of person-environments interaction. In M. P. Lawton, P. G. Windley, & T. O. Byerts (Eds.), *Aging and the environment: Theoretical approaches* (pp. 97–121). New York, NY: Springer.

Kendig, H. (2003). Directions in environmental gerontology: A multidisciplinary field. *The Gerontologist, 43*, 611–615.

Krippendorff, K. (2006). *The semantic turn: A new foundation for design*. Boca Raton, FL: Taylor & Francis.

Kuhn, T. S. ([1962] 1970). *The structure of scientific revolutions*. Chicago, IL: The University of Chicago Press.

Lawton, M. P. (1980). *Environment and aging*. Albany, NY: Center for the Study of Aging.

Lawton, M. P. (1982). Competence, environmental press, and the adaption of older people. In M. P. Lawton, P. G. Windley, & T. O. Byerts (Eds.), *Aging and the environment: Theoretical approaches* (pp. 33–59). New York, NY: Springer.

Lawton, M. P. (1989). Environmental proactivity in older people. In V. L. Bengston & W. Schaie (Eds.), *The course of life: Research and reflections* (pp. 15–23). New York, NY: Springer.

Lawton, M. P. (1990). An environmental psychologist ages. In I. Altman & K. Christensen (Eds.), *Environment and behavior studies: Emergence of intellectual traditions* (pp. 339–363). New York, NY: Plenum Press.

Lawton, M. P. (1998). Environment and aging: Theory revisited. In R. Scheidt and P. Windley (Eds.), *Environment and aging theory: A focus on housing* (pp. 161–185). Springer.

Lawton, M. P., & Nahemow, L. (1973). Ecology and the aging process. In C. Eisdorfer & M. P. Lawton (Eds.), *The psychology of adult development and aging* (pp. 619–674). Washington, DC: American Psychological Association.

Layder, D. (2004). *Social and personal identity*. London: Sage.

Lewin, K. (1951). *Field theory in social science: Selected theoretical papers*. New York, NY: Harper & Row.

Marrow, A. J. (1969). *The practical theorist: The life of Kurt Lewin*. New York, NY: Basic Books, Inc.

Parmelee, P. A. (1998). Theory and research on housing for the elderly: The legacy of Kurt Lewin. In R. J. Scheidt & P. G. Windley (Eds.), *Environment and aging theory: A focus on housing* (pp. 161–185). Westport, CT: Greenwood Press.

Parmelee, P. A., & Lawton, M. P. (1990). The design of special environments for the aged. In J. F. Birren & K.W. Schaie (Eds.), *Handbook of the psychology of aging* (3rd ed., pp. 465–489). San Diego, CA: Academic Press.

Polkinghorne, D. E. (2004). *Practice and the human sciences: The case for a judgment-based practice of care*. New York, NY: State University of New York Press.

Read, R. (2009). On wanting to say 'All we need is a paradigm' In S. P. Upham (Ed.), *All we need is a Paradigm* (pp. 117–134). Chicago, IL: Open Court.

Ruse, M. (1998). Creation-science is not science. In M. Curd & J. A. Cover (Eds.), *Philosophy of science: The central issues* (pp. 38–47). New York, NY: W.W. Norton & Company.

Scheidt, R., & Schwarz, B. (2010). Environmental gerontology: A sampler of issues and applications. In J. C. Cavanaugh & C. K. Cavanaugh (Eds.), *Aging in America. Vol. 1. Psychological aspects* (pp. 156–176). Santa Barbara, CA: ABC-CLIO, Praeger.

Scheidt, R., & Windley, P. (2006). Environmental gerontology: Progress in the post-Lawton era. In J. Birren & K. W. Schaie (Eds.), *Handbook of the psychology of aging* (6th ed., pp. 105–125). San Diego, CA: Academic Press.

Schwarz, B. (2003). M. Powell Lawton's three dilemmas in the field of environment and aging. In I. R. Scheidt & P. Windley (Eds.), *Physical environments and aging: Critical contribution of M. Powell Lawton to theory and practice* (pp. 5–22). New York, NY: The Haworth Press.

Turner, J. H. (1991). *The structure of sociological theory*. Belmont, CA: Wadsworth Publishing Company.

Wahl, H.-W. (2001). Environmental influences on aging and behavior. In J. F. Birren & K. W. Schaie (Eds.), *Handbook of psychology of aging* (5th ed., pp. 215–237). New York, NY: Academic Press.

Wahl, H.-W., & Weisman, G. D. (2003). Environmental gerontology at the beginning of the new Millennium: Reflections on its historical, empirical, and theoretical development. *The Gerontologist, 43,* 616–627.

Weber, M. (1949). *The methodology of the social sciences*. Glencoe, IL: Free Press.

Williams, M. (2000). *Science and social science: An introduction*. New York, NY: Routledge.

The Quest for a New Paradigm: A Need to Rewire the Way We Think

LEON A. PASTALAN

Architecture and Urban Planning, University of Michigan, Ann Arbor, Michigan, USA

This article aims to give a glimpse of what is involved in making changes from traditional constructs to new constructs in three fields: physics, medicine, and communication. It seemed reasonable to start with an understanding of what other disciplines and professions were doing in shifting their paradigms and the problems of abandoning the cozy comfort of familiar ways of thinking and doing things. Suggestions have been made for the environment and aging in terms of how we can proceed and welcome the promise of new and rewarding opportunities.

INTRODUCTION

In an earlier issue of the *Journal of Housing for the Elderly* (From the Editor, *1*(2), p. 1), I characterized the field as lacking a well-developed framework that could provide a systematic direction to the generation of scientific information or formulation of consistent and relevant in-put for policy issues. However, it was also pointed out that this did not mean the field was chaotic because there were recurring themes that give the field a measure of order and predictability. These themes have been couched in historic, scientific practice and advocacy terms and yet, at the core, the themes endure.

In reviewing the literature from the past several decades, some of the work in the areas of shelter needs and its quality, supportive environment, health, psychosocial, economic, and financial issues, and design has been impressive. However, of late, there appears to be a diminishment in the yield of significant outcomes; we seem to be re-ploughing old ground.

Despite of our periodic successes and enthusiasm about what we have done, what we know, and what we can do, I believe that most of us sense our shortcomings and feel that there is something lacking. That it is time for a serious stocktaking of where we go from here. How do we get to the next level? Is it time to seek a new paradigm?

It seems what this calls for is the necessity to "rewire" our way of thinking and doing things. Shifting paradigms seems to be occurring in many scientific fields, as well some professions. If we examine several of these efforts and their struggles and successes, perhaps we can derive some clues to help us begin our own uncertain intellectual adventures. Before we jump into this vast unknown, I can hear some of our colleagues ask what our commitment is. For example, do we have the will and the knowhow to change? Do we really need to undertake such a risky pursuit? What constructs does this new paradigm require? We can't answer these questions at this juncture because we can't predict what will be involved until we're in the process. Whatever we do and whatever in which direction we go, I don't think we have the choice of staying with the status quo—we either change or become irrelevant.

Paradigms seem to be shifting in many scientific fields, as well as the professions such as medicine and engineering. I would like to briefly discuss three fields that have been relatively successful in changing their paradigms or in the process of changing. I believe physics represents the pioneer in radically changing the way they do their science; medicine represents a paradigm change in process; and communication and information are defined broadly, which is changing the way its adherents think about their field and the research they do. It is interesting that they did not necessarily start out with a plan to shift its paradigm. I am hopeful that these models may prove to be informative for us in our efforts to begin thinking about how we might change.

PHYSICS: THE MODEL FOR ALL OF THE EMPIRICAL SCIENCES

To me, physics represents the premiere model in the physical sciences, and it tends to be the model followed in terms of its concepts and methods for all of the empirical sciences, from biochemistry to the behavioral sciences. A brief description of how the field has had to rewire itself over the past 100 years is fascinating, instructive, and inspirational. By the end of the 19th century and in the early 20th century, classical (or Newtonian) physicists were at a point where they had all but solved the big questions in their field, and many wondered what they were to do for new challenges. In his address to the Royal Society in London in 1900, Lord Kelvin stated that the mission of physics was just about completed, and there were only a few minor things that needed to be cleared up (Einstein & Infeld, 1967, pp. 3–9). Then, in

1905 Albert Einstein published his Special Theory of Relativity (his broader Theory of Relativity came later), which radically altered the notion of time and space (Einstein & Infeld, 1967, pp. 3–9). This created a revolution and shattered the old paradigm.

New ideas began to emerge, and quantum mechanics evolved. Fritjof Capra (1982) said that "quantum mechanics was more than a new law of nature, it involved changing the rules of classical physics logic, i.e., the ordering of rules of thought that physicists need to make deductions. There needed to be a change in the way physics presented itself" (p. 18). Chaos followed for several decades until some were able to rewire themselves with a new logic called quantum logic. It was very painful to switch from the Principle of Certainty that characterized Newtonian physics to the Principle of Uncertainty, where probabilistic outcomes characterize quantum mechanics. The problems of trying to apply the concepts of an outdated world view of Newtonian science to a reality that can no longer be understood in terms of these concepts. There apparently are some physicists who really don't understand quantum mechanics to this day or think it is only half the story. Dr. Leonard Suskind (2008) mentioned that Freeman Dyson in a book review declared that "he was happy with the situation in which we have lived for the past 80 years with separate theories for the classical world of stars and planets and the quantum world of atoms and electrons" (p. 20). Although some conceptual differences may exist within the discipline, the reality of what quantum mechanics reveals keeps expanding. For example, Dr. Lisa Randall (2005) has produced experimental outcomes that demonstrate the existence of a reality called String Theory or M Theory, where there is not one universe but multiverses. The paradigm change that was born of necessity has essentially revolutionized our concept of reality.

MEDICINE, BIOSCIENCES, AND CHANGE

Medicine has been a direct beneficiary of modern physics. An on-going change exists in the conceptual basis of medicine and its relation to the new concepts of subatomic physics not from an abstract, theoretical perspective, but rather from the point of view of concrete clinical experience. The major shift in how cancer drugs are developed and patients are treated is a case in point. For the first time, personalized, targeted therapies are becoming possible. Despite breakthroughs such as the above example, Dossey (1982) believed that it wasn't enough, that medicine was still by and large driven by a model of health and illness and birth and death around an outmoded conceptual model of how the universe behaves. He also believed that although physicists had been painfully eliminating the flaws of their own models, medicine was largely ignoring those necessary revisions. He wanted to correct the irony of modern medicine, believing that no medicine could be modern that did not square with the best of contemporary empirical sciences. However, he captured the dilemma that medicine faces in terms of its struggle to change by noting the enormous success modern medicine has had by using the old model, so why change? In some ways, that is a dilemma that our field exhibits because we have had some success, and the belief is that maybe with a little more funding and research we can do even better, so why talk about changing. Actually, the issue of shifting the medical paradigm is still an open question and probably will remain so for a long time. It may be that there will be two separate models for the foreseeable future: the classical medical model and the new quantum model.

I believe that one of the major questions for environment and aging concerns what the biosciences tell us about aging. For example, how do we conceptually incorporate what neurobiology has to say about the constellations of neural networks that change as we age but in some instances can be reordered and change behavior. What types of research methods need to be invented or adapted to provide us with a better grasp of how these on-going discoveries of how the brain works can inform our field and become an essential part of our conceptual frame?

COMMUNICATION AND THE QUANTUM METHOD

There is currently a ground-breaking use of the quantum method in the psychosocial and environmental area. I believe it represents the potential for a new model and has great promise for the environment and aging field. The specific focus of this new method is on social networking. The primary tool is the ever present cell phone, which goes by several names such as iPhone and smart phone. In a recent *Wall Street Journal* article, Hotz (2011) reported that researchers are harvesting a wealth of intimate details from our cell phones, uncovering the hidden patterns of our social lives, travels, risk of disease, and political views on a scale and detail that has been impossible before now.

He further reports that an on-going study at Massachusetts Institute of Technology (MIT) that has tracked the movements, relationships, places, moods, health, calling habits, and financial expenditures of 60 families using sensors and software on their smart phones (with permission). In this wealth of intimate details, the study is showing patterns of human behavior that can reveal how millions of people interact at home, work, and play. Through the use of this type of research methodology, the data that are generated can predict certain behavioral outcomes with uncanny accuracy.

What is emerging here are research tools capable of finding patterns of human dynamics too subtle to detect by other means. Just to give one an idea of the scope of such research regarding the social networks at Northeastern University in Boston, researchers have discovered how predictable people could be by studying the travel routines of 100,000 European cell phone users. After analyzing more than 16 million recorded bits of information, specifically call dates, time, and location, it was determined that people's movements appeared to follow a mathematical pattern. The researchers determined that with enough information about past movements, they could predict someone's future whereabouts with more than 90% accuracy. Northeastern University physicist Albert Barabasi led the study and stated that people look like little particles that move in space and occasionally communicate with each other. He concluded by saying that we have turned society into a laboratory where behavior can be objectively followed on a large scale.

The scale and detail of information that has been demonstrated portends a revolution in the entire world of environment and behavior including of course environment and aging. Since the late 40's to the present our ability to measure information has climbed and is still climbing at an exponential rate and scale. The transition and the way we measure information also plays a vital role. The designation of bit as a unit of measure of information has taken its place along with inch, pound, quart and minute as a fundamental unit of measure. In *Information*, Gleick (2011) said that the measurement of information has gone from bit to byte to mega to giga to tera to peta to exa and currently to yotta, which has one and 24 zeros, or to give you the same in zeros in a figure: 1,000,000,000,000,000,000,000,000. Looking at these zeros, it is hard to comprehend how much data that represents. Of course, the ever increasing ability of the chip to have more information placed on it will probably soon reach its limit, and then we will have the quantum computer that will provide us with an ever-increasing ability to store and measure data.

It is plain that the capacity to store and analyze incredible bits of information offers us an opportunity to raise our field to another level. For the first time, it is possible to track an individual's environment, aging, and aggregate activities at a scale and precision not ever possible before. The Northeastern University researchers did not look at age and place, but the method definitely makes it possible. The study demonstrated that these advanced capabilities made it possible to treat the entire society as a laboratory and not just a subsample of it. It gives us a universe not just a planet. Dossey (1982) stated that we live in interconnected fields in which biological, psychosocial, and environmental phenomena are interconnected.

The cases cited above, I believe, are instructive of the kinds of constructs, research methods, and analytic tools that can provide us with some of the necessary thoughts regarding where we can begin. It is sobering to realize the struggles both physics and medicine had and are still having with paradigm shifts. Change is not ever easy, whether it's a bad habit or a change in the way we do our science. Doesn't this present us with an exciting potential? Although we currently do not have an equivalent Special Theory of Relativity to start a conceptual revolution, it doesn't mean we can't search for new models of thinking and doing things. Looking to the future, I see seismic changes occurring in our field as we search for ways to reach the next level.

Perhaps Dossey (1982) summarized the situation best by using medicine as an example for us to follow. He feels that a feature of a new model of medicine will be its ability to span the heretofore unbridgeable chasm separating a humanistic medicine and a reductionist bioscience. Shouldn't we be a part of this worthwhile goal?

REFERENCES

Capra, F. (1982). Foreword. In L. Dossey (Ed.), *Space, time and medicine* (pp. I–XI). Boston, MA: Shambhala.

Dossey, L. (1982). *Space, time, and medicine*. Boston, MA: Shambhala.

Einstein, A., & Infeld, L. (1967). *The evolution of physics*. New York, NY: Simon & Schuster.

Gleick, J. (2011). *Information*. New York, NY: Pantheon.

Hotz, R. L. (2011, April 23–24). What they know. *Wall Street Journal*, p. c1.

Randall, L. (2005). *Warped passages*. New York, NY: Harvard University Press.

Suskind, L. (2008). *The Black Hole War*. New York, NY: Little Brown.

Out of Their Residential Comfort and Mastery Zones: Toward a More Relevant Environmental Gerontology

STEPHEN M. GOLANT

Department of Geography, University of Florida, Gainesville, Florida, USA

STEPHEN M. GOLANT

Department of Geography, University of Florida, Gainesville, Florida, USA

To advance the field of environmental gerontology and make it more relevant to other social and behavioral scientists, this paper proposes a holistic, emotion-based theoretical model to judge whether older adults occupy residential environments that are congruent with their needs and goals. The model theorizes that older persons achieve this individual-environment fittingness or "residential normalcy" when they have two overall favorable and relevant sets of emotional experiences: (1) pleasurable, hassle-free, and memorable feelings—and are in their residential comfort zones; and (2) competence and in control feelings—and are in their residential mastery zones. Older persons often find that their residential environments have become emotional battlefields because although they are in their comfort zones, they are out of their mastery zones, or vice versa. Distinguishing these constructs becomes critical as we increasingly judge residential settings not just for their home-like qualities, but also for their ability to provide long-term care.

INTRODUCTION

An acknowledged mission of environmental gerontology is to optimize the fit or congruence between aging individuals and their physical and social environments. The belief is that people do not grow old in some situational, contextual, or environmental vacuum, and that it is better, easier, and less costly to grow old in some places than in others (Golant, 1984, 2011a). Thus, seniors may enjoy better health and care outcomes, engage in more rewarding activities, and attain higher levels of life satisfaction by changing, manipulating, or modifying their residential arrangements (Golant, 1985; Golant, Parsons, & Boling, 2010; Moore, 2005; Scheidt & Windley, 1985, 2006; Wahl & Oswald, 2009).

Studies have relied on various constructs or indicators to assess whether the housing environments of older individuals are congruent with their needs and goals. Most have focused on the appropriateness of their dwelling environments, as indicated by measures of affordability, physical condition, architectural and interior design, household composition, and crowding (Golant, 2011a). More recent studies have a stronger applied or evidence-based focus, consistent with the increasing efforts of both the public and private sectors to make aging in place more feasible for vulnerable older adults. For example, architects and interior designers have investigated how to make the dwelling environments occupied by more physically frail individuals safer (e.g., reducing falling accidents), easier to access (e.g., visitability guidelines), and less demanding and have looked for solutions that enable them to more easily perform their daily tasks and manage their health problems (Gitlin, 2000; Gitlin, Hauck, Winter, Dennis, & Schulz, 2006; Gitlin, Liebman, & Winter, 2003; Hiatt, 2004; Iwarsson et al., 2007).

This past decade has also witnessed a surge in scientific and applied research studies focused on the quality of life and care offered in older people's neighborhoods and communities. The more academic investigations have focused on two broad questions (Golant, 2011a). First, how do the physical layout and design of neighborhoods (e.g., density, land uses, walkability, and new urbanism features) influence the mobility, activities, and physical well-being of their older residents? Second, how does the social fabric of neighborhoods (e.g., their socioeconomic status, ethnic and racial composition, support networks, and social disorders) influence the physical and mental health of older occupants?

Joining these more academic efforts have been many planning- and policy-related studies focused on making neighborhoods and communities supportive of less independent older individuals who are seeking to age-in-place. Municipalities are responding by creating elder "friendly," "healthy," or "livable" communities that make it easier and safer for older residents to cope with their age-related losses and declines. The vocabulary of housing experts now includes transit-oriented developments, home- and community-based services, affordable clustered housing-care, adult day care, naturally occurring retirement communities, supportive service programs, and elder villages (such as the Beacon Hill prototype) (Alley, Liebig, Pynoos, Banerjee, & Choi, 2007; Golant, 2011a, 2011b; Golant et al., 2010).

RATIONALE FOR A NEW THEORETICAL PERSPECTIVE

One might expect that environmental gerontologists should celebrate this proliferation of interest in the fittingness or congruence of older people's residential settings. The problem, if we choose to characterize it as such, is that academics or professionals calling themselves environmental gerontologists are not conducting most of the studies. Another way of framing this issue is to ask whether environmental gerontologists can claim any intellectual territory that exclusively belongs to them. At best, we can offer only equivocal responses.

Perhaps the only consistent and widespread acknowledgment of the literature of environmental gerontology is the reference to Powell Lawton's work. We can point to many reasons for the successful diffusion of his ideas, but one explanation is that he used constructs that were widely familiar not just to environmental gerontologists but to other social and behavioral scientists who could readily adopt his discourse in their studies. For example, in his environmental docility hypothesis, he argued that demanding and stressful residential conditions were more likely to explain the behaviors of less competent older individuals. Thus, those with more severe physical or cognitive limitations are more likely to postpone outside activities because of inclement weather. Similarly, in his environmental proactivity hypothesis, he argued that less competent older individuals were less efficacious users of their everyday settings (Lawton, 1989b).

The vocabulary used in these formulations is decidedly multidisciplinary: *adaptive behaviors*, *docility*, *empowered*, *competent*, *environment*, *affect*, *proactivity*, and *efficacious*. Consistently, Scheidt and Windley (1985), using terminology that had broad appeal to those studying successful aging, depicted an ecology of aging focused on "the processes governing the efforts of the aging individual to respond successfully to both endogenous and exogenous changes (needs and demands) occurring over time" (p. 246).

RESIDENTIAL NORMALCY AND ITS UNDERLYING CONSTRUCTS

In this article, I describe one part of a larger theoretical model (Golant, 2011b) that introduces environmental congruence constructs that are also likely to resonate with other social and behavioral science researchers. Its goal is to offer a more holistic framework by which to judge whether older people are occupying residential settings that are consistent with their needs and goals. It theorizes that we must jointly specify and examine two relatively independent, emotion-based constructs—residential comfort and residential mastery emotional experiences. The model theorizes that older people will occupy congruent or fitting residential settings when they report that both sets of these emotional experiences are overall favorable or positive—that is, they achieve residential normalcy (Golant, 2011b):

> Places where older people experience overall pleasurable, hassle-free, and memorable feelings that have relevance to them; and where they feel both competent and in control—that is, they do not have to behave in personally objectionable ways or to unduly surrender mastery of their lives or environments to others. (p. 193)

CONSTRUCT DEVELOPMENT: THEORETICAL PREREQUISITES

Emotional Experiences

Emotions are a recognized subfield of several academic and clinical disciplines, including psychology, psychiatry, neurosciences, sociology, anthropology, and gerontology (Lewis, Haviland-Jones, & Barrett, 2008), and are widely used by advertising and marketing professionals (Morris, Woo, Geason, & Kim, 2002; Poels & Dewitte, 2006). Words that express emotions fill the languages of contemporary and historical populations and cultures all over the world; thus allowing for the possibility of cross-cultural assessments of environmental congruence.

Psychologists have argued that the emotional reactions of individuals represent "the common core of human response to all types of environments" (Mehrabian, 1980, p. 7) and depend on how they perceive, evaluate, and appraise their environments and activities (Barrett, Mesquita, Ochsner, & Gross, 2007). Consequently, they are relevant constructs to explore the individual–environment fit of a wide range of residential environments—whether ordinary dwellings, planned senior housing, or nursing homes—that are occupied by diverse populations of older adults.

Physical scientists believe that all humans are neurobiologically wired to experience emotion and have the universal capacity to experience pleasure and displeasure (Barrett et al., 2007). They have also shown a heightened interest in exploring how people's self-reports of their emotional experiences are linked to their neurophysiological processes, opening up the possibility that we will eventually be able to rely on neuroimaging techniques to assess variations in how older people feel about where they live (Wager et al., 2008).

Gerontologists have argued for the relevance of studying emotional experiences. They were proposed as "the truly significant organizing and motivational forces in human development and functioning" (Izard & Ackerman, 1997, p. 1). When examining the emotions that people experience over their life spans, one scholar emphasized their importance in this way (Magai, 2001):

"They [are] integral to our sense of well-being or lack of well-being. . . . They are what make individuals care about outcomes, and care in particular ways, with fear, revulsion, joy, shame, excitement, guilt, indignation, and so forth." (p. 399)

Early on, Neugarten, Havighurst, and Tobin (1961), focusing on the antecedents of life satisfaction, recognized the importance of older people deriving pleasure from their activities. More recently, the socioemotional selectivity theory of aging by Carstensen (2006) has emphasized that as older adults recognize the finitude of their lives, they attach greater importance to their emotionally significant and rewarding activities and goals. The environmental press model by Lawton, Kleban, Rajagopal, and Dean (1992) also distinguished the affective responses of older people to measure individual–environment congruence; that is, whether they were engaged in adaptive behaviors that achieved the goal of affective optimization.

Interactional Worldview, but Recognition of an Objective Reality

The focus on how older individuals subjectively experience their residential settings is consistent with an interactional worldview perspective on environmental congruence (Golant, 1986). The focus is "not on how the person and situation, as two separate parts of equal importance, interact [but] rather how individuals by their perceptions, thoughts, and feelings, function in relation to the environment" (Magnusson, 1985, p. 117).

However, the theoretical model also acknowledges that older people are living in "an empirical reality, independent of thinking and perceiving human beings, that is capable of being described in rational and detached terms" (Golant, 1998, p. 42). This objective environment comprises a hierarchical array of places including countries, regions, states, communities, neighborhoods, dwellings, and rooms variously distinguished by their natural, physical, social, technological, and organizational features and attributes. The objective conditions of these places have "functional relevance" to their older occupants. That is, they have the "potential of evoking, reinforcing, or modifying an individual's or population's behaviors and experiences" (Golant, 1984, p. 35), and they present opportunities or constraints for them to realize their residential needs and goals. However, consistent with its interactional perspective, the model assumes that "older adults will not have the same encyclopedic awareness and knowledge of their residential setting's contents, nor the same motivations, capabilities, or confidence to use, manipulate, or interact with their features and attributes" (Golant, 2011b, p. 195).

Competence, Mastery and Successful Adaptation

The constructs, competence, control, and environmental mastery are central to the formulation of the theoretical model. Numerous adult development theorists have linked aging successfully with the ability of individuals to achieve higher levels of functioning and to initiate adaptive strategies that selectively maintain or increase their control over their lives and environments. Representative is Richard Schulz's life span theory, in which "control is a central theme for characterizing human development and relates to the human desire to influence the environment to experience events as contingent upon the self's behavior" (Magai, 2001, p. 403). Thus, individuals who judge themselves as more capable of making things happen and of realizing their needs and goals, and who are more efficacious at shaping their surroundings and achieving desired outcomes are more likely than others to experience positive affective outcomes and higher self-worth or self-esteem (Gecas, 1989; Gurin & Brim, 1984; Schulz & Heckhausen, 1996). Theorists have also emphasized that it is the person's actual experience or perceptions of control that may most matter (Abeles, 1991). As Langer (1983) stated:

> The objective reality may be benign. ... [If] the subjective experience of that reality is such that the individual believes no control is available to him or her, then the negative physical and psychological consequences resulting from this belief will exist regardless of the reality. (p. 283)

These constructs are also central to Maslow's hierarchy of human needs. Consider that four of his five levels—physiological needs, safety needs, esteem needs, and need for self-actualization—are predominantly addressing the individual's needs for competence, control, or mastery. Only possibly the third level, belongingness and love needs, speaks to the individual's need for pleasurable emotional experiences (Maslow, 1954).

And let us remind ourselves what the "good life" means to Rowe and Kahn (1998). They organize their prescription for successful aging around three essential principles that require older adults to avoid disease and disability, maintain a high level of mental and physical functioning, and keep actively engaged in life. The first two of these dictums focus on older people's behavioral, cognitive, or physiological indicators of competence.

Environmental gerontologists have theoretically interpreted the competence of older individuals "as an adaptational response to the interactions or confluence of individual and environmental factors" (Golant, 2011a, p. 216). This interactionist perspective was a major focus of a large empirical research project—the Lund's university ENABLE-AGE project—that showed the extent to which the residential environments of older people were usable, accessible, or presented barriers. This depended not just on whether individuals had functional limitations, but also on whether design features in their home environments helped them compensate for these vulnerabilities (Carlsson et al., 2009; Iwarsson, Nygren, Oswald, Wahl, & Tomsone, 2006; Iwarsson et al., 2007).This perspective is also fundamental to the sociomedical model of disability by sociologists (Verbrugge & Jette, 1994). It recognized that functional limitations may restrict the performance levels of individuals, but "disabilities only result, however, when their physical settings, assistive devices and social supports do not mediate or compensate for their limitations" (Golant, 2011a, p. 210).

At the same time, the environment may be too helpful and stifle feelings of competence. For example, Langer (1983) emphasized how "simply helping people may make them incompetent" because "it communicates to the person that he or she is not able to do whatever it is for him- or herself" (p. 285). Parmelee and Lawton (1990) argued that residents may view the introduction of supportive home modifications as assaults on their independence and tangible evidence that they no longer have control over their life and surroundings.

A THEORETICAL MODEL OF INDIVIDUAL–ENVIRONMENT CONGRUENCE

A major premise of the theoretical model is that the residential congruence or the fittingness of residential settings is usually not an all or nothing affair (Golant, 2011a, 2011b). Some subjective experiences will point to older people occupying a highly appropriate place to live, but others will suggest just the opposite conclusion. Consequently, we cannot simply interpret environmental congruence as an alignment of older people's feelings along a single "good-bad" dimension; otherwise, we risk incomplete, or worse distorted, research findings. Rather, the model argues that environmental congruence requires the specification of two relatively independent sets of emotional experiences labeled residential comfort and residential mastery. Together, they holistically depict how older people will feel about their residential settings.

The first category, residential comfort experiences, captures the extent to which older people feel that they are occupying pleasurable, appealing, and enjoyable places to live that are relatively free of hassles and associated with positive memories. These are exemplified by older people's self-reports of their feeling comfortable (vs. uncomfortable), contented (vs. discontented), happy (vs. sad), joyful (vs. pained), elated (vs. heartsick), stimulated (vs. bored), cheerful (vs. glum), delighted (vs. disgusted), and admiring (vs. disgusted). The second category, residential mastery emotional experiences, captures the extent to which they are occupying places where they feel competent and in control of their surroundings. These are exemplified by older people's self-reports of their feeling influential (vs. influenced), dominant (vs. submissive), autonomous (vs. guided), secure (vs. insecure), powerful (or overpowered), strong (vs. helpless), tranquil (vs. anxious), calm (vs. agitated), encouraged (vs. frustrated), confident (vs. uncertain) and feared (vs. fearful).

The model formulates residential comfort and mastery as orthogonal constructs. However, to some extent there will be reciprocal relationships between these two sets of emotional experiences. It is reasonable to expect that feelings of insecurity and vulnerability will dampen the appeal of an older person's residence (Lawton, 1989a). At the same time, older individuals who thoroughly enjoy where they live may be more open to assistance that enables them to function more effectively (Collins, Goldman, & Rodriguez, 2007).

Residential Comfort Emotional Experiences

Older people will differently feel that their residential settings are enjoyable, pleasurable, or appealing places to live. There is no one-size-fits-all place for older individuals to live—paradise will be in the eyes of the beholder. These diverse emotional experiences testify to the diversity of older Americans. Individuals enter old age with different personalities and demographics and assorted life experiences and residential histories. Consequently, they have different residential preferences and expectations and different resources or capabilities to make them happen (Rowles & Ravdal, 2002). How they unequally experience what is often a long period of old age and cope with its vagaries will further fuel their eclectic views of what constitutes an ideal place to live.

To be sure, some residential situations are likely to elicit more similar or shared emotional experiences than others (Magnusson & Torestad, 1992). Most seniors will not relish occupying physically dilapidated dwellings or communities with high crime rates. However, in response to most environmental aspects, older people will feel differently about where they live, variously experiencing their residential settings as rewarding or unrewarding, and they will have more intense feelings about some features than others (Barrett et al., 2007). The result is that older people may occupy an endless array of objectively distinguishable places in which they have favorable emotional experiences:

- For some, it will be places with a warm year-round climate; for others it will be where the seasons change.
- A large and diverse city with lots of restaurants, shops, theaters, and street activity will be appealing to some; others will be happiest in less bustling and less complex rural settings where they are close to nature.

- Some will be content spending their days in their gardens, playing cards, reading books, listening to music, and having quiet gatherings with a few close friends; others will be most uplifted when they spend time outside their dwellings and they are actively involved in their communities participating in religious activities and volunteering (civic engagement) for important causes.
- Some will find places where they continually enjoy new experiences as most appealing; others will enjoy residential situations that allow them to pursue familiar activities and deviate little from their usual social and recreational activity regimens.
- Some will feel that they are inseparable from the treasured stuff that they have collected over their lives; others will dispose of it as junk.
- Some will enjoy being alone; others will feel uplifted only when they are mingling with family and friends.
- Some will enjoy living in active adult communities; others will be disgusted with the prospects of living with people only their own age.

It will be more appropriate to align some residential experiences of older individuals along a negative scale—for example, disagreeable to very disagreeable (as opposed to pleasurable-unpleasurable) because they typically are sources of stress or anxiety. Others have referred to these experiences as the hassles of life, calling attention to "the irritating, frustrating, distressing demands that to some degree characterize everyday transactions with the environment" (Kanne, Coyne, & Schaefer, 1981, p. 3). Once again, what constitutes hassles will be a personal matter, but some residential experiences are more likely candidates: the snow to shovel, the grass to mow, the oversized dwelling to maintain, the annoying neighbor, or the irritating staff person in the assisted living residence.

The temporal origins of their pleasurable residential experiences will also differ (Golant, 2003). Although many will reflect on their current environmental transactions, the etiology of others will be their remembered pasts. Older people often have strong feelings of attachment to their long-occupied dwellings and personal possessions. These have strong autobiographical significance to them and are important reminders of their good past times (Rowles & Ravdal, 2002). This helps explain why some older people describe the places they live in glowing terms, even when they seem so discordant with their present objective realities. When asked about the dilapidated conditions of nearby properties, an 83-year-old woman responded (Rubinstein, 1998):

> I have news for you. I don't see those houses across the street, In my mind's eye those are the houses that I've seen for 40 years, and that's the way I look at them. I remember the people that used to live there. I remember how it used to be in the summer time, and all like that. (p. 99)

Although the literature has predominantly focused on the positive tone of remembered pasts, it is also likely that troubled or unpleasant experiences will dominate the past residential recollections of some older individuals.

Residential Mastery Emotional Experiences

Four sets of environment–behavior interactions are likely to either exacerbate or alleviate the extent to which older people feel incompetent as occupants of where they live. First, with the onset of chronic health problems and physical limitations, they may feel unable to perform various activities. Dwelling upkeep and maintenance tasks become not just hassles, but confirm their inability to live independently, as is their trouble climbing stairs, opening difficult to grasp faucets, and reaching high closet shelves. Neighborhood features also may heighten their feelings of vulnerability. Sidewalks in disrepair or in heavy traffic locations now make walking difficult. They may curtail their outside-the-dwelling activities because they are afraid of their younger and unfriendly neighbors. Older individuals in more remote rural settings will be more anxious about accessing medical assistance.

Second, older people will have heightened feelings of incompetence because of their personal losses—the death of a spouse or the loss of a longstanding friendship. The absence of these significant others may not only simply dampen what were once enjoyable relationships, but also may threaten their perceptions of self-efficacy. As morale boosters or confidants, they assured older people that they had lived relatively successful and productive lives. By assisting them with their everyday activities, they enabled them to temporarily forget about their inability do things on their own. In addition, when older individuals try to find substitutes for these lost relationships, they necessarily must impose on others for help, and they are further reminded of their vulnerabilities.

Third, older people may feel heightened feelings of incompetence when they experience declines in their environmental cognitive abilities. They may feel particularly challenged after losing their driver's licenses because they are unaware of alternative ways of getting to their destinations, they take longer to reach them, or they get lost more often. When they must impose on others for assistance, they are reminded of their failings again.

Fourth, feelings of incompetence may accompany the loss of self-esteem by older individuals because they are less active members in their community or are no longer productive members of the workforce. This lost sense of pride is magnified when their dwellings do not telegraph to others that they have had successful, worthy, or accomplished lives.

Four other sets of environmental transactions will influence whether older people feel in control of their residential circumstances. First, this will depend on whether they are at the mercy of others to perform either their nondiscretionary daily activities (e.g., dressing, bathing, transferring) or their favorite discretionary social, religious, or recreational activities. The frequency and timeliness of their activities now depends on the permission or participation of others. Second, the ability of older individuals to maintain their privacy—whether in their dwellings, neighborhoods, or residential care facilities—will influence their feelings of being in control. They want to decide who sees, hears, and talks to them, and who is monitoring—administratively or technologically—their activities, behaviors, and movements. Third, because they often feel less confident in their ability to live on their own, they seek predictable interpersonal interactions; they feel more in control when they can trust their relationships with friends, family, staff, or professionals, and these individuals treat them honestly, compassionately, and with dignity. Fourth, because older individuals may experience declines in their financial status, they will enjoy enhanced feelings of control when they can pay for their housing expenses without help or difficulty. Homeowners in particular will have confidence that they can rely on their dwelling's equity to pay for future medical or long-term care costs (Golant, 2008b).

Residential Comfort and Mastery Zones

We theorize that older people can represent each of their sets of residential comfort and residential mastery experiences as overall positive or negative. That is, they can sort through and aggregate each of their sets of feelings according to their directions (e.g., their negative feelings will be counterbalanced by their positive feelings, or vice versa) and intensities or arousal levels (how pleasurable or how stressful (Zautra, Potter, & Reich, 1998).

We also assume that older individuals will be able to appraise how relevant or salient their residential experiences are in their lives. Some will weigh more heavily in their overall place assessments. These will have more psychological importance or greater motivational and behavioral significance to them because they will be satisfying more important needs and goals (Stokols, 1985).

This allows for the possibility that even if the majority of their residential experiences are negative, their assessments may be overall positive if they have a few salient and positive residential feelings. By the same reasoning, a large number of positive but irrelevant residential experiences may be more than offset by a few relevant but negative feelings. As one example, the older widow may view everything about her residential situation as unpleasant and expendable except her geographical closeness to a devoted married daughter, who she highly depends on for her everyday needs.

The model theorizes that older people are in their residential comfort zones or residential mastery zones (Figure 1) when they assign overall posi-

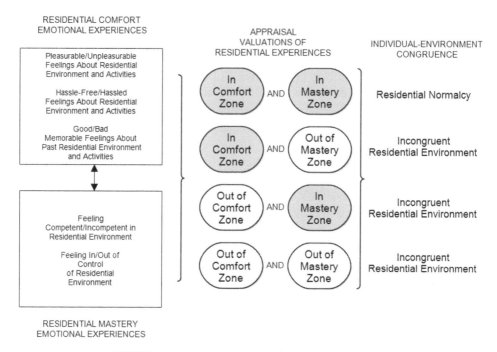

FIGURE 1 Alternative Residential Normalcy Scenarios.

tive appraisal valuations to each of their respective sets of relevant emotional experiences. That is, when in their comfort zones, they will get pleasure and enjoyment predominantly from their place of residence, will not feel hassled, and will have good memories. When in their mastery zones, they will feel mostly competent and in control of their residential surroundings. In the best of worlds, older people will find themselves in both their residential comfort and residential mastery zones. They will have found their sweet spot to live or will have achieved residential normalcy. In the worst of worlds, older individuals will find themselves in incongruent residential settings and out of both their comfort and mastery zones.

OUT OF SYNC RESIDENTIAL COMFORT AND RESIDENTIAL MASTERY EXPERIENCES

Most older people's feelings about where they live will be more equivocal. They will find themselves in their residential comfort zones but out of their mastery zones or vice versa (Figure 1). When confronted with these disparate sets of comfort and mastery experiences, older individuals often find that their housing situations have become emotional battlefields. In particular, those having difficulties managing the declines of old age are often acutely aware of the powerful contradictions between their comfort and mastery feelings. Even as they cling to their desirable home-like settings, they feel increasingly vulnerable and out of control. Pulled in two directions, they feel caught up in what seems like an impossible balancing act. Two prototypical residential scenarios, one played out in ordinary homes and apartments and the other in assisted living residences, help illustrate these conflicts.

Scenario A: Ordinary Homes and Apartments

Longtime older homeowners who are aging-in-place are often squarely in their residential comfort zones. They feel their dwellings are now appealing places to live, recall good memories of their pasts, have found a way to keep their hassles to a minimum, and enjoy the social and recreational opportunities in their neighborhoods and communities. At the same time, the onset of chronic health problems and activity limitations are slowly but unremittingly pushing them out of their mastery zones: they have more difficulties reaching their shopping and medical destinations; a good friend who they relied on for rides has just moved away; they fear showering alone and even simple home maintenance tasks have become burdens; their friends are not calling as often, possibly because they do not want to be around individuals who remind them of their own uncertain vulnerable futures; stairs have become increasingly difficult to negotiate and they have fallen twice in the past month; and because large out-of-pocket medical costs are cutting into their incomes, they are now having difficulty paying for their home mortgage.

Scenario B: The Assisted Living Residence

Assisted-living residences ideally attempt to help their older occupants achieve residential normalcy in two distinctive ways (Golant, 2008a). To keep them in their comfort zones, they offer them home-like and aesthetically pleasing accommodations that mimic the features and ambience of a conventional residence as much as possible (e.g., the creation of smaller scale and more intimate and friendly spaces filled with their furniture and belongings). They offer them restaurant-like dining experiences and outdoor activities and avoid exposing them to an institutional-like environment consisting of nursing stations and medication carts (Calkins & Keane, 2008). To keep them in their mastery zones, they try to respect their privacy, address their self-care needs, and let them participate as much as possible in decisions that affect their activities, care, and well-being.

In practice, the managements of some assisted living fail to meet these ideal goals. It is difficult for them to create home-like and less institutionalized environments in a manner that does not jeopardize their ability to deliver higher quality care and assistance. Consequently, older individuals often feel out of their comfort or mastery zones. Their rooms may be small and uncomfortable; they may have to shower in a common area; they may have to eat at times scheduled by the facility; they are surrounded by very frail residents (who remind them that they too are frail); they find the other residents unfriendly; they must tolerate an errant resident with Alzheimer's disease routinely sleeping in their bed; and they often feel trapped with no other place to go. The assisted-living provider may impose more restrictions on their activities as a way (often well intended) to avoid resident mishaps.

THE NEW REALITY OF ELDERLY HOUSING

In our current scientific and policy worlds, where a proliferation of studies from almost every academic and professional specialty are purporting to study the appropriateness of where older people live, it is increasingly important for environmental gerontologists to effectively claim their intellectual territory. Their contributions must not only be unmistakably driven by an environmental gerontology paradigm, but they must also rely on constructs that are likely to be easily understood and adopted by other social and behavioral researchers and practitioners. The theoretical model proposed in this article attempts to satisfy this mission. It uses an emotion-based framework to conceptualize environmental congruence that recognizes the importance of pleasure, competence, and control in the course of human development.

Elsewhere, I wrote that "older Americans are asking more of their residential environments than any time at history" (Golant, 2011a). This was a recognition that they no longer just view their housing according to how well it realizes traditional outcomes, such as being in good physical condition and affordable, having an attractive architectural and interior design, a home-like ambience, and a convenient location. Rather, in response to threats to their ability to live independently, they are now evaluating their housing not just as a place to live, but also as a long-term care environment enabling them to age in place. They now want the physical design of their dwellings to mollify the effects of their functional limitations and health ailments, their families to help them perform their everyday activities, and their neighborhoods and communities to offer appropriate supportive services and health care.

The proposed theoretical model is a response to the failure of most studies to comprehensively assess or separate out what makes a comfortable, appealing, or enjoyable place to live for their older occupants and what makes a place compatible with their increased vulnerabilities. At the risk of unfairly singling out one body of research, consider the most relied on conceptual framework now guiding investigations of why older people relocate from their residences (Litwak & Longino, 1987). This typology distinguishes three distinctive categories of moves. The first move is amenity, life-style, or want-driven and is typically made by younger retirees seeking a place compatible with their leisure and recreational activities—that is, achieving a more comfortable place to live. On the other hand, the second and third moves are need-based and typically motivated by the onset of physical declines and the loss of significant others—that is, achieving a more competent place to live. Although both are highly relevant moving determinants, the framework explicitly assumes that we can discretely categorize older people into one group or the other and that we can neatly compartmentalize their moving motivations and behaviors.

This analytical divide is no longer consistent with how older Americans view their residential worlds. The increasingly blurred boundaries separating older people's housing and care environments have produced more complex and multidimensional emotional experiences. We now require a more holistic analytical approach to environmental congruence that recognizes the dual importance of both the residential comfort and residential mastery emotional experiences of older Americans. Therein lies their path to residential normalcy.

REFERENCES

Abeles, R. P. (1991). Sense of control, quality of life, and frail older people. In J. E. Birren, J. E. Lubben, J. C. Rowe, & D. E. Deutchman (Eds.), *The concept and measurement of quality of life in the frail elderly* (pp. 297–314). New York, NY: Academic Press.

Alley, D., Liebig, P., Pynoos, J., Banerjee, T., & Choi, I. H. (2007). Creating elder-friendly communities: preparations for an aging society. *Journal of Gerontological Social Work, 49*, 1–18.

Barrett, L. F., Mesquita, B., Ochsner, K. N., & Gross, J. J. (2007). The experience of emotion. *Annual Review of Psychology, 58*, 373–403.

Calkins, M., & Keane, W. (2008). Tomorrow's assisted living and nursing homes: The converging worlds of residential long-term care. In S. M. Golant & J. Hyde (Eds.), *The assisted living residence: A vision for the future* (pp. 86–118). Baltimore, MD: The John Hopkins University Press.

Carlsson, G., Schilling, O., Slaug, B., Fange, A., Stahl, A., Nygren, C., et al. (2009). Toward a screening tool for housing accessibility problems: A reduced version of the housing enabler. *Journal of Applied Gerontology, 28*, 59–80.

Carstensen, L. L. (2006). The influence of a sense of time on human development. *Science, 312*, 1913–1915.

Collins, A. L., Goldman, N., & Rodriguez, G. (2007). *Are life satisfaction and optimism protective of health among older adults?* Princeton, NJ: Princeton Unversity, Office of Population Research.

Gecas, V. (1989). The social psychology of self-efficacy. *Annual Review of Sociology, 15*, 291–216.

Gitlin, L. N. (2000). Adjusting "person-environment systems": Helping older people live the "good life" at home. In R. L. Rubinstein, M. Moss, & M. H. Kleban (Eds.), *The many dimensions of aging* (pp. 41–53). New York, NY: Springer Publishing.

Gitlin, L. N., Hauck, W. W., Winter, L., Dennis, M. P., & Schulz, R. (2006). Effect of an in-home occupational and physical therapy intervention on reducing mortality in functionally vulnerable older people: Preliminary findings. *Journal of American Geriatrics Society, 54*, 950–955.

Gitlin, L. N., Liebman, J., & Winter, L. (2003). Are environmental interventions effective in the management of Alzheimer's Disease and related disorders? *Alzheimer's Care Quarterly, 4*, 85–107.

Golant, S. M. (1984). *A place to grow old: The meaning of environment in old age.* New York, NY: Columbia University Press.

Golant, S. M. (1985). The influence of the experienced residential environment on old people's life satisfaction. *Journal of Housing for the Elderly, 3*(3/4), 23–49.

Golant, S. M. (1986). Subjective housing assessments by the elderly: A critical information source for planning and program evaluation. *The Gerontologist, 26*, 122–127.

Golant, S. M. (1998). Changing an older person's shelter and care setting: A model to explain personal and environmental outcomes. In P. G. Windley & R. J. Scheidt (Eds.), *Environment and aging theory: A focus on housing* (pp. 34–60). New York, NY: Greenwood Press.

Golant, S. M. (2003). Conceptualizing time and space in environmental gerontology: A pair of old issues deserving new thought. *The Gerontologist, 43*, 638–648.

Golant, S. M. (2008a). The future of assisted living residences: A response to uncertainty. In S. M. Golant & J. Hyde (Eds.), *The assisted living residence: A vision for the future* (pp. 3–45). Baltimore, MD: The John Hopkins University Press.

Golant, S. M. (2008b). Low-income elderly homeowners in very old dwellings: the need for public policy debate. *Journal of Aging and Social Policy, 20*, 1–28.

Golant, S. M. (2011a). The changing residential environments of older people. In R. H. Binstock & L. K. George (Eds.), *Handbook of aging and the social sciences* (7th ed., pp. 207–220). New York, NY: Academic Press.

Golant, S. M. (2011b). The quest for residential normalcy by older adults: Relocation but one pathway. *Journal of Aging Studies, 25*, 193–205.

Golant, S. M., Parsons, P., & Boling, P. A. (2010). Assessing the quality of care found in affordable clustered housing-care arrangements: Key to informing public policy. *Cityscape, 12*(2), 5–28.

Gurin, P., & Brim, O. G. (1984). Change in self in adulthood: The example of sense of control. In P. B. Baltes & O. G. Brim (Eds.), *Life-span development and behavior* (vol. 6, pp. 281–334). New York, NY: Academic Press.

Hiatt, L. G. (2004). Environmental design in evoking the capacities of older people. In L. M. Tepper & T. M. Cassidy (Eds.), *Multidisciplinary perspectives on aging* (pp. 63–87). New York, NY: Springer Publishing.

Iwarsson, S., Nygren, C., Oswald, F., Wahl, H.-W., & Tomsone, S. (2006). Environmental barriers and housing accessibility problems over a one-year period in later life in three European countries. *Journal of Housing for the Elderly, 20*(3), 23–43.

Iwarsson, S., Wahl, H.-W., Nygren, C., Oswald, F., Sixsmith, A., Sixsmith, J., et al. (2007). Importance of the home environment for healthy aging: Conceptual and methodological background of the European ENABLE-AGE project. *The Gerontologist, 47*, 78–84.

Izard, C. E., & Ackerman, B. P. (1997). Emotions and self-concepts across the life-span. In K. W. Schaie & M. P. Lawton (Eds.), *Annual review of gerontology and geriatrics* (pp. 1–26). New York, NY: Springer Publishing.

Kanne, A. D., Coyne, J. C., & Schaefer, C. (1981). Comparison of two modes of stress management: Daily hassles and uplifts versus major life events. *Journal of Behavioral Medicine, 4*(1), 1–39.

Langer, E. J. (1983). *The psychology of control.* Beverly Hills, CA: Sage.

Lawton, M. P. (1989a). Behavior-relevant ecological factors. In K. W. Schaie & C. Schooler (Eds.), *Social structure and aging: Psychological processes* (pp. 57–77). Hillsdale, NJ: Lawrence Erlbaum.

Lawton, M. P. (1989b). Environmental proactivity and affect in older people. In S. Spacapan & S. Oskamp (Eds.), *The social psychology of aging* (pp. 135–163). Newbury Park, CA: Sage.

Lawton, M. P., Kleban, M. H., Rajagopal, D., & Dean, J. (1992). Dimensions of affective experience in three age groups. *Psychology and aging, 7,* 171–184.

Lewis, M., Haviland-Jones, J., & Barrett, L. F. (Eds.). (2008). *Handbook of emotions* (3rd ed.). New York, NY: Guilford Press.

Litwak, E., & Longino, C. F. (1987). Migration patterns among the elderly: A developmental perspective. *The Gerontologist, 27,* 266–272.

Magai, C. (2001). Emotions over the life span. In J. E. Birren & K. W. Schaie (Eds.), *Handbook for psychology and aging* (5th ed., pp. 399–426). San Diego, CA: Academic Press.

Magnusson, D. (1985). Implications of an interactional paradigm for research on human development. *International Journal of Behavioral Development, 8,* 115–137.

Magnusson, D., & Torestad, B. (1992). The individual as an interactive agent in the environment. In W. B. Walsh, K. H. Craik, & R. H. Price (Eds.), *Person-environment psychology: Models and perspectives* (pp. 89–125). Hillsdale, NJ: Lawrence Erlbaum Associates.

Maslow, A. (1954). *Motivation and personality.* New York, NY: Harper.

Mehrabian, A. (1980). *Basic dimensions for a general psychological theory: Implications for personality, social, environmental, and developmental studies.* Cambridge, MA: Oelgeschlager, Gunn & Hain.

Moore, K. D. (2005). Using place rules and affect to understand environmental fit: A theoretical exploration. *Environment and Behavior, 37,* 330–363.

Morris, J. D., Woo, C., Geason, J. A., & Kim, J. (2002). The power of affect: Predicting intention. *Journal of Advertising Research, 42*(3), 7–17.

Neugarten, B. L., Havighurst, R. J., & Tobin, S. S. (1961). The measurement of life satisfaction. *Journal of Gerontology, 16,* 134–143.

Parmelee, P. A., & Lawton, M. P. (1990). The design of special environments for the aged. In J. E. Birren & K. W. Schaie (Eds.), *Handbook of the psychology of aging* (3rd ed., pp. 465–488). New York, NY: Academic Press.

Poels, K., & Dewitte, S. (2006). How to capture the heart? Reviewing 20 years of emotion measurement in advertising. *Journal of Advertising Research, 46*(1), 18–37.

Rowe, J. W., & Kahn, R. L. (1998). *Successful aging.* New York, NY: Pantheon.

Rowles, G. D., & Ravdal, H. (2002). Aging, place and meaning in the face of changing circumstances. In R. S. Weiss & S. A. Bass (Eds.), *Challenges of the third age: Meaning and purpose in later life* (pp. 81–114). New York, NY: Oxford University Press.

Rubinstein, R. L. (1998). The phenomenology of housing for older people. In P. G. Windley & R. J. Scheidt (Eds.), *Environment and aging theory: A focus on housing* (pp. 89–110). New York, NY: Greenwood Press.

Scheidt, R. J., & Windley, P. G. (1985). The ecology of aging. In J. E. Birren & K. W. Schaie (Eds.), *Handbook of the psychology of aging* (2nd ed., pp. 245–258). New York, NY: Van Nostrand Reinhold.

Scheidt, R. J., & Windley, P. G. (2006). Environmental gerontology: Progress in the post-Lawton era. In J. Birren & K. W. Schaie (Eds.), *Handbook of the psychology of aging* (6th ed., pp. 105–125). New York, NY: Academic Press.

Schulz, R., & Heckhausen, J. (1996). A life span model of successful aging. *American Psychologist, 51*, 702–714.

Stokols, D. (1985). A congruence analysis of human stress. *Issues in Mental Health Nursing, 7*(1/4), 35–64.

Verbrugge, L. M., & Jette, A. M. (1994). The disablement process. *Social Science & Medicine, 38*(1), 1–14.

Wager, T. D., Barrett, L. F., Bliss-Moreau, E., Lindquist, K. A., Duncan, S., Kober, H., et al. (2008). The neuroimaging of emotion. In M. Lewis, J. M. Haviland-Jones & L. F. Barrett (Eds.), *Handbook of emotions* (pp. 249–267). New York, NY: The Guilford Press.

Wahl, H.-W., & Oswald, F. (2009). Environmental perspectives on aging. In D. Dannefer & C. Phillipson (Eds.), *International handbook of social gerontology* (pp. 111–124). Thousand Oaks, CA: Sage.

Zautra, A. J., Potter, P. T., & Reich, J. W. (1998). The independence of affects is context-dependent: An integrative model of the relationships between positive and negative affect. In K. W. Schaie & M. P. Lawton (Eds.), *Annual review of gerontology and geriatrics: Focus on emotion and adult development* (pp. 75–103). New York, NY: Springer.

Environmental Gerontology for the Future: Community-Based Living for the Third Age

LYN GEBOY

Research and Planning Consultant, Milwaukee, Wisconsin, USA

KEITH DIAZ MOORE

School of Architecture, Design and Planning, University of Kansas, Lawrence, Kansas, USA

ERIN KATE SMITH

Gerontology Center, University of Kansas, Lawrence, Kansas, USA

The viability of the field of environmental gerontology depends upon whether it can make itself practically relevant by helping to resolve some of the urgent, real-world problems facing older adults. Many of the problems relate to which and how residential environments might best forward the goals and aspirations of an aging popu-lation. More attention should be directed toward improving the environments of choice of older adults, which are not institutional settings, but rather their own homes located in neighborhoods and communities. To help direct attention, this article begins by linking the concept of the Third Age with theories of environmental geron-tology and summarizes key empirical understandings of autonomy and security at the community level because these are the essential environmental attributes for the Third Age. Taking into account contextual issues for community-based living for aging suggests that relocation in the pursuit of residential normalcy ought to pro-duce a diversity of environmental responses. We then sketch out the different ways in which three models of community-based liv-ing in the Third Age—the leisure-oriented retirement community, the naturally occurring retirement community, and the villages model—reflect contextual issues as they relate to residential envi-ronments for the Third Age.

INTRODUCTION

Unprecedented growth in the elderly population is washing across the globe. The Population Division of the United Nations projects that by 2050 the world's population will have more people 60 years of age or older than those younger than 15 years of age for the first time in human history (United Nations, 2002). A century of advancements in health and economic prosperity has paved the way for the "longevity dividend" of extended healthy living and delayed aging (Olshansky, Perry, Miller, & Butler, 2006). Enhanced longevity raises profound questions regarding the societal implications of this extraordinary extension in lifespan. What is the role of the older person within the socio-cultural milieu? How might these role expectations affect the built environment? What sorts of environmental design solutions will support the various lifestyle options the older adult cohort is sure to demand? Phenomena related to aging and the manner in which societies respond to aging issues will affect everyone's quality of life. Creating an environmental context that supports successful aging will be a major challenge facing world societies in the coming decades.

The viability of the field of environmental gerontology depends on whether it can make itself practically relevant by helping to resolve some of the urgent, real-world problems of the aging population. Given that 84% of adults age 50 and older want to remain in their own homes while aging (American Association of Retired Persons, 2005), environmental gerontologists' attention should be reapportioned from a focus on institutional environments toward improving the environments of choice of older adults, specifically their own homes located in neighborhoods and communities. To help direct attention, this article begins by linking the concept of the Third Age with theories of environmental gerontology and summarizes key empirical understandings of autonomy and security at the community level because they are the essential environmental attributes for the Third Age. Taking into account contextual issues for community-based living for aging suggests that relocation in the pursuit of residential normalcy ought to produce a diversity of environmental responses. We then sketch out the different ways in which three models of community-based living in the Third Age—the leisure-oriented retirement community (LORC), the naturally occurring retirement community (NORC), and the Village model—reflect contextual issues as they relate to residential environments for the Third Age.

THE THIRD AGE AND ENVIRONMENTAL GERONTOLOGY

Gerontological research, including environmental gerontology, has made important contributions in illustrating the heterogeneity of the aging population. The field has helped to establish that chronological age is only one dimension of aging; lifestyle and life course have emerged as crucial variables in understanding the aging experience. For example, this broader approach is reflected in the concept of the Third Age (Laslett, 1989). In Laslett's four-part conceptualization of the life course, "first comes an era of dependence, socialization, immaturity, and education; second an era of independence, maturity, and responsibility, of earning and of saving; third an era of personal fulfillment; and fourth an era of final dependence, decrepitude and death" (p. 4). The Third Age is the period in the life course when "there is no longer employment and childraising to commandeer time, and before morbidity enters to limit activity" (Weiss & Bass, 2002, p. 3). The Third Age is a time of comparative independence: "freedom from the demands of earlier life, freedom from the need to earn a living, freedom from responsibilities for others" (Weiss & Bass, 2002, p. 4). Paradoxically, it is the responsibilities of family, work, and community that are major determinants of self-identity.

Identity is also shaped by place via place attachment (Rubinstein & Parmelee, 1992). Place attachment is a key concept in environmental gerontology, wherein individual identity and identity of the collective are in perpetual dialogue:

> The fulcrum of the model is identity; life experience, shaped by specific circumstances and personal interpretations, is the single most proximate contributor to sense of place. At the same time, one's position on the collectively defined life course shapes personal experiences, and the meanings one assigns those experiences are, at least in part, derived from and evaluated within the larger socio-cultural context." (Rubinstein & Parmalee, 1992, p. 148)

Yet, juxtapose the place attachment conceptualization of later life and all the richness it entails with the description proffered by Weiss and Bass (2002), in which the Third Age is a phase in human development slotted between one's "life's work" and dependence followed by death. It is not surprising then that the definition for this phase of the life course is ambiguous (Rubinstein, 2002) and invites deliberation regarding which and how residential environments might best forward the goals and aspirations of the Third Age.

Our deliberations will be usefully framed by a recent theoretical contribution that brings a life course perspective to environmental gerontology: Wahl and Lang's (2003) social-physical place over time (SPOT). This model distills the aging adult–environment relationship to two-goal dimensions: agency and belonging. According to the model, these two dimensions are more or less relevant (important) over the life course—with increasing age, belonging becomes more relevant than agency (Table 1). In Early Age/Young Old, the dimensions of agency and belonging are equivalent. The theory's "central assumption is that 'negotiating' SPOT reveals quite different

TABLE 1 Subjective Relevance of Socio-Physical Agency and Belonging over Adulthood and Old Age

Stage of Aging	Relevance of Socio-Physical Agency	Relevance of Socio-Physical Belonging
Middle adulthood	+++	+
Early age/young-old	++	++
Old-old/oldest old	+	+++

Source. Reproduced from Wahl and Lang (2003). Used with permission of Springer Publishing Company, Inc. Permission conveyed through Copyright Clearance Center, Inc.

dynamics across the adult lifespan that are highly relevant for the course and outcomes of aging" (Wahl & Lang, 2003, p. 18).

In linking the SPOT model with the Third Age, two observations are made. First, where Wahl and Lang (2003) defined the transitions in life according to chronological age (e.g., Young-Old and Old-Old), the Third Age perspective moves beyond chronological age and organizes human development according to life stage. Second, regarding goals, Wahl and Lang (2003) adopted language from the field of human development, specifically, the terms agency and belonging. Fortunately, we see undeniable parallels between Wahl and Lang's (2003) terms agency and belonging (which stem from Lang's work on social motivation) and Parmelee and Lawton's (1990) terms autonomy and security, two attributes that are fundamental in the relationship between the older adult and the environment. To wit, where Wahl and Lang (2003) specifically cite autonomy as a correlate concept of agency (p. 18), Parmelee and Lawton (1990) equate autonomy with agency.

The conceptual correspondence extends to the attribute of security, which is, for Parmelee and Lawton (1990), "a state in which pursuit of life goals is linked to, limited by, and aided by dependable physical, social, and interpersonal resources" (p. 465) and means more than physical safety, "but also the communality rather than separateness of the person" (p. 465). Comparably, Wahl and Lang (2003) suggested that belonging involves goal–resource compensation with a focus on the social or communal: "As people experience resource loss, seeking to belong to one's social world (e.g., helping other people or experiencing positive social contact) is expected to obtain greater priority" (p. 18). Extending these ideas specifically to residential environments for those in the Third Age, the interdependence of agency/autonomy and belonging/security is central to the older adult–environment relationship. Furthermore, building on the position of Wahl and Lang (2003), we believe that over time, as agency degenerates with aging, the salience of security intensifies in matters related to the physical environment. We suggest that autonomy is more salient in the Second Age, the Third Age will seek balance between autonomy and security, and

TABLE 2 Subjective Relevance of Autonomy and Security during Life Phases

Life Stage	Relevance of Autonomy	Relevance of Security
Second Age	+++	+
Third Age	++	++
Fourth Age	+	+++

the Fourth Age will be willing to accept sacrifices in autonomy for greater security (Table 2).

AUTONOMY AND SECURITY IN THE THIRD AGE

In considering the array of environmental needs of those in the Third Age, we see the principal issues as relating to those person–environment transactions that produce the place attributes of autonomy and security. This section summarizes key empirical understandings on autonomy and security at the community level of analysis.

Autonomy

At the community level of environment, accessibility (physical distance and mobility) has considerable influence over personal autonomy. For example, the presence of amenities or services, such as pharmacies and grocery stores, plays a role in location selection for older adults (Golant, 2002; Hunt, 2001; Kahana, Lovegreen, Kahana, & Kahana, 2003). Hunt and Ross (1990) found that older residents indicated proximity to grocery stores was an important element in the attractiveness of a location; those stores located within a half-mile facilitated residents' walking to use the amenities and services. Given that many amenities and services may not be located within a half mile of a residence, transportation becomes a related factor in accessing basic amenities and services. Hoehner, Brennan Ramirez, Elliott, Handy, and Brownson (2005) discovered that the proximity and availability of public transportation were positively associated with use, although Walters (2002) cautioned that the proximity of public transportation and libraries only influences use by those who require those services.

The presence of certain social and physical characteristics in a community has a beneficial effect on the health of older residents (Masotti, Fick, Johnson-Masotti, & MacLeod, 2006). This work recognizes that older people are at higher risk for inactivity-associated health problems, and thus promotion of physical activity should be an imperative (AHRQ, 2002). For example, a study by King et al. (2003) suggested that "women who lived within walking distance to a biking or walking trail; department, discount, or hardware store; or park had significantly higher pedometer readings than women who did not" (p. 78). Research in this area should serve to broaden our understanding of the importance of neighborhood-based resources.

With the declines in competency (e.g., physical, cognitive) that accompany aging, the salience of the environment increases (Lawton & Simon, 1968). Thus, when an individual is of marginal competence, access to "neighborhood-based supportive services may make the difference between a positive and a negative outcome" (Lawton, 1980, p. 51). Indeed, Oswald, Schilling, Wahl, and Gäng (2002) found that 43% of relocation motives arose from concerns about the physical environment, not due solely to either personal or social reasons; the researchers conclude that maintenance of autonomy is one of the primary reasons for relocation. When the goal is autonomy maintenance, the older adult may look for ways to compensate for losses or barriers (the selection-optimization-compensation model [Baltes, 1996]). According to Haas and Serow (1993), efforts to compensate may arise from push and pull factors embedded in the relocation decision. For Bekhet, Zauszniewski, and Nakhla (2009), push factors related to relocation include the loss of autonomy in maintaining one's home, and pull factors include proximity to family, services, or amenities that may compensate for perceived losses. In a study of relocations to a continuing care retirement community, Krout, Moen, Holmes, Oggins, and Bowen (2002) detected access to needed services as a pull factor, and not being a burden on family as a push factor. The discrepancy between push and pull factors has been found to negatively affect psychological well-being (Ryff & Essex, 1992). Furthermore, the effect of this discrepancy may be exacerbated when relocations are involuntary (Lawton, 1980).

Security

The topic of the personal safety of community-dwelling older adults is effectively summed up in Lawton's (1980) statement that "the many types of vulnerability associated with aging undoubtedly potentiate the growth of fear" (p. 46). Neighborhood satisfaction is strongly influenced by perceived safety in general (Nasar & Fisher, 1993), especially among elderly residents (Christensen & Carp, 1987). Neighborhood characteristics linked with perceived safety include neighborhood deterioration (Krause, 1998), unattended dogs (King et al., 2000), police inadequacy (Lawton & Hoover, 1979), familiarity with neighborhood social structure (Merry, 1976), and exhibited mobilization behaviors (e.g., bars on windows) (Sundeen & Mathieu, 1976). A perceived sense of safety is a key pull factor in residential decisions of the elderly (Bekhet et al., 2009; Krout et al., 2002).

Variations in perceived safety may relate to differences in place attachment, defined as "a set of feelings about a geographic location that emotionally binds a person to that place as a function of its role as a setting for experience" (Rubinstein & Parmelee, 1992, p. 139). According to Brown and Perkins (1992), place attachment involves a sense of belonging, the expression of self, and feelings of psychological security. Years of social exchanges produced over the course of long-time residency give rise to a strong orientation toward the expectations of a place and a support system of mutual reciprocity (McHugh & Mings, 1996; Rowles & Ravdal, 2002). With respect to rural settings in particular, Norris-Baker and Scheidt (2005) observed that "community culture (or that of an identifiable subgroup within the community) can provide a milieu, including aspects of the physical and social environment, in which late-life developmental changes can be experienced safely and in a psychologically healthy way, supporting needs for community, security, and self continuity" (p. 283).

The need for security (and its correlate territoriality—which promotes security through predictability, order, and stability [Brown, 1987])—is a main factor underlying the desire to age in place (Rowles & Ravdal, 2002). As Lawton (1990) stated, aging in place is "a transaction between an aging individual and his or her residential environment that is characterized by changes in both person and environment over time, with the physical location of the person being the only constant" (p. 288). Thus, although the proximate setting is static, the contextual environment may change over time, and often does. Recognition of the dynamic, multidimensional, and transactional nature of aging-in-place is at the core of much of the critique of the fixed definition of aging in place often referenced in public policy discussions (Golant, 2008).

CONTEXTUAL ISSUES IN COMMUNITY-BASED LIVING FOR THE THIRD AGE

Although the previous section reviewed the key empirical understandings of autonomy and security for the elderly in the community, in everyday life people engage in various strategies to navigate the autonomy–security dialectic. These strategies are shaped not only by the activities that occur in places, but also by the cognitive–emotional meaning that one constructs in relation to the place (Rubinstein & Parmelee, 1992).

Residential Normalcy

This activities-and-meanings notion is central to Golant's (2011) concept of residential normalcy, with its dual interdependent constructs of older adults' experiences of the residential environment: the zone of comfort and the zone of mastery. An individual is thought to be in the zone of comfort when the general experience of the environment is pleasurable, hassle-free, and memorable, and to be in the zone of mastery when one feels competent and in control. When the elderly find themselves out of their comfort or mastery zones, they initiate accommodative (mental management of expectations) strategies or assimilative (action management) strategies for coping to restore residential normalcy. The resources they draw on to enact the necessary strategies are idiosyncratic and predicated on life experience (e.g., an individual may want to move but not have the physical competency or the economic resources to do so).

Relocation

One of the more dramatic assimilative strategies is relocation. Researchers have distinguished the relocations of older adults in terms of first, second, and third moves (Haas & Serow, 1993; Litwak & Longino, 1987). First moves are typically made by younger, healthier, wealthier older adults seeking specific amenities; second moves are motivated by desires to be in a more urban area or closer to family due to increased needs for assistance; and third moves refer to relocation to institutional settings, usually as the result of declining physical or mental health (Litwak & Longino, 1987). Note that first moves reflect agency in seeking personal fulfillment, the goal of the Third Age, whereas second and third moves reflect the increased dependence indicative of the Fourth Age. Because the focus of this article relates to community-based living options for the Third Age, the remainder of this article will concentrate on environmental choices related to first moves, which Bradley and Longino (2009) have recently described as moves that occur "in early retirement ... driven by lifestyle considerations" (p. 325).

As it happens, most community-based living options for older adults come to be recognized have primarily for the retirement aspect of the relocation, and thus are usually referred to as retirement communities. Retirement communities are characterized by four qualities: a retirement element (i.e., the majority of the population is actively retired); a community element (i.e., a geographically bounded area in which the group of residents is of the same age); a collective spirit (i.e., the group acts together with respect to activities, interests, and within the same facilities); and support of residents' desires to remain autonomous but secure (Phillips, Bernard, Biggs, & Kingston, 2001). Note the dialectic portrayal of autonomy and security in the fourth quality of retirement communities—the essential attributes of the older adult–environment relationship described by Parmelee and Lawton (1990) and referred to by Wahl and Lang (2003) as agency and belonging.

Diversity in Third Age Residential Environments

Given the possible range of life experiences of older adults, we can assume that the diversity of residential environments for individuals in the Third Age will be as heterogeneous as that of the Second Age. By merging our life stage adaptation of the SPOT theory (Table 2) with the aforementioned definition of retirement community (Phillips et al., 2001), we can anticipate that Third Age individuals pursue a balance between autonomy and security issues compared with the agency-directed Second Age and the belonging-directed Fourth Age. Mixing the life stage-adapted SPOT theory with the concept of residential normalcy, we can hypothesize that as Third Agers seek balance in autonomy and security, the strategies they use to achieve that balance in their residential environments will vary considerably.

Furthermore, our thinking follows Rubinstein and Parmelee's (1992) suggestion that place experience is shaped by an individual's position in their life course relative to the larger sociocultural context. Thus, although we see a general trend among Third Agers' searches for residential balance between autonomy and security, we envisage diversity—some individuals will be pulled toward retaining autonomy whereas others will feel compelled to seek greater security. As such, we would expect to see a range of options that demonstrate the interdependence of autonomy and security, which in turn reflects Third Agers' efforts to maintain residential normalcy. The following section focuses on three existing models of community-based living that illustrate this diversity.

THREE MODELS OF COMMUNITY-BASED LIVING FOR THE THIRD AGE

Community-based living options for the Third Age can be initially classified in terms of their intentional natures: planned and unplanned. Although many variations exist, we will limit our review to three exemplar models that reflect this continuum. Among planned communities is the LORC model. Among the unplanned, the most common model is the NORC. The Village model, a hybrid, has emerged in more recent times.

Leisure-Oriented Retirement Communities

As the label implies, leisure activities are the main focus of planned LORCs (Folts & Muir, 2002; Folts & Streib, 1994; Streib, Folts, & Peacock, 2007). First appearing in the early 1960s, the LORC concept came to be epitomized by mega-developments such as Sun City and Leisure World (Strevey, 1989). LORCs appeal to older adults interested in an active lifestyle in an age-restricted, secure environment; these features are marketed heavily to this audience by their project developers, regions, or municipalities. Although many residents of LORCs elect to move on the basis of amenities (Blakely & Snyder, 1997) such as shops, services, sport facilities (golf courses, swimming pools), and communal buildings (i.e., club houses), supportive personal and health care services are generally not part of the LORC proposition (Folts & Streib, 1994). Security is often manifest in the gated community form, in which the perimeter of the community area is bounded by walls or fences with controlled entrances for motorized traffic, bicycles, and pedestrians. Residents of LORCs indicate the gated community feature provides a sense of security (McHugh & Larson-Keagy, 2005).

Naturally Occurring Retirement Communities

NORCs are "housing developments that are not planned or designed for older people but that attract a preponderance (over 50 percent) of residents at least 60 years or older" (Hunt & Gunter-Hunt, 1985; Hunt & Ross, 1990, p. 667). NORCs are located in rural and urban environments (Golant, 2003; Lawton, 1980) and in warm and cool climates, although they appear to be more prevalent in warm climates (Longino & Bradley, 2006). NORCs are formed through residential continuity (i.e., an initially pre-elderly population remaining in their homes beyond age 60 and aging in place) or the in-migration of older adults in search of more convenient locations or amenity-oriented lifestyles (but not specifically planned or designed for an older population) (Golant, 1992).

In contrast to purpose-built residential communities such as LORCs, NORCs are not specifically designed for older people; they are age-integrated, often located in single buildings of fewer than 500 residents, and are not marketed as communities for older adults (Hunt & Ross, 1990). For NORC residents, the three most important aspects of their community are proximity to services, access to social groups, and "the surrounding neighborhood and its characteristics" (Hunt & Gunter-Hunt, 1985, p. 13).

The Village Model

The Village is a hybrid model of planned and unplanned in that older adults remain in their homes in the community, and pay to become a member of an organization that coordinates and delivers programs and services (health and wellness care, home repair, groceries, transportation, social events), which helps members maintain their independence (Beacon Hill Village, 2011; Thomas & Blanchard, 2009). The model was developed in 2001 by a group of older adults residing in the Beacon Hill neighborhood of Boston (McWhinney-Morse, 2009) as an alternative to having to move to retirement or assisted living communities (Beacon Hill Village, 2011). To create a "virtual retirement community" for members, Beacon Hill Village founders focused on three areas for older adults: community building, support services, and healthcare (Boston Channel, 2002; McWhinney-Morse, 2009). The goal of Beacon Hill Village is to "offer programs and services [via reliable vendors] that address not only medical and housing needs but social, physical, emotional, and intellectual needs as well" (McWhinney-Morse, 2009, p. 85).

Comparison of Models of Community-Based Living Across Contextual Issues

The three models of community-based living for the Third Age differ in terms of their characteristics with respect to the key contextual issues summarized earlier (Table 3).

RELOCATION

The LORC model presumes relocation. Third Agers must have the financial means to relocate to support their leisure interests. They must have the physical and mental health competencies that allow them to participate in their leisure interests to their personal levels of satisfaction. Those Third Agers who lack the financial, physical, or mental means to support relocation are unlikely to choose the LORC model as their environmental context for aging. The NORC model does not demand relocation for the mode of residential continuity, but it does require relocation for the in-migration mode. The Village model presumes residential continuity, which precludes relocation. Indeed, the model was purposely developed to help older adults avoid relocation from their own homes in the community.

AUTONOMY

LORCs offer autonomy via the lifestyle and recreational amenities that facilitate social and physical activities. However, LORCs restrict residents' autonomy to the degree that the environment is secure. NORCs offer autonomy via community-based living. Indeed, autonomy is a defining characteristic of living in community. The Village model offers autonomy via community-based living that is supplemented by lump-sum membership and fee-for-service programs and services that help to sustain independence.

SECURITY

Security in the LORC model is literal, manifest in real and hidden barriers such as eligibility requirements, controlled gate entries, walls, and fences that separate the community from the surrounding area. The security of a NORC is literal and perceptual. Literally, physical security is provided via community-

TABLE 3 Contextual Characteristics of Community-Based Living Models for the Third Age

Model	Relocation	Autonomy	Security	Residential Normalcy (Coping Strategies)
LORC	Requires relocation that is presumed to be voluntary, as residents are assumed to be making a conscious choice to reside in the LORC	Via leisure amenities that facilitate social and physical activities	In a literal way, via eligibility requirements, physical barriers such as controlled gate entries, walls, and fences	Relocation to the LORC is a demonstration of an assimilative strategy to achieve residential congruence
NORC	In residential continuity mode, does not require relocation. In in-migration mode, requires relocation	Via community-based living	Literally, physical security is provided via community-based resources such as police and through individual measures to ensure home security. Perceptual security is facilitated via familiarity with the community (residential continuity) and as evidenced by selection (in-migration)	NORC residency via residential continuity likely entails accommodative coping in order to reconcile loss of residential mastery over the environment with preference for residential comfort. In-migration to a NORC is a demonstration of an assimilative strategy to achieve residential congruence
Village	Presumes residential continuity, thus precluding relocation	Via community-based living that is supplemented by lump-sum membership and fee-for-service programs and services that sustain independence	Literally, physical security is provided via community-based resources such as police and through individual measures to ensure home security. Perceptually, via the membership fees that entitle members to become part of an organized community whose sole purpose is to provide programs and services that support the range of needs of aging adults	Election to join the organization demonstrates an assimilative strategy in order to maintain residential congruence

Note. LORC = leisure-oriented retirement community; NORC = the naturally occurring retirement community.

based resources, such as police, and through individual measures to ensure home security. Perceptual security of the NORC is facilitated via familiarity with the community (in the case of residential continuity) and as evidenced by selection (in the case of in-migration). The security of the Village model stems from the support received from the programs and services offered to its paying members.

RESIDENTIAL NORMALCY

Relocation to a LORC is a demonstration of an assimilative strategy to achieve residential congruence. NORC residency via residential continuity likely entails accommodative coping to reconcile loss of residential mastery over the environment with preference for residential comfort. NORC in-migration is a demonstration of an assimilative strategy to achieve residential congruence. In the Village model, election to join the member organization demonstrates an assimilative strategy to maintain residential congruence.

CONCLUSION

In this article, we have outlined some of the essential details of our position—that in order for the field of environmental gerontology to succeed in the future, environmental gerontologists must redirect their attention toward the residential environments of choice of older adults, which are not institutional settings, but rather their own homes located in neighborhoods and communities. In the future, environmental gerontologists must approach residential environments for aging with a nuanced awareness of the Third Age experience. Apropos is Rubinstein's (2002) observation that the Third Age is still understood as a post period (e.g., post child-rearing, post wage-earning). Whether this post condition is viewed as loss or freedom establishes a rhetorical frame for the choices and adaptations the older adult makes and the assessments of quality of life that follow. If the Third Age is viewed as an age of loss, we must be able to ascertain how uncertainty in the various domains of life might lead to increased needs or desires for security and belonging in the person's relationship with the environment, a reflection of what Lawton (1989) refers to as the maintenance function of the environment. Conversely, if the Third Age is perceived as an age of freedom, environmental support for autonomy and provision of stimulation may be particularly salient. In this regard, we would do well to note Rubinstein's (2002) reflection that from a developmental perspective, freedom may foster narcissism or generativity, each orientation involving different sets of sociophysical relationships as determined by dissimilar goals.

Where the variety in Third Age goal orientation is undeniably shaped by the life stages that preceded, so will the Third Age be tied to the Fourth. In her socio-emotional selectivity theory, Carstensen (1995) suggested that the elderly, having shrinking time horizons, become increasingly selective in placing their energy and resources, focusing on emotionally meaningful goals and related activities. For the Third Age, selectivity reflects the negotiation between one's sequential development through First and Second Ages and the inevitability of the shrinking time horizon in the Fourth Age.

The theoretical ambiguity of the Third Age at both the individual and collective levels of analysis introduces intriguing prospects for environmental gerontology research. We believe our examination posits four likely conclusions for the next phase of research in environmental gerontology:

1. There will be increasing innovation in the community-based living models that serve the diverse Third Age demographic. As described in this article, three models of community-based living for the Third Age—the LORC, the NORC, and the Village—show promise as exemplary options for community-based living for older adults. Further innovations should be driven by robust, theory-based research.
2. We believe the dialectic between residential continuity and relocation is fundamentally driven by the complementary needs of autonomy and security in conjunction with the individual's ability to achieve and maintain residential normalcy. These are the critical dimensions of environmental concern for the Third Age.
3. Future research on existing and emerging models of community-based living should draw on the many relevant theoretical approaches from environmental gerontology, including the competence-press model found in the Ecological Model of Aging (Lawton & Nahemow, 1973), approaches to the concept of place (Weisman, Chadhury, & Diaz Moore, 2000), and the effects of change over time on the relationship between the person and environment (Wahl & Lang, 2003). Given the ambiguity regarding the Third Age, lateral connections to developmental theories such as the socio-emotional selectivity theory (Carstensen, 1995) should be considered (the SPOT model is an excellent example in this regard).
4. A caveat—although place experience is individualistic, we recognize that places must be designed for groups of people. As such, analysis of place at the consensual level of understanding is essential to inform better environmental design (Weisman et al., 2000).

The unprecedented global aging arc has set the stage for environmental gerontology to become a force in understanding and creating residential environments for aging. Environmental gerontologists would do well to shift the historical focus from institutional settings and the needs of the Fourth Age to community-based living options for the Third Age. Rest assured that our value position is unwavering; as Lawton (1980) stated, "the right to a decent environment is an inalienable right and requires no empirical justification" (p. 160). We proffer these suggestions not only to enhance the viability of the field of environmental gerontology, but also with the goal of enhancing environments for the elderly in this leisure emergent, exciting period of the life course we refer to here as the Third Age.

REFERENCES

Agency for Healthcare Research and Quality. (2002). *Physical activity and older Americans: Benefits and strategies.* Rockville, MD: Author. Retrieved from http://www.ahrq.gov/ppip/activity.htm

American Association of Retired Persons. (2005). *Beyond 50.05: A report to the nation on livable communities: Creating environments for successful aging.* Retrieved from http://assets.aarp.org/rgcenter/il/beyond_50_communities.pdf

Baltes, M. M. (1996). *The many faces of dependency in old age.* Cambridge, UK: Cambridge University Press.

Beacon Hill Village. (2011). Retrieved from http://www.beaconhillvillage.org/

Bekhet, A., Zauszniewski, J., & Nakhla, W. (2009). Reasons for relocation to retirement communities. *Western Journal of Nursing Research, 31,* 462–479.

Blakely, E. J., & Snyder, M. G. (1997). *Fortress America: Gated communities in the United States.* Washington, DC: The Brookings Institution.

Boston Channel. (2002, April 22). *Virtual retirement allows seniors to stay home.* Boston, MA: WCVB. Retrieved from http://www.thebostonchannel.com/news/1412801/detail.html

Bradley, D. E., & Longino, C. F. (2009). Geographic mobility and aging in place. In P. Uhlenberg (Ed.), *International handbook of population aging* (vol. 1, pp. 319–339). Dordrecht, The Netherlands: Springer-Verlag.

Brown, B. B. (1987). Territoriality. In D. Stokols & I. Altman (Eds.), *Handbook of environmental psychology* (pp. 505–531). New York, NY: Wiley.

Brown, B. B., & Perkins, D. D. (1992). Disruptions in place attachment. In I. Altman & S. Low (Eds.), *Place attachment* (pp. 279–304). New York, NY: Plenum.

Carstensen, L. (1995). Evidence for a life-span theory of socioemotional selectivity. *Current Directions in Psychological Science, 5,* 151–156.

Christensen, D., & Carp, F. (1987). PEQI-based environmental predictors of the residential satisfaction of older women. *Journal of Environmental Psychology, 7*(1), 45–64.

Folts, W.E., & Muir, K.B. (2002). Housing for older adults: New lessons from the past. *Research on Aging, 24*(1), 10–28.

Folts, W. E., & Streib, G. F. (1994). Leisure-oriented retirement communities. In W. E. Folts & D. E. Yeatts (Eds.), *Housing and the aging population: Options for the New York Center* (pp. 121–144). New York, NY: Garland.

Golant, S. M. (1992). *Housing America's elderly: Many possibilities, few choices.* Newbury Park, CA: Sage Publications.

Golant, S. (2002). Deciding where to live: The emerging residential settlement patterns of retired Americans. *Generations, 26*(11), 66–73.

Golant, S. M. (2003). Conceptualizing time and behavior in environmental gerontology: A pair of old issues deserving new thought. *The Gerontologist, 43*, 638–648.

Golant, S. (2008). Commentary: Irrational exuberance for the aging in place of vulnerable low-income older homeowners. *Journal of Aging and Social Policy, 20*, 379–397.

Golant, S. (2011). The quest for residential normalcy by older adults: Relocation but one pathway. *Journal of Aging Studies, 25*, 193–205.

Haas, W. H., & Serow, W. J. (1993). Amenity retirement migration process: A model and preliminary evidence. *The Gerontologist, 33*, 212–220.

Hoehner, C. M., Brennan Ramirez, L. K., Elliott, M. B., Handy, S. L., & Brownson, R. C. (2005). Perceived and objective environmental measures and physical activity among urban adults. *American Journal of Preventative Medicine, 28*, 105–116.

Hunt, M. E. (2001). Settings conducive to the provision of long-term care. *Journal of Architectural and Planning Research, 18*, 223–233.

Hunt, M. E., & Gunter-Hunt, G. (1985). Naturally-occurring retirement communities. *Journal of Housing for the Elderly, 3*, 3–21.

Hunt, M. E., & Ross, L. E. (1990). Naturally-occurring retirement communities: A multi-attribute examination of desirability factors. *The Gerontologist, 30*, 667–674.

Kahana, E., Lovegreen, L., Kahana, B., & Kahana, M. (2003). Person, environment, and person-environment fit as influences on residential satisfaction. *Environment and Behavior, 35*, 434–453.

King, A. C., Castro, C., Wilcox, S., Eyler, A. A., Sallis, J. F., & Brownson, R. C. (2000). Personal and environmental factors associated with physical inactivity among different racial-ethnic groups of U.S. middle aged and older aged women. *Health Psychology, 19*, 354–364.

King, W., Brach, J. S., Belle, S., Killingsworth, R., Fenton, M., & Kriska, A. M. (2003). The relationship between convenience of destinations and walking levels in older women. *American Journal of Health Promotion, 18*, 74–82.

Krause, N. (1998). Neighborhood deterioration, religious coping, and changes in health during late life. *The Gerontologist, 38*, 653–664.

Krout, J. A., Moen, P., Holmes, H. H., Oggins, J., & Bowen, N. (2002). Reasons for relocation to a continuing care retirement community. *The Journal of Applied Gerontology, 21*, 236–256.

Laslett, P. (1989). *A fresh map of life: The emergence of the third age*. London, England: Weidenfled & Nicholson.

Lawton, M. P. (1980). *Environment and aging*. Monterey, CA: Brooks/Cole.

Lawton, M. P. (1989). Three functions of the residential environment. *Journal of Housing for the Elderly, 5*, 35–50.

Lawton, M. P. (1990). Knowledge resources and gaps in housing the aged. In D. Tilson (Ed.), *Aging in place* (pp. 287–309). Glenview, IL: Scott Foresman.

Lawton, M. P., & Hoover, S. (1979). *Housing and neighborhood: Objective and subjective quality*. Philadelphia, PA: Philadelphia Geriatric Center.

Lawton, M. P., & Nahemow, L. (1973). Ecology and the aging process. In C. Eisdorfer & M. P. Lawton (Eds.), *The psychology of adult development and aging* (pp. 619–674). Washington, DC: American Psychological Association.

Lawton, M. P., & Simon, B. (1968). The ecology of social relationships in housing for the elderly. *The Gerontologist, 8*, 108–115.

Litwak, E., & Longino, C. F. (1987). Migration patterns among the elderly: A developmental perspective. *The Gerontologist, 27*, 266–272.

Longino, C. F., & Bradley, D. E. (2006). Internal and international migration. In R. H. Binstock & L. K. George (Eds.), *Handbook of aging and social sciences* (6th ed., pp. 76–93). San Diego, CA: Elsevier.

Masotti, P., Fick, R., Johnson-Masotti, A., & MacLeod, S. (2006). Healthy naturally-occurring retirement communities: A low-cost approach to facilitating healthy aging. *American Journal of Public Health, 96*(7), 1–8.

McHugh, K., & Mings, R. (1996). The circle of migration: Attachment to place in aging. *Annals of the Association of American Geographers, 86*, 530–550.

McHugh, K. E., & Larson-Keagy, E. M. (2005). These white walls: The dialectic of retirement communities. *Journal of Aging Studies, 19*, 241–256.

McWhinney-Morse, S. (2009). Beacon Hill Village. *Generations, 33*, 85–86.

Merry, S. (1976, November). The management of danger in a high-crime urban neighborhood. Paper presented at the annual meeting of the American Anthropological Association, Washington, DC.

Nasar, J., & Fisher, B. (1993). "Hot spots" of fear and crime: A multi-method investigation. *Journal of Environmental Psychology, 13*, 187–206.

Norris-Baker, C., & Scheidt, R. (2005). On community as home: Places that endure in rural Kansas. In G. D. Rowles & H. Chaudhury (Eds.), *Coming home: International perspectives on place, time and identity in old age* (pp. 279–296). New York, NY: Springer.

Olshansky, S. J., Perry, D., Miller, R. A., & Butler, R. N. (2006). In pursuit of the longevity dividend. *The Scientist, 20*, 28–36.

Oswald, F., Schilling, O., Wahl, H., & Gäng, K. (2002). Trouble in paradise? Reasons to relocate and objective environmental changes among well-off older adults. *Journal of Environmental Psychology, 22*, 273–288.

Parmelee, P., & Lawton, M. P. (1990). The design of special environments for the aged. In J. Birren & K. W. Schaie (Eds.), *Handbook of the psychology of aging* (3rd ed., pp. 464–488). New York, NY: Academic Press.

Phillips, J., Bernard, M., Biggs, S., & Kingston, P. (2001). Retirement communities in Britain: A 'third way' for the third age? In S. M. Peace & C. Holland (Eds.), *Inclusive housing in an ageing society: Innovative approaches* (pp. 189–214). Bristol, England: The Policy Press.

Rowles, G. D., & Ravdal, H. (2002). Aging, place and meaning in the face of changing circumstances. In R. Weiss & S. A. Bass (Eds.), *Challenges of the Third Age: Meaning and purpose in later life* (pp. 81–114). New York, NY: Oxford University.

Rubinstein, R. (2002). The third age. In R. Weiss & S. Bass (Eds.), *Challenges of the third age: Meaning and purpose in later life* (pp. 81–114). Oxford, England: Oxford University Press.

Rubinstein, R., & Parmelee, P. (1992). Attachment to place and representation of life course by the elderly. In I. Altman & S. Low (Eds.), *Human behavior and environment: Volume 12: Place attachment* (pp. 139–163). New York, NY: Plenum.

Ryff, C., & Essex, M. (1992). The interpretation of life experience and well-being: The sample case of relocation. *Psychology and Aging, 7*, 507–517.

Streib, G. F., Folts, W. E., & Peacock, J. (2007). The life course of leisure-oriented retirement communities. *Journal of Housing for the Elderly, 20*(4), 39–59.

Strevey, T. E. (1989). *The first 25 years of Leisure World, Laguna Hills*. Laguna Hills, CA: The Leisure World Historical Society.

Sundeen, R., & Mathieu, J. (1976). The fear of crime and its consequences among elderly in three urban communities. *The Gerontologist, 16*, 211–219.

Thomas, W. H., & Blanchard, J. M. (2009). Moving beyond place: Aging in community. *Generations, 33*(2), 12–17.

United Nations. (2002). *World population ageing: 1950–2050*. New York, NY: United Nations.

Wahl, H.-W., & Lang, F. (2003). Aging in context across the adult life course: Integrating physical and social environmental research perspectives. *Annual Review of Gerontology and Geriatrics, 23*, 1–33.

Walters, W. H. (2002). Later-life migration in the United States: a review of recent research. *Journal of Planning Literature, 17*(1), 37–66.

Weisman, G. D., Chaudhury, H., & Diaz Moore, K. (2000). Theory and practice of place: Toward an integrative model. In R. Rubinstein, M. Moss, & M. Kleban (Eds.), *The many dimensions of aging: Essays in honor of M. Powell Lawton* (pp. 3–21). New York, NY: Springer.

Weiss, R., & Bass, S. (2002). *Challenges of the Third Age: Meaning and purpose in later life*. Oxford, England: Oxford University Press.

PART II: METHODS AND MEASURES: ISSUES AND APPLICATIONS

Implementation of Research-Based Strategies to Foster Person–Environment Fit in Housing Environments: Challenges and Experiences during 20 Years

SUSANNE IWARSSON

Department of Health Sciences, Lund University, Lund, Sweden

Since the early 1990s, we have engaged in the development of methodology for the assessment of person–environment fit in housing and the determination of how such dynamics interact with aspects of health. Ultimately, all projects are aimed at practice implementation. Our research efforts represent methodology development, problem-oriented studies among older people and individuals with disabilities, and solution-oriented projects in interaction with users and practitioners, aimed to implement research-based solutions and evaluate their effects. The aim of this article is to provide an overview of the strategies used, challenges met, and experiences gathered while implementing research-based strategies to overcome housing accessibility problems.

Together with Björn Slaug, the author holds the copyright for the Housing Enabler methodology. The instrument, software, and related methodology courses are marketed and sold by Iwarsson and Slaug via their private enterprises. According to current Swedish legislation, after individual probation this arrangement has been formally approved by Lund University.

The author thanks Professor E. Steinfeld, University at Buffalo, NY, for permission to translate and develop his original idea; B. Slaug and A. Johannisson for fruitful collaboration through the years; staff at the Centre for Ageing and Supportive Environments (CASE) for continuous contributions to the methodological development of the instrument; practicing occupational therapists and others for stimulating cooperation and for providing information to assist in the methodological development; partners in various countries for their valuable opinions and rewarding collaboration. This article was prepared within the context of CASE at Lund University, financed by the Swedish Research Council on Social Science and Working Life. Financial support was also granted by the Swedish Research Council and the Ribbing Foundation, Lund, Sweden.

INTRODUCTION

Concern about relationships between the housing and health has been recorded over several centuries by architects, health care practitioners, and social reformists. Today, following the results of studies in a range of disciplines, the residential environment is known to be an important determinant of quality of life and well-being (Lawrence, 2010). For example, the role of the home environment for maintaining independence in daily life among older people and individuals with disabilities is widely recognized in research and practice (Wahl, Oswald, Schilling, & Iwarsson, 2009) and constitutes an important facet of environmental gerontology.

Interventions targeting individual needs for housing adaptation are initiated by rehabilitation specialists, most often occupational therapists. In some countries, such adaptations are being supported by national legislation providing individual grants, whereas in many countries it is up to the individual to finance such interventions (Iwarsson, 2009). At the societal level, the responsibility to provide all citizens with appropriate housing designed to support daily activities of living, despite frailty and disability, rests with politicians and community planners. Against this background, it seems reasonable to assume that gains could be made by an integration of the knowledge and experience of health care staff specialized in housing adaptation case management and societal actors engaged in housing provision.

Guidelines and standards for designing accessible built environments have been gradually developed, especially in the past 25 years, but housing still shows serious deficiencies regarding accessibility. The measures that are taken in practice contexts are rarely based on systematic assessment, and there is often insufficient consideration for the different perspectives that should be included in the analysis preceding the measures (Iwarsson & Slaug, 2010). Methods targeting accessibility problems should give a measure of the degree to which a particular physical environment can prevent or support daily activities of living and participation in society (Steinfeld & Danford, 1999). According to an extensive literature review on housing and health (Wahl et al., 2009), few psychometrically sound tools exist in this field, and it is challenging to derive valid and reliable home measurement tools.

Since the early 1990s, we have been engaged in the development of methodology for the assessment of accessibility in housing and immediate neighborhoods (Iwarsson & Slaug, 2010) and how person–environment fit dynamics interact with aspects of health (Oswald et al., 2007). The aim of this article is to provide an overview of the strategies used, challenges met, and experiences gathered during 20 years of efforts aiming for implementation of research-based strategies to overcome housing accessibility problems.

CONCEPTUAL AND THEORETICAL FOUNDATION

Constituting the core of environmental gerontology, theoretical models that illuminate the relationship between the individual's capacity and the demands of the environment emphasize that maladaptive behavior and functioning arise in the relationship between the individual and the environment. Lawton and Nahemow's (1973) ecological model is the most cited in person–environment studies. In 1968, Lawton and Simon stated the docility hypothesis (Lawton, 1986), which says that a balance between the individual's competence and environmental press can be achieved by changing either component or both. Even if the individual's functional competence deteriorates, the capacity for activity can be improved by lowering the demands made by the environment. Another assumption is that individuals with lower competence are more sensitive to the demands of the environment than individuals with higher competence.

Regarding accessibility, theory, practical experience, and research findings support a definition of the term as the relationship between the individual's functional capacity and the demands of the physical environment. Accessibility can be viewed as an aspect of person–environment fit and a relative concept comprising two components: the personal component and the environmental component (Iwarsson & Ståhl, 2003). The term is objective by nature, and the environment is described on the basis of guidelines and standards (Preiser & Ostroff, 2001).

CORE METHODOLOGY

The Housing Enabler instrument is based on approximately 20 years of method development, teaching, and research in cross-national collaboration involving researchers and practitioners, with a systematic synthesizing of knowledge and experiences used to nurture a continuous process of optimization (Iwarsson & Slaug, 2010). The Housing Enabler is one of the few instruments demonstrating the possibility and utility of a person–environment fit assessment approach (Mitty, 2010) and rests theoretically on Lawton and Nahemow's (1973) ecological model. During the 1990s, we introduced the instrument as a method with potential to support practitioners in producing reliable and valid analyses as a basis for interventions targeting housing accessibility problems (Iwarsson, 1999). The Housing Enabler is distinguished by a three-step assessment and analysis approach (Figure 1) based

First mark the functional limitations and dependence on mobility devices that you have observed. Then transfer the crosses to all the rating forms concerning environmental barriers.

Yes No

☐ ☒ A. Difficulty interpreting information A
☐ ☒ B1. Visual impairment B1
☐ ☒ B2. Blindness B2
☒ ☐ C. Loss of hearing C
☒ ☐ D. Poor balance D
☐ ☒ E. Incoordination E
☐ ☒ F. Limitations of stamina F
☐ ☒ G. Difficulty in moving head G
☐ ☒ H. Reduced upper extremity function H
☒ ☐ I. Reduced fine motor skill I
☐ ☒ J. Loss of upper extremity function J
☐ ☒ K. Reduced spine and/or lower
    extremity function **A B C*** K
☒ ☐ L. Dependence on walking aid(s) ☒ ☒ ☒ L
☐ ☒ M. Dependence on wheelchair ☐ ☐ ☐ M

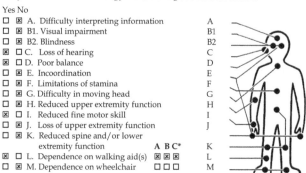

*Section in the environmental component: A. Exterior surroundings. B. Entrance. C. Indoor environment

Mark the observed environmental barriers with a cross. Then circle the scoring points (1–4) found at the intersections between functional limitations etc. and environmental barriers. The total of these scores is a quantification of the magnitude of accessibility problems.

Personal component / functional profile	Yes / No	Bygg ikapp	A	B1	B2	C	D	E	F	G	H	I	J	K	L	M	RATING
Personal component /	Yes					×	×					×			×		
functional profile	No	×	×	×		×	×	×	×	×		×	×		×	
A. Exterior surroundings	Bygg ikapp	A	B1	B2	C	D	E	F	G	H	I	J	K	L	M	RATING
General **A1.** Paths narrower than 1.5 m. *A width of 1.0 m is acceptable provided there are* 1.5 m turning zones at least every 10 m.		p. 304					3	3							3	3	☐ Yes ☒ No ☐ Not rated
A2. Irregular/uneven surface. *(irregular surfacing, joins, sloping sections* cracks, holes; 5 mm or more).		p. 305		2	3		1	1		3				1	3	3	☒ Yes ☐ No ☐ Not rated
A3. Unstable surface (loose gravel, sand, clay, etc). *Mark if it causes difficulties e.g. when using a* wheelchair or rollator.				2	3		3	3	2					1	3	4	☐ Yes ☒ No ☐ Not rated

FIGURE 1 Example illustrating the three-step assessment and analysis procedure of the Housing Enabler (Iwarsson & Slaug, 2010). Reprinted with permission.

on one checklist of functional capacity in the individual (personal component) and one checklist of environmental barriers (environmental component), followed by an analysis of person–environment fit resulting in a quantitative accessibility score. This construction implies that the administration and analysis procedure requires health-related and technical competence, coming with advantages and disadvantages for interdisciplinary implementation ambitions.

STRATEGY

Over the years, a series of projects has been accomplished in an integrated and cumulative manner. The projects represent different types and levels of scientific ambition, ranging from practice-based, small pilot studies (Iwarsson, Slaug, & Malmgren Fänge, 2011) and PhD student projects

(Fänge & Iwarsson, 2005; Helle et al., 2010; Iwarsson, Isacsson, & Lanke, 1998; Slaug, Schilling, Iwarsson, & Carlsson, 2010) to large-scale longitudinal, cross-national studies (Iwarsson et al., 2007; Oswald et al., 2007). Ultimately, all projects aim at practice implementation.

Our strategy builds on three types of activities:

1. Methodology development to create a tool-kit feasible not only for research, but also for structuring practices in community-based health care and in housing provision and city planning (Iwarsson, 1999; Iwarsson & Isacsson, 1996; Iwarsson, Nygren, & Slaug, 2005; Iwarsson et al., 2011; Mitty, 2010).
2. Problem-oriented studies aimed to describe person–environment dynamics and influences on health, among older (Iwarsson, 2005; Iwarsson et al., 2007; Oswald et al., 2007) and younger individuals with disabilities (Fänge, Iwarsson, & Persson, 2002; Iwarsson et al., 2004).
3. Solution-oriented projects in interaction with users and practitioners aimed to implement research-based solutions and evaluate their effects (Fänge et al., 2007; Iwarsson et al., 2004).

Based on the conviction that research in this field requires an explicit interdisciplinary approach, the core research team consists of senior and junior scientists representing gerontology, occupational therapy, research engineering, traffic planning, education, sociology, and statistics. A practicing architect experienced in accessibility and universal design issues serves as a consultant. Over the years, we have expanded our research cooperation to include additional individual researchers, practitioners, research teams, and representatives for institutes of higher education, not only in European countries but also in the United States and China.

With the Housing Enabler as the core instrument, we have made numerous attempts to implement the use of research-based methodology in different types of practice contexts (Fänge & Iwarsson, 2007; Fänge, Risser, & Iwarsson, 2007; Helle et al., 2010; Iwarsson et al., 2011). Most of the projects and studies were concentrated on housing environments, but to expand our knowledge a few projects targeted other environmental arenas, such as public facilities in the local community (Fänge et al., 2002; Iwarsson, 2005). Our studies rest on a platform of mixed methodologies (Creswell & Plano Clark, 2007), using quantitative and qualitative approaches in combination (Nygren & Iwarsson, 2009). Another type of study concerns the process of implementation, focusing on attitudes among practitioners and organizational aspects fostering or hindering implementation (Fänge et al., 2007; Fänge & Dahlin Ivanoff, 2009). Different strategies have been used, all aiming to support the process of implementation:

- Methodology courses targeting practitioners such as occupational therapists, architects, and technicians, as well as university teachers.

- Methodology teaching included in university education for professionals (Carlsson, Slaug, Johannisson, Fänge, & Iwarsson, 2004).
- Publication of books and information material, and presentations at numerous conferences, in popular and scientific formats.
- Structured, systematic comparisons of standards for housing design between countries, engaging interdisciplinary expert panels, paralleled with structured linguistic translation, involving researchers and practitioners (Helle et al., 2010; Iwarsson et al., 2005).
- Validity and reliability studies, involving students, teachers, practitioners, and researchers (Helle et al., 2010; Iwarsson & Isacsson, 1996, Iwarsson et al., 2005).
- Piloting of research-based assessment instruments in health care, housing provision, and city planning contexts, foremost in the Nordic countries (Fänge & Iwarsson, 2003; Helle et al., 2010; Iwarsson et al., 2011).
- Definition of needs for environmental measures, involving individuals with disabilities and different stakeholders (Fänge et al., 2002; Iwarsson et al., 2004).
- Follow-up studies of different types of effects of environmental interventions based on research-based methodology, such as adherence to advices given and user satisfaction (Iwarsson et al., 2004).
- Studies about attitudes to evidence-based practices and barriers to implementation (Fänge & Dahlin Ivanoff, 2009; Fänge et al., 2007).
- Collaboration with private companies (e.g., software development, housing provision) (Iwarsson et al., 2011).

CHALLENGES EXPERIENCED

Based on our research studies and systematic documentation of collaboration with different actors over our approximate 20-year process, five interrelated themes summarizing the challenges of implementation we have experienced so far appeared.

The first theme is related to the fact that practitioners and researchers have different missions, with practitioners mostly concentrated on doing a decent work and earning a living and researchers driven by forces such as scientific inquiry and scientific merit. This is manifested by differences in attitudes, where researchers take for granted that the use of research-based methods and results are positive and a driver of quality improvement, even if it necessitates a change of traditional practices. This is often in contrast to the attitudes not only of practitioners, but also of policymakers and politicians. It should also be emphasized that, based on the difference in missions, it is not at all self-evident among researchers to be willing to work in an integrated manner, involving practitioners and end-users from the start of a research project. That is, researchers are not always willing to make compromises as regards scientific rigor. The second theme is communication, where obvious but insufficiently reflected on differences in use of terminology and language, as well as the critical stance, often result in communication breakdown. The third theme is competence issues, which represent a distinctive challenge because practitioners and researchers must develop specific skills to be able to interact efficiently in implementation processes. For neither of these groups of actors, knowledge about the facts is sufficient; they also have to develop an understanding of the context in which they are acting. Moreover, both groups need to be creative in how to apply research results to practice (i.e., in how to adapt their well-known practices to new circumstances). The fourth theme is awareness of the influence of project context as both a facilitator and a barrier to success. Because the research described in this article involves complex structures, the power of factors such as staff discontinuity, weak leadership commitment, and complex organizations cannot be overestimated. The fifth theme, funding, plays a major role. As yet, it is difficult for researchers to get sufficient funding for communication and implementation beyond the traditional dissemination of results. For example, funders and reviewers lack competence and routine to review applications involving higher levels of implementation ambitions, but they may also be prejudiced against the scientific merits of implementation science.

FUTURE PROSPECTS

For the future, we have ambitions for further optimization of the Housing Eanbler methodology. During 2012, two PhD theses based on methodological articles will be completed. Issues under study are methodology for identification of core items in large item pools (Carlsson et al., 2009), inter-rater reliability in complex assessment situations (Helle et al., 2010), type profiles of functional limitations (Slaug et al., 2011), problems and examples of the consequences of a lack of research-based standards for accessible housing (Helle, Brandt, Slaug, & Iwarsson, 2011), and scoring principles for the quantification of person–environment fit.

We also have ambitions to enter the emerging field of social innovations, using the Housing Enabler as the platform for the development of tools fostering user-driven housing provision. The bearing idea behind this initiative is to combine the Housing Enabler with computerized tools for city planning already being used by architects and building constructors, and 3D technology. An interactive computer interface will be developed based on active end-user involvement, allowing older people with disabilities to identify their current profiles of functional limitations and identify which types of existing and future housing units they would have the best possibilities to live an active everyday life. Such initiatives are in line with the ambitions of environmental gerontology, influencing research and practice to the benefit of the ageing population.

CONCLUSIONS

When starting this journey in the early 1990s, no literature on what we now know as implementation science was available. With that in mind, it is nevertheless reasonable to conclude that it would have been beneficial if we had adopted a more systematic approach to document and study the complex process of development we have experienced so far. In retrospect, our learning process could have been more structured and efficient, but it might still be valuable to share some of our experiences with others. We conclude our research has informed policies and practices in Sweden and other European countries, while obvious, direct, and sustainable effects in practice contexts still are scarce. With ambitious prospects for the future based on our previous results and experiences, we envision that we will be able to continue to contribute to the development of environmental gerontology and to the development of social innovations.

REFERENCES

Carlsson, G., Schilling, O., Slaug, B., Fänge, A., Ståhl, A., Nygren, C., Iwarsson, S. (2009). Towards a screening tool for housing accessibility problems: A reduced version of the Housing Enabler. *Journal of Applied Gerontology, 28,* 59–80.

Carlsson, G., Slaug, B., Johannisson, A., Fänge, A., & Iwarsson S. (2004). The Housing Enabler: Integration of a computerised tool in occupational therapy undergraduate teaching. *CAL-laborate, 11,* 5–9.

Creswell, J. W., & Plano Clark, V. L. (2007). *Designing and conducting mixed-methods research.* Thousand Oaks, CA: Sage.

Fänge, A., & Dahlin Ivanoff, S. (2009). Integrating research into practice. A challenge for local authority occupational therapy. *Scandinavian Journal of Occupational Therapy, 16,* 40–48.

Fänge, A., & Iwarsson, S. (2003). Accessibility and usability in housing: Construct validity and implications for research and practice. *Disability and Rehabilitation, 25,* 1316–1325.

Fänge, A., & Iwarsson, S. (2005). Changes in ADL dependence and aspects of usability following housing adaptation: A longitudinal perspective. *American Journal of Occupational Therapy, 59,* 296–304.

Fänge, A., & Iwarsson, S. (2007). Challenges in the development of strategies for housing adaptation evaluations. *Scandinavian Journal of Occupational Therapy, 14,* 140–149.

Fänge, A., Iwarsson, S., & Persson, Å. (2002). Accessibility to the public environment as perceived by teenagers with functional limitations in a south Swedish town centre. *Disability and Rehabilitation, 24,* 318–326.

Fänge, A., Risser, R., & Iwarsson, S. (2007). Challenges in implementation of research methodology in community-based occupational therapy: The Housing Enabler example. *Scandinavian Journal of Occupational Therapy*, *14*, 54–62.

Helle, T., Brandt, Å., Slaug, B., & Iwarsson, S. (2011). Lack of research-based standards for accessible housing design: examples and consequences. *International Journal of Public Health*, *56*(6), 635–644.

Helle, T., Nygren, C., Slaug, B., Brandt, Å., Pikkarainen, A., Hansen, A.-G., et al. (2010). The Nordic Housing Enabler: Inter-rater reliability in cross-Nordic occupational therapy practice. *Scandinavian Journal of Occupational Therapy*, *17*, 258–266.

Iwarsson, S. (1999). The housing enabler: An objective tool for assessing accessibility. *British Journal of Occupational Therapy*, *62*, 491–497.

Iwarsson, S. (2005). A long-term perspective on person-environment fit and ADL dependence among older Swedish adults. *Gerontologist*, *45*, 327–336.

Iwarsson, S. (2009). Housing adaptations: Current practices and challenges for the future. In I. Söderback (Ed.), *International handbook of occupational therapy interventions* (pp. 63–69). New York, NY: Springer.

Iwarsson, S., Fänge, A., Hovbrandt, P., Carlsson, G., Jarbe, I., & Wijk, U. (2004). Occupational therapy targeting physical environmental barriers in buildings with public facilities. *British Journal of Occupational Therapy*, *67*, 29–38.

Iwarsson, S., Isacsson, Å., & Lanke, J. (1998). ADL dependence in the elderly: The influence of functional limitations and physical environmental demand. *Occupational Therapy International*, *5*, 173–193.

Iwarsson, S., & Isacsson, Å. (1996). Development of a novel instrument for occupational therapy assessment of the physical environment in the home: A methodologic study on "The Enabler." *Occupational Therapy Journal of Research*, *16*, 227–244.

Iwarsson, S., Nygren, C., & Slaug, B. (2005). Cross-national and multi-professional inter-rater reliability of the Housing Enabler. *Scandinavian Journal of Occupational Therapy*, *12*, 29–39.

Iwarsson, S., Slaug, B., & Malmgren Fänge, A. (2011). The housing enabler screening tool: Feasibility and inter-rater reliability in a real-estate company practice context. *Journal of Applied Gerontology*. doi: 10.1177/0733464810397354.

Iwarsson, S., & Slaug, B. (2010). *Housing Enabler: A method for rating/screening and analysing accessibility problems in housing. Manual for the complete instrument and screening tool*. Lund & Staffanstorp, Sweden: Veten & Skapen HB and Slaug Enabling Development.

Iwarsson, S., & Ståhl, A. (2003). Accessibility, usability, and universal design: Positioning and definition of concepts describing person-environment relationships. *Disability and Rehabilitation*, *25*, 57–66.

Iwarsson, S., Wahl, H.-W., Nygren, C., Oswald, F., Sixsmith, A., Sixsmith, J., et al. (2007). Importance of the home environment for healthy aging: Conceptual and methodological background of the European ENABLE-AGE Project. *Gerontologist*, *47*, 78–84.

Lawrence, R. J. (2010). Housing and health promotion: moving forward. *International Journal of Public Health*, *55*, 145–146.

Lawton, M. P. (1986). *Environment and aging*. Albany, NY: Center for the Study of Aging.

Lawton, M. P., & Nahemow, L. (1973). Ecology and the aging process. In C. Eisdorfer & M. P. Lawton (Eds.), *The psychology of adult development and aging*. Washington, DC: American Psychological Association.

Mitty, E. (2010). An assisted living community environment that optimizes function: Housing Enabler assessment. *Geriatric Nursing, 31*, 448–451.

Nygren, C., & Iwarsson, S. (2009). Negotiating and effectuating relocation to sheltered housing in old age: A Swedish study over 11 years. *European Journal of Ageing, 6*, 177–189.

Oswald, F., Wahl, H.-W., Schilling, O., Nygren, C., Fänge, A., Sixsmith, A., et al. (2007). Relationships between housing and healthy ageing aspects in very old age: Results from the European ENABLE-AGE Project. *Gerontologist, 47*, 96–107.

Preiser, W. F. E., & Ostroff, E. (Eds.). (2001). *Universal design handbook*. New York, NY: McGraw-Hill.

Slaug, B., Schilling, O., Iwarsson, S., & Carlsson, G. (2011). Defining profiles of functional limitations in groups of older persons: How and why? *Journal of Aging and Health, 23*, 578–604.

Steinfeld, E., & Danford, G. S. (1999). Theory as a basis for research on enabling environments. In E. Steinfeld & G. S. Danford (Eds.), *Enabling environments. Measuring the impact of environment on disability and rehabilitation*. New York, NY: Kluwer Academic/Plenum.

Wahl, H-W., Oswald, F., Fänge, A., Gitlin, L., & Iwarsson, S. (2009). The home environment and disability-related outcomes in aging individuals: What is the empirical evidence? *Gerontologist, 49*(3), 355–367.

On the Quantitative Assessment of Perceived Housing in Later Life

FRANK OSWALD and ROMAN KASPAR

Interdisciplinary Ageing Research, Goethe University Frankfurt, Frankfurt, Germany

Person-environment relationships become particularly important in later life. Our discussion of challenges in the assessment of experiential person-environment exchange processes is grounded on a four-domain model of perceived housing. We present empirical findings from an iterative process of instrument revision seeking optimization of both reliability and validity issues regarding control-related and meaning-oriented domains of perceived housing. Our initial reconstruction, however, was not confirmed to represent a consistent and reliable measure for the suggested dimensions of housing-related identity, privacy, and autonomy. Exploratory post-hoc analyses of the pilot pool of indicators suggests six holistic facets, such as "daily independence" "neighborhood belonging", "mirror of self", "continuity and remaining in place" and "being alone and at peace". Plausible content-related interpretation and relations to major background characteristics encourage the continuous task of tailoring assessment instruments to meet the holistic character of housing experiences in later life.

INTRODUCTION

Environmental gerontology emphasizes the relationship between the person and the physical and social environment in old age (Lawton, 1977; Scheidt

The authors thank all study participants of the student project on perceived housing assessment in old age and are grateful for the creative contribution of our student co-researchers.

& Windley, 2006; Wahl, 2001; Wahl & Gitlin, 2007). Due to behavioral and experiential reasons, person–environment relationships become particularly important in later life. For instance, the ecological theory of aging (Lawton, 1982, 1998; Lawton & Nahemow, 1973; Scheidt & Norris-Baker, 2004) describes the interaction between levels of competence (e.g., functional limitations) and settings with different levels of environmental stress (e.g., barriers at home) that both lead to outcomes in zones of behavioral adaptation (or person–environment fit) and comfort versus maladaptation (or person–environment misfit) and negative affect. Thus, from a behavioral perspective, theoretical concepts and empirical data address the need for people of very old age to maintain daily independence despite an inevitable reduction of physical and cognitive competence. The environment may exert increasing levels of environmental pressure that forces the individual to adapt to ever-new barriers and obstacles. However, from an experiential perspective, cognitive and emotional representations of the environment may hold different layers of meaning for the individual, which may foster place attachment, reflecting facets of bonding and contributing to place identity in later life (Rowles, Oswald & Hunter, 2004; Rowles & Watkins, 2003; Rubinstein, 1989).

The aim of this article is to address methodological issues of environmental gerontology. The leading question is how to properly assess experiential person–environment exchange processes, emphasizing particular aspects of perceived housing. That is, we will not focus on the assessment of objective environmental conditions and barriers or on behavioral processes of environmental accessibility, use, or adaptation. Instead, we will focus on existing measurement options for person–environment experience in later life and report an illustrating four-domain model of perceived housing based on data from a European research project (Oswald et al., 2006). Finally, we want to exemplify one way to reconsider existing quantitative assessments and to introduce first steps ahead for two of the four domains of perceived housing—that is, housing-related control beliefs and meaning of home (based on pilot data not yet published). However, note that some of the presented data are based on prior work and publications generated together with other fellow researchers (Iwarsson et al., 2007; Nygren et al., 2007; Oswald et al., 2006; Oswald, Wahl, Schilling, Nygren, Fänge, Sixsmith et al., 2007; Wahl & Oswald, 2010; Wahl, Fänge, Oswald, Gitlin, & Iwarsson, 2009; Wahl, Iwarsson, & Oswald, 2012; Wahl, Oswald, Schilling, & Iwarsson, 2009).

THEORETICAL CONCEPTS OF PERSON–ENVIRONMENT EXCHANGE

Concepts of Person–Environment Exchange with a Focus on Environmental Behavior

Although we will emphasize perceived housing, it is necessary to also address environmental behavior to better understand person–environment experience from an environmental gerontology perspective in general. The focus in these concepts is on functional person–environment exchange processes, observed behavior, and objectively measured environmental characteristics; however, one may nevertheless agree that environmental behavior is closely linked to some unobserved experiential processes, such as cognitions and evaluations, which precede adaptive or proactive behavior aimed to regulate person–environment dynamics as people age.

A prominent construct in this vein is psychological control theory (Lachman, 1986; Lachman & Burack, 1993), which has found further specification for the environmental domain of housing (Oswald, Wahl, Schilling, & Iwarsson, 2007; Oswald, Wahl, Martin, & Mollenkopf, 2003). Housing-related control beliefs trigger interpretations of housing as either contingent on one's own behavior (internal control) or on luck, chance, fate, or powerful others (external control). The argument is that control beliefs related to the regulation of person–environment exchange become increasingly important in old age. Longitudinal data show that external control beliefs are especially sensitive to age-related changes due to health and functional ability losses; thus, they are crucial in explaining age-related outcomes, such as autonomy or well-being (Baltes, Freund, & Horgas, 1999; Clark-Plaskie & Lachman, 1999).

Concepts of Person–Environment Exchange with a Focus on Environmental Experience

In addition to the behavioral notion of person–environment exchange, person–environment exchange processes have been addressed on the experiential level in terms of residential satisfaction, place attachment, or meaning of place and are related to identity and well-being in later life (Rowles et al., 2004; Rowles & Watkins, 2003; Rubinstein, 1989). Among these concepts, residential satisfaction addresses a subjective global evaluation of the congruence between the individual and his or her living environment (Pinquart & Burmedi, 2004), often assessed by single-item self-evaluations (Oswald, Wahl, Mollenkopf, & Schilling, 2003). Concepts of place attachment and identity (Altman & Low, 1992; Lalli, 1992; Neisser, 1988; Proshansky, 1978; Stedman, 2002) emphasize experiential processes of person–environment exchange in a more differentiated way. Place attachment is not only related to attitudes, but also to a gamut of processes operating when people form affective, cognitive, behavioral, and social bonds to the environment (Brown & Perkins, 1992), thereby transforming space into place (Altman & Low, 1992; Rowles & Watkins, 2003). In this regard, the concept of the meaning of place or, more specifically, the meaning of home, deals with the most frequent manifestation of bonding (Oswald & Wahl, 2005). For instance, because older adults have often lived a long time in the same residence, cognitive and emotional aspects of the meaning of home are often strongly linked to biography. Such social, cognitive, and emotional links may manifest through processes of reflecting on the past, symbolically represented in certain places and cherished objects within the home. Thus, the experience of place covers non–goal-oriented cognitive and emotional aspects of bonding. Moreover, it covers behavioral and physical bonding because familiarity and routines have been developed over time.

Aspects of bonding and meaning have been assessed by global evaluations (e.g., on indoor vs. outdoor place attachment) (Oswald, Hieber, Wahl, & Mollenkopf, 2005), as well as from a more qualitative empirical in-depth approach (Haak, Fänge, Iwarsson, & Ivanoff, 2007; Peace, 2005). Often, data were drawn from case studies or qualitative in-depth interviews in the fields of geography, ethnography, sociology, or psychology. They dealt with small numbers of participants, transcribed verbal data sets, and heuristic or explorative analyses with only limited possibilities to be interpreted in relation to objective assessments of environmental characteristics or of extensive assessments of person–environment fit or accessibility (Rowles, 1983; Rubinstein, 1989; Sixsmith & Sixsmith, 1991), but promising efforts have also been made of quantifying meaning-of-home aspects (Oswald et al., 2006).

THE MULTIDIMENSIONALITY OF PERCEIVED HOUSING

The label of perceived housing is used to cover issues of person–environment experience with relation to the socio-physical home environment. We refer to a four-domain model of perceived housing, introduced as a comprehensive set of assessments based on four conceptual domains: housing satisfaction, usability in the home, meaning of home, and housing-related control beliefs (Oswald et al., 2006). The model was tested with a subset of the European ENABLE-AGE Project (Iwarsson et al., 2007), i.e., 1,223 community-dwelling very old individuals (80-89 years old) who lived alone in Sweden, the United Kingdom, and Germany. Four instruments on perceived housing were administered in individual face-to-face sessions at home visits, after several rounds of translation and pilot testing.

Housing Satisfaction

To address this basic evaluation, a single-item measure (five-point rating scale) from the Housing Options for Older People questionnaire (Heywood, Oldman, & Means, 2002) was used, which specifically targeted satisfaction with the condition of the house ("Are you happy with the condition of your home?").

Usability in the Home

Usability addresses the degree to which the physical home environment supports the performance of activities at home, based on individual ratings, assessed with the Usability in My Home Questionnaire (Fänge & Iwarsson, 1999, 2003) (five-point rating scale). Although this instrument was originally introduced with three subdomains—addressing activity aspects, personal and social aspects, and physical environmental aspects of usability—only two subscales were used in the four-domain model due to psychometric analyses: activity aspects (4 items; Cronbach's α = .67, e.g., "In terms of how you normally manage your cooking/heating of food or preparation of snacks, to what extent is the home environment suitably designed in relation to this?") and physical-environmental aspects (6 items; Cronbach's α = .75, e.g., "How usable do you feel the entrance to your home is?").

Meaning of Home

The development of the Meaning of Home Questionnaire (Oswald, Mollenkopf, & Wahl, 1999) was derived from open-ended examinations of a broad scope of contents for four areas of theoretical importance (physical, behavioral, cognitive/emotional, and social), representing the heterogeneity of perceived housing (Oswald & Wahl, 2005). To assess subjective meaning, participants were instructed to judge to what extent they agreed or disagreed with statements on an 11-point scale (range, 0-10). Psychometric analyses indicated acceptable internal consistency (Cronbach's α > .50) in three of four subscales: physical aspects (6 items, Cronbach's α = .60, e.g., "Being at home means for me living in a place which is well-designed and geared to my needs"), behavioral aspects (6 items, Cronbach's α = .67, e.g., "Being at home means for me being able to change or rearrange things as I please"), and cognitive/emotional aspects (10 items, Cronbach's α = .62, e.g., "Being at home means for me feeling comfortable and cosy/homey"). The subscale on social aspects (5 items, Cronbach's α = .44) was discarded due to its low reliability.

Housing-Related Control Beliefs

The assessment of domain-specific control beliefs is based on the conceptual distinction between internal control, which means that housing-related events are highly contingent upon a person's own behavior (where personal responsibility implies that one is responsible for what happens) versus external control, which means either some other person is responsible or things happen by mere luck, chance, or fate. The Housing-related Control Beliefs Questionnaire was developed as a 24-item questionnaire based on the psychological dimensions of internal control, external control: powerful others, and external control: chance to be judged on a five-point rating scale (Oswald, Wahl, Schilling, & Iwarsson, 2007; Oswald, Wahl, Martin, & Mollenkopf, 2003). However, psychometric analyses indicated poor levels of internal consistency in the internal control subscale and only medium internal consistency in both external control subscales. To improve the psychometric qualities of this instrument and in accordance with the conceptual argument that housing-related external control is of particular interest in perceived housing in very old age (Baltes et al., 1999), the internal control subscale was removed. Both external subscales were combined, resulting in sufficient reliability (Cronbach's α = .67, e.g., "Where and how I live has happened more by chance than anything else," "Other people have told me how to arrange the furnishings in my home").

What was found in ENABLE-AGE was a confirmation of the hypothetically proposed four factor model by means of multi-group analysis (multi-sample Structural Equation Model). Without going into detail, perceived housing was best displayed by the selected four constructs, reflecting four different domains, each uniquely contributing to the understanding of perceived housing in old age. In addition, cultural differences or similarities in terms of structural relationships between the four domains were revealed in the multi-group analysis for the three subsamples (i.e., Germany, Sweden, and the United Kingdom), showing little variability. Although personal and environmental background variables and objective living conditions could vary within and between the samples in the three countries, findings revealed comparable patterns of relationships, indicating a certain level of universality of perceived housing patterns in very old age across research sites.

FIRST STEPS TOWARD A MORE HOLISTIC MEASURE OF PERCEIVED HOUSING

In this section, we want first to briefly revisit some issues that may keep the current measurements of perceived housing from unfolding their full potential for representing person–environment experience. Second, we will present first results from the piloting of an approach to the measurement of perceived housing in later life that aims at addressing aspects of meaning of home and housing-related control beliefs in a holistic way. Note that we exclude the concepts of housing satisfaction and usability in this article. The reason is that the concept of housing usability is about to be further developed in close relation to objective housing accessibility from an occupational therapy perspective. As housing satisfaction is concerned, the concept draws its importance from its inclusiveness and generality but appears to be less promising to further deepen our understanding of person–environment experience processes in later life.

Shortcomings of Measures on Housing-Related Control Beliefs and Meaning of Home

Apart from the general supporting evidence for a conceptually multidimensional model with both considerable overlap and substantial uniqueness of the four concepts of perceived housing reported so far, previous analyses indicated some challenges to most existing measures. These measures should be addressed from both a substantive and a methodological perspective to further enrich the discussion on proper assessments of perceived housing in later life.

CEILING EFFECTS

Our previous studies revealed a substantial amount of ceiling apparent in many items that ask for perceived housing aspects. With respect to the concept of housing-related control beliefs, most individuals acknowledge their own responsibility for their living situation (i.e., internal control focus), with, on average, more than three of four respondents choosing the highest category. Likewise, the living environment is considered to hold a high amount of meaning with respect to the individuals' social, physical, or cognitive and emotional demands. Therefore, current instruments do not discriminate well among the majority of people that do not experience substantial problems with their living conditions.

HETEROGENEITY OF HOUSING-RELATED ISSUES

The rationale for many of the proposed scale developments was to deliberately include many different connotations of perceived housing into scale construction to address the heterogeneity of living conditions and lifestyles apparent in old age. Similarly, introducing domain-specific content may result in a loss of generalizability in attitudinal response. For instance, in the assessment of domain-specific control beliefs, a danger is that the concrete domain-specific content is taking the lead, so the control beliefs cannot be "put to work" in answering the questions to a sufficient degree. However, because some aspects are only represented by a restricted set of items, psychometric requirements are hard to meet for many of the proposed instruments. As a consequence, subscales with low scale consistency have been discarded from subsequent analyses, and conceptually distinct aspects of perceived housing have been merged into a single indicator.

STRUCTURAL VALIDITY

In a related vein, the plethora of different meanings of housing, the complex structure of responsibilities and potentials for continuity and change in living conditions, and the diverse activities supported or restricted by the living environment have been segmented and ordered using global categories drawn from the respective disciplinary dictionaries (e.g., physical, behavioral, cognitive, emotional, social). However, it is unclear how these analytic categories relate to the experience of housing and the living environment. Salient perceptions of housing in old age may incorporate emotional, cognitive, and behavioral reactions to physical and social aspects of the living environment, representing a more holistic experience of living circumstance than the sum of its parts may indicate. Elaborating on valid themes of perceived housing, variation in question content could tap emotional, cognitive, and behavioral aspects, thereby transposing the existing structure but retaining much of the analytical framework used so far.

ECOLOGICAL VALIDITY

Even with a higher percentage of time spent indoors in old age, the perception of housing may nevertheless be strongly influenced by subjective appraisals of the immediate outdoor environment, the neighborhood, or even larger spatial expenses; this would be due to their enabling, supporting, or self-referencing characteristics. Therefore, the current focus on the indoor housing environment may be unduly narrow and miss both important aspects of housing as a fundamentally social human experience and targets for housing interventions on a neighborhood or community level.

Reconsidering Concepts of Housing-Related Control Beliefs and Meaning of Home

To address some of these challenges, we revisited our conceptual framework of housing-related control beliefs and meaning of home by seeking empirical evidence for an alternative—possibly even more holistic—underlying structure of perceived housing indicators. In other words, driven by the assumption that the current partitioning of the housing experience, both within and across proposed instruments, may blur more holistic pictures of main themes in housing-related person–environment exchange, explorative factor analysis was used to identify possible consistent content areas or themes of perceived housing in the German ENABLE-AGE dataset. Results from these analyses indicated the meaning questionnaire and the control beliefs questionnaire to address common themes.

In this article, we present findings of a research-oriented seminar at the Goethe University Frankfurt, where a group of students followed-up these themes of perceived housing in later life by generating an extended list of items that capture both indoor (respectively home) and out-of-home (respectively neighborhood) housing-related experiences. The extended pool of 47 items was intended to represent three meta-categories supposed to be at the core of perceived housing in old age: identity-related aspects of perceived housing, issues of privacy and familiarity at home, and autonomy-related aspects of perceived housing. Although behavioral and experiential aspects of person–environment exchange are reflected in all three domains, identity-related aspects of perceived housing, as well as privacy and familiarity, more explicitly cover components of thinking and feeling. Conversely, autonomy-related aspects of perceived housing cover more behavior-related items and issues of housing-related control beliefs. To assure content validity of these versatile and broadly defined target concepts, three to four subdomains have been proposed for each category, and multiple indicators (items) were sought for each of these subscales. In addition, half of the items were designed to explicitly refer to the indoor environment, whereas the other half aimed at addressing meaning held by individuals' immediate out-of-home environment. This initial pool of items has been piloted with a total of 232 participants in a mixed paper-pencil self-report, a face-to-face interview, and an online survey (Table 1).

RESULTS

Sample Description

Basic characteristics of the convenience sample for the pilot study are given in Table 2. Mean age for the total sample was approximately 65 years, with a range of 50 to 96 years. Somewhat less than two-thirds of the participants were women. Self-reported health status used the full range of answering options. The average self-rated health was expectedly good. Because most of the participants had been recruited from an adult education mailing list, a high share of respondents (more than 50%) had an academic educational background. In line with this finding, approximately 40% of respondents reported their monthly income as ranging above 2,500 Euros. A 30% minority of respondents lived in single-person households. Two-thirds of participants indicated that they live in their own houses or apartments (or on a rent-free basis). Respondents' spread over urban, suburban, and rural regions was surprisingly balanced, with a somewhat higher proportion of respondents living in suburban areas. As could be expected for this age segment, on average participants had a history of living in the same place both with respect to the current city or town (36.5 years) and with respect to the

TABLE 1 Item Pool for Three Conceptual Meta-Categories of Perceived Housing (Examples)

Sub-domains	Example items
	Domain "Identity-related aspects of perceived housing"
Design	- The furnishing of my home tells a lot about me.
	- The composition of my neighborhood matters a lot to me.
Continuity	- Many things in my home have their specific places.
	- I am a regular customer in many shops in my neighborhood.
Social	- I am a part of the social community in this building.
	- I can just be myself in my neighborhood.
Physical	- I would lose a lot of myself if I were to move away from here.
	- This building's style and shape means a lot to me.
	Domain "Issues of privacy and familiarity"
Familiarity	- I know my home like the back of my hand.
	- I am well-acquainted to streets and walkways in my neighborhood.
Comfort	- My home is a place to relax.
	- I feel safe and secure in my neighborhood.
Retreat	- I have the opportunity to be by myself at home.
	- I know places in my neighborhood where I can be by myself if I want to.
Intimacy	- What I do at home is nobody's business but my own.
	- There are places in my neighborhood that hold private memories.
	Domain "Autonomy-related aspects of perceived housing"
Independence	- I can handle my daily housekeeping routines myself.
	- I do not need anybody's help to get from A to B in my neighborhood.
Freedom of choice	- I myself decide how to structure my day.
	- I myself decide which options in the neighborhood I will use.
Self-responsibility	- Whether I can stay at home or not depends on luck and circumstance (recoded).
	- I can contribute my share to the neighborhood life.

current house or apartment (21.6 years). Not surprisingly, overall satisfaction with the current housing situation was high for most of the participants.

The majority of participants ($n = 179$, 84.4%) rated the statements on their housing experiences in an online questionnaire, whereas a total of 33 (15.6%) participants rated the items either on their own or as a part of a face-to-face interview. The participants who were recruited and participated in the study in person were substantially older and rated their health as significantly lower than the participants who completed the online questionnaire (differences and tests not reported in Table 2). Moreover, participants in the online questionnaire were well-educated and reported a high level of financial resources. With regard to housing, the personally addressed participants lived more often in rural areas, had on average significantly more years (approximately 9.5 years) of residency in the current city or town, and reported significantly lower overall housing satisfaction. As was planned, the

TABLE 2 Characteristics of Pilot Study Sample

Background variables	Total Sample ($N = 212$)		
	No.	Mean ± SD or %	(Range)
Age, years	212	64.8 ± 8.5	(50–96)
Female sex	135	63.7%	
Self-rated health (1–5)[a]	208	3.3 ± 1.0	(1–5)
Education (selected categories)			
Elementary school	20	9.8%	
University	103	50.5%	
Net income (combined categories)			
Less than 2,500 € per month	93	44.7%	
Refused to answer	29	13.9%	
Housing tenure			
Owner (own house or no rent)	135	65.9%	
Household composition			
Living alone	62	29.4%	
Area of residency			
Urban	68	32.7%	
Suburban	78	37.5%	
Rural	62	29.8%	
Living duration			
Years of residency (city/town)	210	36.5 ± 19.5	(0–89)
Years in current house/apt.	210	21.6 ± 12.9	(0–76)
Housing satisfaction (1–5)[a]	209	4.4 ± 0.7	(2–5)

[a]Lower scores indicate better perceived health or lower housing satisfaction.

multi-method sampling approach yielded a more diverse sample of individuals aged 50 years or older for the pilot than any single approach would have captured. Although we did not aim for generalizability of our convenience sample for this pilot study, we would nevertheless like to see this added heterogeneity as an advantage toward our goal of developing an instrument for perceived housing that may correspond with a variety of lifestyles apparent in current and future cohorts of older individuals.

SCALE ANALYSIS

Major indices for the psychometric properties of the proposed instrument that have been investigated for the full study sample are given in Table 3. Although we carefully sought items that may help to discriminate also in the upper range of the respective domains, a considerable share of respondents still lingered in the highest category. However, ceiling effects appeared to be limited to the familiarity and comfort subdomains of the privacy component and the independence in daily routines subdomain of autonomy. The latter finding may not come as a surprise with this relatively young, healthy, and

TABLE 3 Psychometric Properties of Perceived Housing Pilot Instrument

Domains and Sub-domains	Number of items	Percent in highest category	Cronbach's Coefficient alpha		
			Overall	Indoor	Outdoor
"Identity-related aspects of perceived housing"	17	40.2	.79	.65	.71
Design	5	45.8	.60		
Continuity	4	50.6	.51		
Social	4	35.6	.65		
Environment	4	28.8	.39		
"Issues of privacy and familiarity"	16	61.5	.82	.79	.72
Familiarity	4	76.9	.67		
Comfort	4	70.3	.70		
Retreat	4	53.4	.64		
Intimacy	4	45.4	.40		
"Autonomy-related aspects of perceived housing"	14	65.5	.88	.73	.85
Independence	5	86.1	.88		
Freedom of choice	5	64.3	.75		
Self-responsibility	4	46.2	.44		

proactive sample. However, some items do not elicit a more balanced spread of responses (e.g., "I know my home like the back of my hand").

On the level of the primary domains of perceived housing, scale consistency—with estimates between .79 and .88—seems sufficient throughout. Because the relatively large number of items per dimension is foremost a result of our attempt to cover a broad content field, one might consider these scales as efficient. However, on the subscale level, reliability cannot be regarded as satisfactory for several subscales, but note that each subscale only comprises a maximum of 5 items that are designed to capture both indoor- and outdoor-related aspects of perceived housing that may not be congruent in each respect.

Responses to the autonomy-related items appeared to be substantially more homogeneous when considering aspects of the out-of-home environment compared with an indoor focus of appraisal. Apparently, elders' daily indoor home routines and expectations to age in place are affected by various potential influences in a much more heterogeneous way than they are with respect to the out-of-home environment.

CONFIRMATORY MODEL TEST

Confirmatory factor analysis has been used for a more rigid testing of the assumed structure of the item pool. However, results for the three-domain model indicated substantial misfit to the empirical data, regardless of whether single indicators or aggregated sub-domain scores were considered. More specifically, outbound parameter estimates for the relationship between the identity- and privacy-related components indicate that these factors could not be separated. Introducing method factors for indoor and outdoor indicators did not result in a more appropriate representation of the empirical data.

These findings preclude us from suggesting the proposed instrument as a consistent and reliable estimate for the three conceptually holistic dimensions of perceived housing in later life. The results indicate that people may not perceive issues of privacy and identity as separate experiential entities of person–environment exchange. Moreover, the multi-dimensional space of perceived indoor housing appears to be only partly congruent with the perception of the neighborhood home environment.

POST-HOC EXPLORATORY ANALYSIS

In an attempt to inform further conceptual reasoning and scale development, we present results from post hoc analyses of the pilot pool of perceived housing indicators.

Exploration of Item Interrelationships

In concordance with the aforementioned results of both conventional scale analysis and confirmatory factor analysis, principal component analysis suggests the need to consider more than three (overarching) but less than 11 subcomponents to account for the observed variance in perceived housing. According to the Kaiser criterion, up to 12 components could be extracted. However, visual inspection of the eigenvalues indicates a comparably good representation by 6 major components (Table 4).

Interpretation of the pattern of item loadings yields a clear daily independence factor (factor 1, 15 items) that, apart from the vast majority of both indoor and out-of-home autonomy indicators, also includes the privacy aspect familiarity with the out-of-home environment. The second and third components are characterized by indicators from both the identity and privacy domain. Because the second component is dominated by references to the out-of-home environment with respect to 6 of the 8 proposed identity- and privacy-related meanings of housing, this experiential component may be interpreted as neighborhood belonging (factor 2, 10 items). On the contrary, although it also shows a considerable spread over the presupposed subdimensions, the third factor is characterized by references that express the perceived home environment as a mirror of self (factor 3, 9 items), using a term borrowed from Markus (1995). Indicators that may define the fourth component share a connotation of continuity and remaining in place (factor 4, 7 items) and incorporates some of the indicators from the initially proposed autonomy domains, especially those that explicitly refer to chances

TABLE 4 Exploratory Factor Structure of Item Pool

Factor loading (only > .30 displayed)	One: Daily independence	Two: Neighborhood belonging	Three: Mirror of self	Four: Continuity and remaining in place	Five: Being alone and at peace	Six (...)
35[1] I can handle daily routines of my personal hygiene alone at home.	0.83					
42 How to move around in my neighborhood is up to my decision.	0.82					
21 I know all the places I need to run errands.	0.81					
37 If I need medical help, I can go to the doctor alone.	0.81					
34 I can handle my daily housekeeping routines myself.	0.79					
38 I don't need anybody's help to get from A to B in my neighborhood.	0.75					
36 I need help from others for my daily shopping.	−0.75					
43 I myself decide which opportunities in the neighborhood I will use.	0.67					
20 I am well—acquainted to streets and walkways in my neighborhood.	0.64					
39 I myself decide how to structure my day.	0.62					0.38
44 I have a lock on my daily routines.	0.61					0.52
46 I can contribute my share to neighborhood life.	0.58				0.41	
41 I myself decide what I do in my neighborhood.	0.46				0.36	
5 I would take part in initiatives to design my neighborhood.	0.45					
8 I am a regular customer in many shops in the neighborhood.	0.37					
12 I feel myself attached to the people in my neighborhood.		0.69				
33 There are places in my neighborhood that have shaped me.		0.68				
32 There are places in my neighborhood that hold private memories.		0.66				
7 I would like to stay in this neighborhood in the future.		0.65	0.33			
11 Familiar faces in the neighborhood make me feel a part of it.		0.63				
17 Changes in the neighborhood do affect me.		0.57				
24 I feel good in my neighborhood.		0.57	0.35			
16 The neighborhood has nothing to do with me.		−0.51				
4 The condition of my neighborhood matters a lot to me.	0.37	0.48				
15 I would lose a lot of myself if I were to move away from here.		0.46	0.31	0.31		
19 I feel attached to my home.			0.77	0.30		
22 I feel at home in my apartment.			0.69			
30 At home I can just be what I am.			0.68			

(Continued on next page)

TABLE 4 (*Continued*)

#	Factor loading (only > .30 displayed)	One: Daily independence	Two: Neighborhood belonging	Three: Mirror of self	Four: Continuity and remaining in place	Five: Being alone and at peace	Six (...)
9	Since I live here, my home has become an important point of reference to me.			0.61			
23	My home is a place to relax.					0.38	
25	I feel secure in my neighborhood.			0.53			
2	I do care much about personal objects in my home.			0.42	0.40		
1	The furnishing of my home tells a lot about me.	0.39		0.42	0.34	0.34	
10	I can be myself in my neighborhood.			0.39			
6	Many things in my home have their specific places.				0.61		
31	What I do in my home is nobody's business but my own.				0.61		
27	I have the opportunity to be myself at home.				0.59		
40	Everything in my home will stay the way it is, no one is going to tell me what to do.				0.50		
45	Whether I can stay in my home or not depends on luck and circumstance.				0.41		
18	I know my home like the back of my hand.	-0.39			0.39		
47	Whether or not I will be able to stay in my home will probably depend on other people.			-0.31	0.39		0.37
28	I know places in my neighborhood where I can be alone and at peace with the self if I want to.					0.68	
29	There are places in my neighborhood where I can be undisturbed although being among people.					0.68	
26	At home I have the opportunity to be undisturbed.			0.40		0.52	
3	I do not follow the advice of others when it comes to the layout of my home.					0.36	-0.33
13	I am a part of the social community in this building.		0.32			0.57	
14	This building's style and shape means a lot to me.					-0.36	

Note. Items are sorted according to factor loading. Highest factor loadings for indicators with substantial cross-loadings are underlined. The translation of the German word "Quartier" may cover neighborhood, quarter, or even district; we emphasized the word "neighborhood," although it is characterized by social and physical entities.

[1] Numbers indicate the order of appearance in the questionnaire.

and risks of remaining in place. Factor 5 is best represented by indicators that express experiences of undisturbed and autonomous housing with respect to both the immediate indoor and adjoining out-of-home environment. Different from the functionally coined daily independence component, this domain appears to be more strongly related to a notion of being alone and at peace (factor 5, 4 items). As a consequence of the implied method, any additional component extracted will be more specific to connotations represented by only a small set of indicators. Thus, the last factor (not separately labeled) represents covariation in two items that address social ties to the neighborhood and that participants don't care much about the style of the building one lives in.

Descriptives for Hypothetical Components of Perceived Housing

Given the post hoc character of the identified empirical meanings of housing in later life, we will present differentiations of these components for various individual background characteristics in a purely descriptive way and refrain from any statistical testing. The hints to the potential validity of different connotations of perceived housing in different subgroups of the pilot sample may inform a more tailored generation of additional indicators to use in future scale development. Table 5 gives correlations and mean differences with respect to the individual factor scores on all six hypothetical aspects of perceived housing.

Substantial relationships between chronological age and perceived housing aspects are suggested by a moderate negative correlation for factor 1 only. The plausibility of this relationship, and hence the validity of the interpretation of this hypothetical factor, is further supported by the relatively large positive correlation with respondents' self-rated health. With respect to other sociodemographic background variables, those participants from urban and suburban residential areas hold higher values of factor 1 than those living in more remote areas. Moreover, because financial and educational resources are vital ingredients to independence in later life, we were not surprised to find more of these resources to come with higher reported levels on this factor. Factor 2 shows the highest correlation with living duration with respect to both house/apartment and neighborhood (i.e., town, city). However, relationships to chronological age are small in magnitude. High attachment to the neighborhood context of housing is positively associated with higher overall housing satisfaction. Nevertheless, motivations or options to relate to the surrounding housing area appear to be smaller in urban areas compared with rural settings, as well as for those participants who do not own the house or flat they live in. Apart from these differences, financial resources do not appear to play a major role for attachment to the neighborhood. Because higher educational backgrounds are often related to flexibility

TABLE 5 Individual Factor Scores by Sociodemographic Background Variables

N, r (Pearson) or Mean value within category	No.	Factor					
		One: Daily independence	Two: Neighborhood belonging	Three: Mirror of self	Four: Continuity and remaining in place	Five: Being alone and at peace	Six (...)
Age, years	157	**-.52**	**.15**	**.08**	**.14**	**<.01**	**.20**
Sex							
Male	58	0.04	0.09	-0.12	-0.14	-0.14	0.10
Female	99	-0.02	-0.05	0.07	0.09	0.08	-0.06
Self-rated health (1–5)	155	**.41**	**-.11**	**.18**	**-.14**	**.10**	**.10**
Household composition							
Living alone	62	-0.01	-0.16	0.05	0.10	0.19	-0.35
Living together with others	149	-0.01	0.06	-0.03	-0.05	-0.08	0.13
Home ownership							
Tenant	57	0.06	-0.17	-0.13	0.03	0.06	-0.12
Own house/no rent	97	-0.05	0.01	0.06	<-0.01	-0.03	0.07
Area of residency							
Rural	48	-0.40	0.33	0.09	-0.09	-0.10	0.19
Suburban	55	0.09	-0.15	-0.08	0.22	0.05	0.12
Urban	52	0.25	-0.11	-0.02	-0.11	0.09	-0.30
Net income (comb. cat.)							
Less than 2,500 € per month	70	-0.28	0.01	-0.09	0.18	-0.06	-0.09
2,500 € or more per month	64	0.20	0.02	0.07	-0.17	0.09	0.03
Refused to answer	21	0.27	-0.07	0.02	-0.06	-0.05	0.26
Education (selected cat.)							
No university	75	-0.21	0.18	0.06	0.04	<0.01	0.09
University	77	0.18	-0.15	-0.04	-0.03	<-0.01	-0.08
Living duration (in city/town)	156	**-.07**	**.27**	**.14**	**-.02**	**-.15**	**.11**
Living duration (house/app.)	156	**-.05**	**.30**	**.13**	**.10**	**-.18**	**.16**
Housing satisfaction (1–5)	156	**.13**	**.31**	**.47**	**-.02**	**.14**	**.04**

Note. Numbers in bold indicate correlations between factors and approx. continuous background characteristics.

with respect to housing, participants with academic background hold lower positions on this perceived housing component. A less diverse picture can be found with respect to potential individual characteristics' effect on factor 3. Somewhat higher mean factor scores for women compared with men and owners compared with tenants support the validity of our interpretation. Moreover, slightly higher positions for participants who live in rural settings, possess more financial resources, or are less educated may be regarded as further support for this perceived housing aspect. Finally, substantial positive relationships with overall housing satisfaction can be found for this factor. Being a woman, living in a suburban place, and having to get along with compromised health or a limited amount of financial resources seem to be background characteristics that may affect factor 4. This housing-related experience may also capture some of the more problematic feelings related to housing in old age. Also for factor 5, only small tendencies can be found with respect to different background characteristics. Being a man, living in rural areas, and having less money and a longer history of living in a place appears to be inversely related to the experience of positive withdrawal and autonomy. Finally, the hypothesized more social component of perceived housing is also found to be positively related to chronological age and the duration of living in the current home. The most prominent experiential differences can be found with respect to living area and household composition: participants from single households and urban residential areas perceive their housing much less as a matter of social issues. Even when taking into account their low scientific virtue, we would argue that these findings can make a point for considering more holistic components of experiences to better address the heterogeneity of perceived housing in old age.

DISCUSSION

In this article, we tried to emphasize content-related and methodological aspects of the assessment of experiential person–environment exchange processes (in particular, aspects of perceived housing). Starting from a four-domain model of perceived housing developed in the project ENABLE-AGE, we identified challenges in the existing measures and presented preliminary data to continue the discussion on valid assessment of perceived housing. In this regard, we were able to at least address some of the challenges with existing perceived housing measures. In particular, the new indicators were less susceptible to show ceiling effects and captured the out-of-home environment as an important area of perceived housing, strengthening claims for structural and ecological validity. Moreover, identity-related aspects of perceived housing, issues of privacy and familiarity at home, and autonomy-related aspects of perceived housing have been assessed in a methodological mix of face-to-face assessment and an online survey that may allow for a better coverage of the diversity of housing arrangements in old age. Finally, instead of relying on the acceptable Cronbach's alpha scores for the three overarching scales and concepts, we used a rigid testing of our conceptual model by using confirmatory factor analysis that revealed substantial misfit to the empirical data on the subscale level. However, from a substantive point of view, investigation of areas not fitting well with the conceptual model turned out to be informative in its own right. This is particularly true for the disparity of indoor and outdoor perceptions of housing aspects. To proceed from this step of analysis, we finally presented results from exploratory post-hoc analyses of the pilot pool of perceived housing indicators, further underlining a more holistic perspective on perceived housing that may incorporate behavioral, cognitive, and emotional aspects. Descriptive findings for six extracted facets of perceived housing showed plausible relationships to major background characteristics of this pilot sample that encourage us to continue with further steps of method development.

However, this first step ahead toward further method development has several limitations. Concerning the data assessment, there was only little control over sample composition and validity of information given (especially within the online survey). Although some of the mentioned methodological shortcomings of the former instruments have been addressed, psychometric problems, such as the heterogeneity of subscales—as well as ceiling effects—are partially still there. In terms of the assumption to balance out the home and the out-of-home environment, at least in German, the term "home" appears to be easier to define than the term "Quartier," which refers to both the neighborhood and the district. Finally, and most importantly, this study considered only parts of the former four-domain model and did not include any cross-cultural replication.

In conclusion, asking how to address the overarching question "Environmental Gerontology: What Now?," we would argue that with this article we tried to shed some light on the ongoing struggle for empirically sound quantitative assessment of perceived person–environment processes in the field of housing. Moreover, presenting first findings may show that measurement development in environmental gerontology includes work in progress to further strengthen this perspective also for future cohorts of older adults.

REFERENCES

Altman, I., & Low, S. M. (Eds.). (1992). *Human behavior and environment, Vol. 12: Place attachment.* New York, NY: Plenum Press.

Baltes, M. M., Freund, A. M., & Horgas, A. L. (1999). Men and women in the Berlin aging study. In P. B. Baltes & K. U. Mayer (Eds.), *The Berlin aging study* (pp. 259–281). Cambridge, UK: Cambridge University Press.

Brown, B. B., & Perkins, D. D. (1992). Disruptions in place attachment. In I. Altman & S. M. Low (Eds.), *Place attachment* (pp. 279–304). New York, NY: Plenum Press.

Clark-Plaskie, M., & Lachman, M. E. (1999). The sense of control in midlife. In S. L. Willis & J. D. Reid (Eds.), *Life in the middle: Psychological and social development in middle age* (pp. 181–208). San Diego, CA: Academic Press.

Fänge, A., & Iwarsson, S. (1999). Physical housing environment–development of a self-assessment instrument. *Canadian Journal of Occupational Therapy, 66,* 250–260.

Fänge, A., & Iwarsson, S. (2003). Accessibility and usability in housing–Construct validity and implications for research and practice. *Disability and Rehabilitation, 25,* 1316–1325.

Haak, M., Fänge, A., Iwarsson, S., & Ivanoff, S. D. (2007). Home as a signification of independence and autonomy: Experiences among very old Swedish people. *Scandinavian Journal of Occupational Therapy, 14,* 16–24. doi: 10.1080/11038120601024929

Heywood, F., Oldman, C., & Means, R. (2002). *Housing and home in later life.* Buckingham, UK: Oxford University Press.

Iwarsson, S., Wahl, H.-W., Nygren, C., Oswald, F., Sixsmith, A., Sixsmith, J., ... & Tornsone, S. (2007). Importance of the home environment for healthy aging: Conceptual and methodological background of the European ENABLE-AGE project. *The Gerontologist, 47,* 78–84. doi: 10.1093/geront/47.1.78.

Lachman, M. E. (1986). Locus of control in aging research: A case for multidimensional and domain-specific assessment. *Journal of Psychology and Aging, 1,* 34–40.

Lachman, M. E., & Burack, O. R. (Eds.). (1993). Planning and control processes across the life span: An overview. *International Journal of Behavioral Development, 16,* 131–143. doi: 10.1177/016502549301600203

Lalli, M. (1992). Urban-related identity: Theory, measurement, and empirical findings. *Journal of Environmental Psychology, 12,* 285–303.

Lawton, M. P. (1977). The impact of the environment on aging and behavior. In J. E. Birren & K. W. Schaie (Eds.), *Handbook of the psychology of aging* (pp. 276–301). New York, NY: Van Nostrand Reinhold.

Lawton, M. P. (1982). Competence, environmental press, and the adaptation of older people. In M. P. Lawton, P. G. Windley, & T. O. Byerts (Eds.), *Aging and the environment* (pp. 33–59). New York, NY: Springer.

Lawton, M. P. (1998). Environment and aging: Theory revisited. In R. J. Scheidt & P. G. Windley (Eds.), *Environment and aging theory. A focus on housing* (pp. 1–31). Westport, CT: Greenwood Press.

Lawton, M. P., & Nahemow, L. (1973). Ecology and the aging process. In C. Eisdorfer & M. P. Lawton (Eds.), *The psychology of adult development and aging* (pp. 619–674). Washington, DC: American Psychological Association.

Markus, C. C. (1995). *House as a mirror of self: Exploring the deeper meaning of home.* Berkley, CA: Conari Press.

Neisser, U. (1988). Five kinds of self-knowledge. *Philosophical Psychology, 1,* 35–59, doi: 10.1080/09515088808572924

Nygren, C., Oswald, F., Iwarsson, S., Fänge, A., Sixsmith, J., Schilling, O., . . . & Wahl, H.-W. (2007). Relationships between objective and perceived housing in very old age. *The Gerontologist, 47*, 85–95.

Oswald, F., & Wahl, H.-W. (2005). Dimensions of the meaning of home in later life. In G. D. Rowles & H. Chaudhury (Eds.), *Home and identity in later life. International perspectives* (pp. 21–46). New York, NY: Springer.

Oswald, F., Hieber, A., Wahl, H.-W., & Mollenkopf, H. (2005). Ageing and person-environment fit in different urban neighbourhoods. *European Journal of Ageing, 2*(2), 88–97. doi: 10.1007/s10433-005-0026-5

Oswald, F., Mollenkopf, H., & Wahl, H.-W. (1999). *Questionnaire on the meaning of home*. Unpublished manuscript, The German Centre for Research on Ageing.

Oswald, F., Schilling, O., Wahl, H.-W., Fänge, A., Sixsmith, J., & Iwarsson, S. (2006). Homeward bound: Introducing a four domain model of perceived housing in very old age. *Journal of Environmental Psychology, 26*, 187–201. doi: 10.1016/j.jenvp.2006.07.002

Oswald, F., Wahl, H.-W., Martin, M., & Mollenkopf, H. (2003). Toward measuring proactivity in person-environment transactions in late adulthood: The Housing-related Control Beliefs Questionnaire. *Journal of Housing for the Elderly, 17*, 135–152.

Oswald, F., Wahl, H.-W., Mollenkopf, H., & Schilling, O. (2003). Housing and life-satisfaction of older adults in two rural regions in Germany. *Research on Aging, 25*, 122–143.

Oswald, F., Wahl, H.-W., Schilling, O., & Iwarsson, S. (2007). Housing-related control beliefs and independence in activities of daily living in very old age. *Scandinavian Journal of Occupational Therapy, 14*, 33–43. doi: 10.1080/11038120601151615

Oswald, F., Wahl, H.-W., Schilling, O., Nygren, C., Fänge, A., Sixsmith, A., . . . & Iwarsson, S. (2007). Relationships between housing and healthy aging in very old age. *The Gerontologist, 47*(1), 96–107. doi: 10.1093/geront/47.1.96

Peace, S. M. (2005). *Environment and identity in later life*. Berkshire, UK: Open University Press.

Pinquart, M., & Burmedi, D. (2004). Correlates of residential satisfaction in adulthood and old age: A meta-analysis. In H.-W. Wahl, R. Scheidt, & P. G. Windley (Eds.), *Annual review of gerontology and geriatrics* (pp. 195–222). New York, NY: Springer.

Rowles, G. D. (1983). Geographical dimensions of social support in rural Appalachia. In G. D. Rowles & R. J. Ohta (Eds.), *Aging and milieu. Environmental perspectives on growing old* (pp. 111–129). New York, NY: Academic Press.

Rowles, G. D., Oswald, F., & Hunter, E. G. (2004). Interior living environments in old age. In H.-W. Wahl, R. Scheidt, & P. G. Windley (Eds.), *Annual review of gerontology and geriatrics* (vol. 22, pp. 167–193). New York, NY: Springer.

Rowles, G. D., & Watkins, J. F. (2003). History, habit, heart and hearth: On making spaces into places. In K. W. Schaie, H.-W. Wahl, H. Mollenkopf, & F. Oswald (Eds.), *Aging independently: Living arrangements and mobility* (pp. 77–98). New York, NY: Springer.

Rubinstein, R. L. (1989). The home environments of older people: A description of the psychosocial processes linking person to place. *Journal of Gerontology: Social Sciences, 44*, S45–S53. doi: 10.1093/geronj/44.2.S45

Scheidt, R. J., & Norris-Baker, C. (2004). The general ecological model revisited: Evolution, current status, and continuing challenges. In H.-W. Wahl, R. Scheidt, & P. G. Windley (Eds.), *Aging in context: Socio-physical environments* (pp. 35–48). New York, NY: Springer.

Scheidt, R. J., & Windley, P. G. (2006). Environmental gerontology: progress in the post-Lawton era. In J. E. Birren & K. W. Schaie (Eds.), *Handbook of the psychology of aging* (6th ed., pp. 105–125). Amsterdam, The Netherlands: Elsevier.

Sixsmith, A. J., & Sixsmith, J. A. (1991). Transition in home experience in later life. *Journal of Architectural and Planning Research, 8*, 181–191.

Stedman, R. S. (2002). Toward a social psychology of place. Predicting behaviour from place-based cognitions, attitude and identity. *Environment & Behavior, 34*, 561–581.

Wahl, H.-W. (2001). Environmental influences on aging and behavior. In J. E. Birren & K. W. Schaie (Hrsg.), *Handbook of the psychology of aging* (5th ed., pp. 215–237). San Diego, CA: Academic Press.

Wahl, H.-W., & Gitlin, L. N. (2007). Environmental gerontology. In J. E. Birren (Ed.), *Encyclopedia of gerontology* (2nd ed., pp. 494–502). Oxford, UK: Elsevier.

Wahl, H.-W., & Oswald, F. (2010). Environmental perspectives on aging. In D. Dannefer & C. Phillipson (Eds.), *International handbook of social gerontology* (pp. 111–124). London, England: Sage.

Wahl, H.-W., Fänge, A., Oswald, F., Gitlin, L. N., & Iwarsson, S. (2009). The home environment and disability-related outcomes in aging individuals: What is the empirical evidence? *The Gerontologist, 49*, 355–367. doi: 10.1093/geront/gnp056

Wahl, H.-W., Iwarsson, S., & Oswald, F. (2012). Aging well and the environment: Toward an integrative model and a research agenda for the future. *The Gerontologist, 1*, 306–313. doi: 10.1093/geront/gnr154

Wahl, H.-W., Oswald, F., Schilling, O., & Iwarsson, S. (2009). The home environment and quality of life related outcomes in advanced old age: Findings of the ENABLE-AGE project. *European Journal of Ageing, 6*, 101–111.

Building a "Practice-Based" Research Agenda: Emerging Scholars Confront a Changing Landscape in Long-Term Care

MIGETTE L. KAUP

Department of ATID, College of Human Ecology, Kansas State University, Manhattan, Kansas, USA

MARK A. PROFFITT

School of Architecture and Urban Planning, University of Wisconsin, Milwaukee, Wisconsin, USA

ADDIE M. ABUSHOUSHEH

Association of Households International, Manhattan, Kansas, USA

This article examines issues related to the research–practice divide in long-term care and offers insights on why environmental geron-tology has had a variable effect on the larger long-term care system, specifically nursing homes. A Delphi survey technique, a form of action-based research, is a viable solution to assist in bridging the divide. A discussion follows of the key research agendas gleaned by the authors from a recent Delphi study that engaged multiple stakeholders involved in transformative practices in long-term care. This article calls for systemic research agendas that are rooted in the context of practice.

INTRODUCTION

A fundamental divide between research and practice has existed in the field of environmental studies, as well as in the more narrowly defined field of

---

The authors would like to acknowledge Dr. Gerald Weisman for his continued guidance and support.

environmental gerontology (Weiner & Ronch, 2003; Weisman, 2001; Windley & Weisman, 2004). Among the limits that this divide produces is the application of research and theory into practice, policy, and design guidance. Therefore, the ability for environmental gerontology to inform the creation of more appropriate settings and programs for older adults has been variable. Such a divide calls for a pragmatic and applied environmental gerontology to inform the creation of more appropriate settings and programs for older adults. Nowhere is this divide more prevalent than in the rapidly changing long-term care industry and the place-type referred to as nursing homes. Pioneering practitioners have instigated a culture change revolution that is consumer-driven and has increasingly gained traction as a moral imperative, rather than emerging from evidence-based research (Zimmerman & Cohen, 2010). For environmental gerontology to remain relevant, bridging the research–practice divide should be paramount in future research agendas.

This article first examines issues related to the research–practice divide in long-term care. A brief literature review historically situates the divide and offer insights on why environmental gerontology has improved the design of dementia care settings but has had a limited effect on other components of the long-term care system, specifically the nursing home. A Delphi survey technique, a form of action-based research, is presented as a viable solution to assist in bridging the divide. A discussion follows of key research agendas from a recent Delphi study that engaged multiple stakeholders involved in transformative practices in long-term care. This article calls for systemic research agendas that are rooted in the context of practice.

THE HISTORIC RESEARCH–PRACTICE DIVIDE:

Although the purpose of research is to expand knowledge or solve problems, the application of research-based knowledge is generally slow (Rogers, Singhal, & Quinlan, 2009). According to Schneekloth (1987), the transfer of knowledge between research and practice (in many fields of study) is limited due to an institutional separation. Those in the research community have a different knowledge base and priorities for conducting research than those in practice. Academic researchers are highly trained specialists who use rigorous methods to conduct studies and author publications in peer-reviewed journals, which are primarily read by other researchers (Sommer, 1997). In contrast, practitioners are faced with immediacy when solving the problems that research often attempts to understand and dissect to solve (Sommer, 1997). Consequently, practitioners often rely on a pragmatic knowledge base that places them in the position of drawing on many scenarios of what has and has not worked.

One of the fundamental distinctions in the way information from research is transferred into practice lies in the origin of the research questions. Although basic research is done to inform theory, applied research investigates questions posed by a client (Sommer, 1997). Thus, applied research generates knowledge that is intended to be put into practice. However, much of this information is proprietary and, because it may improve a client's competitive advantage, it is not often widely disseminated. Furthermore, the outcomes are not always generalizable to other settings and situations. Therefore, what is learned through applied research is often not easily accessible or transferred into the wider field of practice.

Another key reason for the lack of transferability is that researchers may not be familiar with the resources required to implement findings or recommendations. Indeed, policy-based research often overlooks the resources available to the practitioner as it prioritizes the wants, needs, and welfare of society (Finkler & Ward, 2003). This presents special challenges when applying research to organizations with fixed resources, such as nursing homes that offer the highest level of care within the continuum of long-term care. For example, institutional buildings, which have become synonymous with the nursing home place-type, are typically constructed based on current programs and operations that may quickly outgrow the space allocated or evolve in such a way that the building becomes restrictive; however, these structures are one of the slowest building types to change, which is partially due to limited resources (Brand, 1994). Framing research questions from a resource and application-based perspective requires a paradigm shift with an emphasis on the practical use of knowledge.

Windley and Weisman (2004) addressed the transference of knowledge from research to practice through the assembly of a framework, which is based on Schneekloth's (1987) six categories of transfer. Within this framework, they argue that one solution is moving from passive forms of transfer (i.e., trickle down and communication dissemination) to more active forms such as applied research and action-based research (Figure 1).

Weisman (1983) argued that an action-based paradigm requires rethinking the research purpose toward addressing a specific problem. An action-

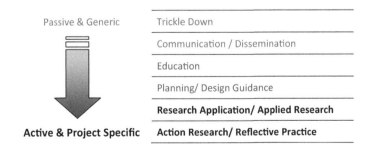

FIGURE 1 A Continuum of Research Application Strategies (Windley & Weisman, 2004).

based research design obliges the researcher to engage in the dual purpose of facilitating change and generating knowledge (McNiff, 2002; McNiff & Whitehead, 2002). Therefore, action-based research has a cyclical approach of planning, acting, observing, and reflecting, with a generative cycle in which a feedback loop starts the process over again (McNiff, 2002). Systematic collection techniques—including experiencing (observing and taking field notes), inquiring (asking people for information), and examining (using and making records)—are used to engage in action research and to gather quantitative and qualitative data to address changes in a setting, approach, or outcome. However, action-based research has proved challenging within the context of the organization, who may be unwilling to adopt the method or is concerned with the overall outcome[1] (Sommer, 1997). The transferability of knowledge between project-specific studies is also potentially limited, making it less attractive for addressing larger theoretical problems. However, the authors contend that the action-based research paradigm holds promise for generating new research agendas, which will be discussed further in the article.

PAST AND PRESENT RESEARCH AGENDAS FOR LONG-TERM CARE

At its earliest inception, the field of environment-aging studies was rooted in solving practical problems. One of the key founders, M. Powell Lawton, was committed to improving the quality of life for elders. Lawton believed that research should inform practice, and that research, service delivery, and policy could develop in a mutually reinforcing fashion (Lawton, 1980; Weisman & Diaz Moore, 2003). Although nursing homes have received considerable attention in the field of environmental gerontology (Koncelik, 1976; Perkins, Hoglund, King, & Cohen, 2004; Schwartz, 1996), the environments and practices of long-term care have remained relatively static since 1965, when Medicare and Medicaid were established (Braithwaite, 1993; Schwartz, 1996; Talerico, O'Brien, & Swafford, 2003; Vitaliano & Toren, 1994; Vladeck, 1980, 2003; Winzelberg, 2003). The following section outlines some of the key reasons research has had little effect on these care settings.

Minimal Effect of Research on Nursing Home Environments

Much of the environmental gerontology research conducted takes a trickle-down dissemination approach, in which information is transferred through discrete mechanisms (e.g., they are "trickling down" through the research journals, and are only occasionally translated into common language for trade sources or widely publicized); therefore, applicability and accessibility to the practitioner is limited. This is further compounded by the significant resources and the long-range planning time it takes to construct the built environment. By the time a building is occupied, new research may exist, operators might have lost sight of the reasons for the original design decisions, or organizational turnover can result in a new group of operators who are unaware or uninterested in initial priorities.

Environmental gerontology research has traditionally attempted to isolate variables specifically related to the older adult and the environment (Lawton & Nahamow's, 1973; competence press model) competence press model. Such research rarely considers the role of the organization or its available resources. Furthermore, a disconnect continues to exist between the expectation of how an organization should meet the policy changes that reflect shifting societal goals and expectations (Kane, 2005). For example, although expectations for quality of life for nursing home residents was included in the Nursing Home Reform Act, as part of the Omnibus Reconciliation Act of 1987, Talerico et al. (2003) stated, "research suggests that current health care systems fail to reward high quality person-centered care and reinforce financially standardized care" (p. 14). Because nursing homes are rewarded for providing more extensive healthcare, penalized for poor clinical outcomes, and not incentivized for advancing quality of life, their focus tends to remain on the quality of their clinical care delivery. Concerns for nursing home quality at the policy level have shifted from creating a safe and efficient structure to emphasizing medical processes to validating outcomes (Capitman, Leutz, Bishop, & Casler, 2005). These shifts have occurred through limited policy reactions responding to adverse reports of nursing home quality, which have rarely attempted to address the entire long-term care system. Walshe (2001) noted that many of the quality problems that spurred increased regulation in the 1970's and 1980's are still endemic throughout the nursing home industry today (p. 128).

Finally, the potential of the environment is rarely considered a key contributing factor in long-term care fields interested in quality besides environmental gerontology. For example, recent work addressing nursing home quality has considered the implications of nursing staff roles, hierarchy of staff, staff quality, and organizational factors associated with management, but little attention was paid to the physical setting where these staff work (Barry, Brannon, & Mor, 2005; Brannon, Zinn, Mor, & Davis, 2002; Rantz et al., 2004; Siegel, Young, Mitchell, & Shannon, 2008; Zhang & Grabowski, 2004). Recent research agendas posited by Rahman and Schelle (2008) identified quality outcomes in transformative care settings but were also void of a significant environmental component, focusing more specifically on the behavioral implications of staff and residents.

Effect on Care Settings for People with Dementia

In contrast to nursing homes in general, significant advances have been made specifically in the area of dementia care environments, which are also situated within the continuum of long-term care and may be located in a nursing home (Calkins, 1988; Cohen & Day, 1993; Cohen & Weisman, 1991; Day, Carreon, & Stump, 2000;). Research in this particular field has been instrumental in formally acknowledging the role of the environment in care practices but has been directed at and used by a relatively small component of the larger long-term care system. The changes were able to be instituted without a wholesale adjustment to the underlying set of values and the system of meaning that defines what the long-term care industry in America looks and acts like (Johnson & Grant, 1985). However, the changes to physical settings that altered care practices demonstrated what is possible through changing a paradigm and have undoubtedly contributed to the current shifts that are being advocated by practitioners.

Early research on environments for people with dementia was aided by the clear boundaries inherent in special care settings, which facilitated comparisons with institutional settings and offered opportunities for before and after comparisons (Day et al., 2000). The observable behaviors of people with dementia (i.e., wandering, exit seeking, wayfinding, incontinence) provided opportunities to test environmental hypothesis; therefore, research justified using one strategy over another, which offered immediate insight into resolving existing problems (Namazi & Johnson, 1991; Namazi, Rosner, & Rechlin, 1991; Nolan, Mathews, Truesdell-Todd, & VanDorp, 2002). Furthermore, research provided long-term care facilities with a clear conceptualization of the place where people with dementia were cared for as a home (Cohen & Weisman, 1991). The use of place as a guiding goal for special care settings suggested altering the entire system, which considered the broad context of the organization, residents, program, and physical environment (Briller & Calkins, 2000). Such a clarity of focus in nursing homes and the advancement of the environment as a research agenda has not existed until the more recent Culture Change movement.

Culture Change in Long-Term Care

Since the late 1990s, advocates of Culture Change initiatives have argued for the reconceptualization of long-term care into a consumer-focused setting for service provision. The Culture Change movement in long-term care is still in a state of development and reflects multiple initiatives that assume a similar trajectory, which emphasizes an individual's overall well-being and personal engagement more than their conformity and adherence to care-based interventions (Weiner & Ronch, 2003). The term "Culture Change" in long-term care refers to replacing a medical model of care with a social model of care through a shift in the organizational objectives of the nursing home setting that radically revise staff configurations and transform physical environments. Proponents of the movement typically seek to alter the institution into a home, which embodies inherent physical features and the sociocultural attributes related to meaning and place experience. Thus, the emphasis is on a holistic milieu that includes the acknowledgment of place and a good quality of life for residents, as well as quality health care for chronic conditions (Kane, Lum, Cutler, Degenholtz, & Yu, 2007; Lustbader, 2001; Rabig, Thomas, Kane, Cutler, & McAlilly, 2006; Shields & Norton, 2006). As it has gained traction, this initiative has thrust rapid change throughout the long-term care system, advancing significant modifications in the design of buildings, user roles and expectations, and the organizational models that these facilities subscribe to (White-Chu, Graves, Godfrey, Bonner, & Sloane, 2009). The shift has also forced adjustments in the policy structures that oversee this highly regulated setting.

Unlike the more measured advancements in dementia care, all of this has happened at such a pace that little research or evidence-based design has been attributed to the process or outcomes (Rabig et al., 2006). In essence, each pioneering practitioner is engaging in a quasi-action-based research process, with a cyclical process of acting, reflecting, and acting again. However, this information is done on an ad hoc basis and is rarely systematically collected or shared, which results in ambiguity and conjecture. However, the long-term care community's growing awareness of these pioneering providers has created an increased demand for the dissemination of information that will inform best practices and strategies for change. Publications, such as those by Shields and Norton (2006), and assessment instruments, such as those by Grant and Norton (2003), are promoted as guides for initiating the change. Rahman and Schelle (2008) looked at the rapid advancement of Culture Change within the field of long-term care. They state that "culture-change interventions are often advocated with little mention of their mostly untested premises. Instead, case studies and anecdotal reports are often presented as evidence of success, typically with no mention of the prudence needed when one is attempting to generalize from this information" (Rahman & Schelle, 2008, p. 144). Some models for Culture Change are not clearly defined and offer much ambiguity. One example is the Household Model, which suggests the subdivision of the nursing home and disbursement of services and functions similar to that of a domestic home for smaller groups of residents. Because the Household Model has been used to describe fundamentally different environments, organizational structures, and places with different daily routines, it is challenging for researches to evaluate the model even though it is frequently referred to in the Culture Change literature.

Although researchers attempt to catch up to the rapidly emerging process of Culture Change, they have not always considered the role of the physical environment. For example, measures targeted at empirically testing person-directed care practices have recently been explored through The Better Jobs Better Care demonstration program funded by the Atlantic

Philanthropies and Robert Wood Johnson Foundation, with limited consideration of the built environment. White, Newton-Curtis, and Lyons (2008) identified five central dimensions of person-directed care: personhood, knowing the person, autonomy and choice, comfort care, and nurturing relationship. They acknowledged that a sixth dimension, a supportive environment, also appeared to be critical for supporting person-directed care practices (p. 116) but did not directly link the environment with care outcomes. Although this work attempts to bridge the practice–research divide, from an environmental perspective it continues to treat the role of the built environment as a separate and isolated variable, suggesting that environmental gerontology research expertise in this area is needed to provide a cohesive perspective.

To fill this identified void, some research has looked at the new long-term place type of physically detached or interconnected households for small groups of residents, which are currently heralded in the Culture Change literature (Grant & Norton, 2003; Weiner & Ronch, 2003). Kane et al. (2007) investigated the effects of the physically detached households (i.e., Green Houses®, Small Houses, cottages). However, the measured variables focused only on those that could be ascertained through clinical metrics. The physical features of the settings and the behavioral patterns of residents and staff were not described such that insight could be gleaned into the specific factors that contributed most significantly to the outcomes. The researchers (Kane et al., 2007) acknowledge that this is a limitation of study based on a specific environmental program and change. When considering the complex nature of a place-based program, it is not always possible to isolate, control, predict, or decipher the interaction of specific components. However, there is a danger if research only considers or reports outcomes because this lacks the systemic focus needed to inform practice about the inner workings of various strategies and models.

Long-term care Culture Change providers are increasingly adopting an open-systems approach—looking outside their own organizations and geographic regions to other provider's models and place types, learning and adapting as they evolve (Unruh & Wan, 2004). Popular or well-publicized Culture Change models offer some guidance for those wishing to begin. However, a recent review of the research literature related to the implementation of long-term care Culture Change households by Zimmerman and Cohen (2010) found limited premises for the models. The significant changes suggested for Culture Change increase the risks that an organization must assume as they attempt to be more innovative with their service and housing options. With no theoretical foothold for change and limited evidence-based protocols, decisions are based primarily on practice-based acumen and empathetic intuition and with approaches and evaluations that are somewhat stochastic. Great interest exists within the industry to reduce these risks by acquiring information about best practices and the impact of investing resources. Although practice-based knowledge is a rich resource, it also is inherently limited by an organization's scope of interaction and awareness of strategies being implemented. Thus far, few research studies have been conducted that offer a cross-industry view such as traditional surveys, which engaged specific audiences in determining the degree to which Culture Change strategies are being employed by providers throughout the United States (Doty, Koren, & Sturla, 2008). However, few research studies have asked long-term care stakeholders to express their opinions about the Culture Change movement and its associated practices.

USE OF THE DELPHI METHOD TO BRIDGE THE RESEARCH PRACTICE DIVIDE

A means of exploring emerging topics across a field of practice is the Delphi technique (Mitchell, 1991, p. 337), which, as one strategy within action-based research, is situated in the praxis paradigm where practice and knowledge have a reciprocating information generating relationship (O'Brien, 2001). The RAND Corporation developed the Delphi method in the 1950s with the purpose of obtaining expert consensus (Dalkey & Helmer, 1963). As such, the Delphi technique explores the common experience of individuals attempting to associate or relate variables that reveal collective patterns of understanding and actionable information (Creswell, 2008a, 2008b). The objective of most Delphi applications is the reliable and creative exploration of ideas or the production of suitable information for decision making where there is uncertainty on both the nature of a problem under investigation and the possible measures for addressing it effectively and efficiently—order from chaos. Rather than wait for the derivation of an adequate theory based on tested scientific knowledge, the Delphi technique attempts to systematically obtain the relevant intuitive insights of experts. Participating in an action-based research Delphi panel offers participants the opportunity to bypass the trickle-down approach of traditional research and immediately discover and learn from different views.

As an iterative process, the Delphi method provides structure for communication among experts that allows them to deal with a complex problem systematically, with feedback related to individual contributions, assessment of group judgment, and opportunities for experts to revise views and reassess previous contributions (Adler & Ziglio, 1996). This process is hallmarked by multiple waves of input using a multidisciplinary panel with the objective of achieving consensus on a particular topic (Linstone & Turoff, 2002). The Delphi method is dependent on the participation of contributors who have intimate knowledge of the topic of exploration because they are asked to individually respond to questions and submit results to a host or coordinator who looks for central, extreme, and conflicting tendencies. This information is summarized and shared with all of the respondents, who are then asked to weigh in on the results. The coordinator continues the process until consensus appears to be reached (Grisham, 2008). Unlike traditional action-based research where the researcher may have a clear bias, the coordinators of a Delphi technique are expected to stay neutral and encourage the equal participation of all panelists, even if their initial premise for engaging participants in the Delphi technique may be to evoke change.

Because individuals participate and provide feedback anonymously, the process allows for a reduced bias that can sometimes occur when experts meet face-to-face and avoid domination by a particular profession, vested interest, or personality. If carefully guided, this can allow researchers to identify where theory development and further investigation are needed. The iterative process of the Delphi technique is also reflected in the cyclical actions of action-based research in which the researcher reflects on the results of previous actions and reacts with new questions. Action research projects are contextually specific but rarely generalizable to the context of other situations; however, knowledge gained from a Delphi study offers an opportunity to explore future research directions from the field of practice. The remainder of this article describes a Delphi study that was conducted to explore the field of Culture Change in nursing homes broadly that generated several key research agendas for the field of environmental gerontology.

PURPOSE OF THE CULTURE CHANGE HOUSEHOLD MODEL SURVEY

Recognizing the need to tap into the divergent but practice-based knowledge of the authors, three emerging scholars conducted a Delphi study to engage a broad range of long-term care Culture Change stakeholders in a discussion to determine if and how different approaches to Culture Change were being operationalized by those who were actively engaging in some aspect of implementation. The Culture Change Household Model Survey took an action research approach that was both contextually specific to the place-type of long-term care in regard to applicable goals and generally broad with regard to actual strategies being used. The survey was designed to identify: (1) which strategies were most commonly associated with Culture Change and the household model; (2) the feasibility of the strategies; (3) the perceived outcomes for the strategies; (4) the key barriers to adoption strategies; and (5) the measurement strategies for progress in Culture Change. This participatory process was based on the premise that the most applicable and actionable knowledge would arise thorough the process of a national community of practitioners addressing problematic, real-life situations that were occurring within long-term care. This research was seen as a foundational step for the research team, whose individual research agendas are collectively situated within the household model in long-term care as part of the Culture Change movement, as well as for the broad constituency of practitioners engaging in Culture Change who were also interested in coming to a collective understanding of the changing and emerging field.

The process allowed for multiple world views on the redefinition of the entire long-term care system (at the macro scale), seeking input on the inter-relationships of the environment, which included multiple dimensions. The Delphi technique is well-suited not only for when the resources required to assemble an appropriate representation of experts together is not feasible, but also for situations in which exploring emerging and divergent opinions when a face-to-face meeting might result in more posturing than productive discussion (Linstone & Turoff, 2002). The Culture Change movement in long-term care could not have come as far as it has without the powerful personalities and personal conviction of many individuals, who often prioritize strategies differently. Because the literature on long-term care is wide ranging and crosses multiple disciplines, the Delphi technique also allows for a cross-disciplinary panel to contribute to the current application of practice-based knowledge. The complexities confronting the rapidly changing health care setting result in many types of experts voicing their opinions, often with competing priorities, either in both practice or and research. Both of these conditions were relevant factors as the research team considered suitable research strategies.

The Culture Change Household Model survey incorporated multiple viewpoints that drew on multiple theoretical lenses, highlighting those of practitioners, as it attempted to reexamine the assumptions and questions of what constitutes desired and undesirable attributes of the environment milieu and the behaviors enacted within these settings. The belief was that by engaging directly with practitioners as part of the larger care system, practices being implemented can be better understood and more appropriate research agendas can be established. Unlike other survey-based research projects that have queried for awareness of Culture Change or the general adoption of Culture Change practices (Doty et al., 2008; Miller, Mor, & Clark, 2009), this action research strategy attempted to explore the efficacy of asserted Culture Change practices as well evaluative strategies to measure outcomes.

THE CULTURE CHANGE HOUSEHOLD MODEL SURVEY

The development of the Culture Change Household Model Survey required assembling a targeted panel of experts and the construction of an instrument that would engage these panelists in a discussion focused on the most relevant Culture Change issues confronting long-term care settings.

Expert Panel

Participation of a broad range of stakeholders engaging in the advancement of Culture Change strategies was seen as critical to process. For the three planned waves of the Delphi survey, 219 experts representing practitioners and providers (consistently comprising approximately 60% of the sample), researchers (approximately 12%), designers and consultants (approximately 18%), policy regulators (approximately 8%), and vendors (approximately 2%) were asked to contribute their professional perspectives. Participants were identified using a variation of snowball sampling using key experts in the field. Priority was given to enlisting long-term care providers who were engaged in Culture Change and those who were nationally recognized for their active interest in Culture Change.

Identifying the Key Strategies for Culture Change in the Literature

A literature review was conducted to identity various assertions of industry experts and pioneers for the panelist to discuss. Because long-term care Culture Change practice literature is not prevalent in the scholarly literature, the research team also consulted a wide array of resources that practitioners might consult while launching or implementing Culture Change in their own care communities. Criteria were derived from a review of the Culture Change literature in long-term care published before January 2010, which included scholarly publications (Angelelli, 2006; Eppelheimer & Sheahan, 2009; Flesner, 2009; Kane et al., 2007; Rabig et al., 2006; Rahman & Schnelle, 2008; Weiner & Ronch, 2003), and white papers, reports, and conference presentations (Bowman & Schoeneman, 2006; Calkins, 2008; Chance, 2008; Cutler, 2008; Dotyet al., 2008; Grant & Norton, 2003; Nelson, 2008; Tellis-Nayak, 2009). Popular and trade publications as well as newsletters that are especially relevant to practitioners were also reviewed (e.g., *Culture Change Now; Long-term Living Magazine; Provider Magazine; LeadingAge;* and *Pioneer Networking*), as well as World Wide Web sources that provided documented assertions made by long-term care stakeholders (e.g. Centers for Medicare and Medicaid Services; Center on Age and Community; Leading Age; and Pioneer Network).

Some notable examples in the literature concerning areas which reflect differences of opinion regarding what are central or tangential elements to the success of Culture Change include; emphasis on the physical environment and roles that staff play. Another example that is often discussed in the literature but is sometimes questioned by practitioners when they come together is residents' level of autonomy. The influence of the built environment is considered by some to be absolutely essential in establishing a different expectation; other providers feel strongly that Culture Change is possible regardless of the setting (e.g. Rabig et al., 2006; Kehoe & Van Heesch, 2003;

Calkins, 1997). There are diverse opinions expressed in the literature and by providers about the role of staff. Some advocate for the universal worker, others feel that care practices will decline if there isn't a full complement of staff on duty at all times (e.g. Hagy, 2003; Rabig et al., 2006). Regarding residents' level of autonomy, there are those who assert that residents should be able to make choices, even if those choices are considered to be counter to their own well-being (e.g. Shields & Norton, 2006; Calkins & Brush, 2009). While it wasn't easy to locate literature that would argue otherwise, discussions with practitioners reveals that others feel strongly that there is a clear custodial role in care settings that trumps the residents' decision making priority as a matter of health and safety.

Organization of the Strategies

The assertions derived from the literature review (including personal communications) were sorted into 95 key strategies that were grouped into five domains to organize the panelist discussion (Table 1). These domains also reflect a systemic view of the nursing home as a place (Lawton, 1980, 1998; Wahl & Weisman, 2003). Four of these domains are encompassed within traditional long-term care settings—organizational, operational, financial, and environmental. The fifth domain—household—is unique to Culture Change facilities that have made a purposeful deviation from institutional architecture and created a distinct environment that is patterned after a residential structure. Table 1 provides more detail, including the number of individual strategies for each domain of the study. Using multiple sources provided an opportunity to test popular assumptions, novel approaches, and competing ideas of Culture Change among the panelist.

As presented in Table 1, individual strategies were clustered within each of the five identified domains. The panel was asked to weigh in on each individual strategy and indicate their level of agreement on the desirability and feasibility of the particular item. Table 2 provides an example of three

TABLE 1 Five Domains of the Culture Change Household Model Survey

No. of Strategies	Domain	Description
13	Organizational	The roles of individuals or how the nursing home is organized
20	Operational	The daily routines or operations of the nursing home
17	Environmental	The alterations of utilization of the built environment
14	Financial	Obtaining resources or cost centers for Culture Change
31	Household	Organization, operation, or the built environment of a Household Model

TABLE 2 Examples of Strategies within the Domains of the CCHHM Survey

Examples of Strategies within Five Key Domains
Organizational
Culture Change should strive to increase staff longevity and tenure (retention, full time, non-use of agency staff).
The same staff should consistently works with the same residents.
Culture Change requires shifting the emphasis from a medical diagnosis to the holistic needs of the residents.
Operational
Culture Change should include a way to evaluate progress.
Culture Change should encourage personal relationships between staff and residents.
Culture Change should utilize current technologies to enhance quality of care, communication, and documentation.
Environmental
Residents should be encouraged to personalize their own rooms however they choose (furniture, accessories, photos, paint).
Outdoor areas should be visible and accessible to residents.
Audible call alarms and overhead paging systems should be replaced by silent communication systems.
Finance & Cost
Culture Change improves the nursing home's competitive advantage.
The nursing home should invest in additional staff training related to Culture Change.
Non-managerial staff should be paid to attend off-campus educational conferences/workshops or other care settings to advance their culture change movement
Household
Individual staff or household teams should have the authority to carry out daily decisions and activities in their household.
Each household should have consistent staff assigned exclusively to that household.
Residents who live in a household should be encouraged to personalize shared spaces.

strategies within each of these domains. These items were the initial foundation of the discussions and feedback by the panel.

CULTURE CHANGE HOUSEHOLD MODEL SURVEY OVERVIEW OF THE PROCESS

The three waves of the Culture Change Household Model Survey were administered and completed over a 10-month period from March through December in 2010. DatStat Illume™, an electronic web-based survey instrument, was used to distribute and collect each wave. The DatStat Illume™ program generated descriptive statistics for closed-ended quantitative question responses. A thematic analysis was conducted by the research team on the open-ended responses. Wave one of the Culture Change Household Model Survey asked participants to rate the 95 identified Culture Change and household strategies and to rank their top five Culture Change and household themes according to importance. For the rating exercise, participants were asked to review each strategy and rate its desirability (importance to Culture Change or the household) and its feasibility (ease of implementation). After providing a quantitative rating, panelists were encouraged to share comments, suggest clarifications, argue in favor of against issues, ask questions, or provide examples, as well as suggest other strategies that might be considered vital to Culture Change or the Household Model.

Wave two provided the Delphi participants with a report on the descriptive statistics that indicated the degree of desirability, perceived feasibility, and the extent of agreement among the entire participant panel for each assertion, as well as a brief summary of the open-ended comments from wave one. Participants were also asked to review four key Culture Change goals and three key household goals derived from wave one and suggest barriers to adoption, solutions, positive and negative outcomes, and measurement strategies. A final task for this wave included responding to a list of four controversial issues noted from wave one in an open-ended format.

Wave three reported the summarized responses for four Culture Change goals and three goals for the Household Model. These summaries shared the level of agreement that had been reported through waves one and two and provided related comments on the assertion that were shared by participants who felt that more clarification on the exactness of the assertion was needed.

CULTURE CHANGE HOUSEHOLD MODEL SURVEY IMPLICATIONS FOR FUTURE RESEARCH

The results of the Culture Change Household Model Survey[2] provide a rich resource for understanding the field of practice in long-term care and suggest some clear areas for environmental gerontology to pursue for future research agendas. These targets (as outlined in Table 3) represent opportunities in multidisciplinary fields of gerontology, as well as related fields of environment and behavior studies.

Integrating the Resource System into Research

The limitation of resources was cited as a preventive factor for engaging in Culture Change. Panelist ranked most assertions for Culture Change and the Household Model with a high degree of desirability (i.e., importance), with an average rating indicating moderate (score of 3) to definite (score of 5) desirability. Participants also demonstrated a high degree of consensus for these ratings, as evidenced by standard deviations of less than 1 (Abushousheh, Proffitt, & Kaup, 2011). However, feasibility ratings were almost always rated lower than desirability ratings, and the summative comments from panelist

TABLE 3 Five Targets for Future Research

Targets	Contributions		
	Researchers	Practitioners	Implications
1 **Integrating the Resource System in Research**: Researchers must consider resources available to providers when framing questions, studies, or drawing implications	Familiarity with incentives or grant-sponsored programs to lend financial assistance as well as increased access to and familiarity with imperial research	Tacit knowledge of context, products, reimbursement systems and participants that will contribute to or restrain efforts	Practitioners want practical ideas that consider the available resource structures.
2 **Incorporating the Environment through the Power of Place**: Using familiar, socially relevant place types are a means to promote deep systems change to both the physical environment & social environment	Awareness of other fields of practice, historical underpinnings, and potential implications for abstract associations	Expertise gained through personal history, sense of purpose, diversity of experience and knowledge of successful practices that deviate from the norm	A deeper acknowledgement of the role of the setting could inform decision making about other practices.
3 **Understanding the HH Model Socially & Operationally**: The Household Model must work both socially for residents, staff and family members as well as operationally for the organization to achieve integrity that enables sustainability.	Knowledge of theoretical constructs and concepts that contribute an understanding of social behaviors.	Recognition that some products and environments reinforce behavior, but that desired behavior must also be supported by policy and procedure	Relationships between the people in these settings are influenced by many factors.
4 **Developing Measurement and Training Tools for Culture Change**: Creating benchmarking tools to guide change are essential to demonstrate the contribution of a strategy and determine progress.	Understanding of valid and reliable measurement strategies that may be tailored and are sensitive to a particular intervention	Experience with realistic tactics to obtain information or provide education regarding particular goals	Assessment of outcomes is of interest to practitioners and policy makers.
5 **Engaging in the Field of Practice**: Collaborations between practitioners and researchers are a means to generate practical knowledge	Fluency with theoretical and methodological strategies for interventions as well as strategies for reporting outcomes	Provides access and collaboration in a setting where interventions may be applied and guided by internal goals	Knowledge derived from research will be more rapidly adopted if practitioners assist in setting the research agendas.

demonstrated a wide spectrum of perspectives on the resources required to implement changes, with some panelists arguing that costs should not be barriers. It should be noted that less than 30% of the assertions put forth require significant financial resources, such as substantial changes to the physical environment; however, time (as a resource) is required for creative adaptation and education. Participants confident in their own progress toward Culture Change felt strongly that it was possible to use existing resources in a different way to initiate a deep systems change.

In evaluating the degree of panel consensus for desirability and feasibility of the 95 strategies, the highest degree of consensus was established when responding to the desirability of strategies (78%) in comparison with their degree of consensus related to the feasibility of implementing strategies (58%). Only 2% of the 95 strategies elicited high-panel divergence related to the desirability and feasibility for Culture Change or the Household Model. On average, the degree of consensus was greater for the desirability of a particular strategy than the feasibility, with the only exception relating to the domain of financial strategies for Culture Change. The researchers believe that this reinforces the need for the business case for Culture Change, which has plagued the industry since its inception.

Managing the organization financially during a change process is a practical concern. The reallocation of resources to focus on achieving resident quality of life was projected to result in the potential negative outcomes of reduced efficiency of operations in delivering necessary services. The interrelationships between the dimensions of resident quality of life and the aspects of quality of care present as a reoccurring theme to respondent comments. This suggests an area of environmental gerontology research that may be largely unexplored; the relationship between the larger organizational (and service) component in long-term care and the opportunity for elders to actualize personal autonomy and meaning. This seems to also be especially relevant when objectives turn specifically toward the household model. Research that considers how an organization uses resources or reconsiders resources should clearly be addressed in the future.

Incorporating the Environment through the Power of Place

Environmental assertions were seen as the most costly expenditure, and thereby were less feasible. Several respondents indicated that it was more feasible and essential to alter the people within their environment than it was to alter the environment itself. However, several participants stated that the effect of the environment can help an organization live its intention of providing autonomy to residents. This appears to be especially relevant for interior environments that most closely surround residents and staff (Rowles, Oswald, & Hunter, 2004). A critical area of need exists for long-term care practices and environmental gerontology research agendas to advance education related to the role of the environment. Moreover, environmental gerontology also needs to explore low-cost and budget-neutral improvements to the physical setting that address quality of life for elders.

For the field of environmental gerontology, the perceptions of the environmental components are inherently tied to the established place-type of nursing homes, and the associated architecture establishes a strong perception of how people are expected to behave and what elders should expect from the services of long-term care. A medical atmosphere conveys that those receiving services are sick and need to be acted upon. In this scenario, those individuals providing the treatments hold a position of power and authority. However, the physical environment has the potential to greatly influence the sense of control and autonomy experienced by elders, a stated objective of the Culture Change mantra. If we focus on the complexities specific to long-term care, we can identify the multiple variables and interrelationships in the environment, as well as diverse user-groups and organizational factors that must be considered when understanding this place-type and its effect on quality of life and quality of care. The sociophysical environment must be considered from several vantage points (Wahl & Weisman, 2003). The use of place as a guiding direction can be essential for setting a goal for Culture Change (Briller & Calkins, 2000). What the place of long-term care will be in the future has yet to be completely understood.

Understanding the Household Model Socially and Operationally

New models of care that reflect deep systems change, such as the Household Model, must be evaluated from the resident's perspective, as well as the organization's frame of reference. Numbers of residents in a household have far reaching implications for operations, as well as daily life for residents. Although the consensus among the Delphi panel was that 24 residents should be the maximum number of individuals living together, household size and configuration became an area in which participants agreed to disagree. The variability of responses indicate that the scale of the living environment and its direct relationship to the organizational, operational, and financial domains is an area that largely unknown. Another area that is largely undocumented is the distinctions between independent, free-standing household structures versus interconnected households that are embedded within a larger facility. Delphi participants rated free-standing households less feasible compared with the connected households. The uncertainty of the panelist echoes recent research and reports. Little is known about the effect on resident socialization and community engagement of small groups of highly frail residents living together in separated household settings versus a connected household (Kane & Cutler, 2008; Zimmerman & Cohen, 2010). Furthermore, the uncertainty also reflects the limited information available about how these operate with limited staff resources.

Measurement and Training Tools for Culture Change

The research team was interested in knowing how the practice community evaluates, measures, and determines their progress toward stated objectives of Culture Change. Responses in this area first identified what the measurable targets were and then how or which measurement strategies should be used. Participants identified user satisfaction (staff's and residents') as a component of each of the measurable targets with surveys and interviews consistently listed as the measurement strategies. Other targets included clinical or psychosocial measures that might be available through clinical reporting. However, it should be noted that these specific types of targets (quality of care and quality of life) were secondary for the objectives of Culture Change, but primary for the objectives of the Household Model. In some instances, it was suggested that environmental strategies should be evaluated based on their presence or absence but failed to identify or establish connections for what the environmental feature might afford. The lack of widely known measurement tools to evaluate Culture Change progress and training was also apparent. Therefore, a research agenda that focuses on providing long-term care with the tools to evaluate and train for Culture Change should be considered.

Engaging in the Field of Practice

The Culture Change Household Model Survey also demonstrated the effectiveness of examining Culture Change from the field of practice. This article argues that the rapid application of research requires collaboration among stakeholders, including communication and dissemination, as well as action research strategies (Windley & Weisman, 2004). Application and evaluation models may be most appropriate at this juncture in the development of a new place-type for long-term care that is beginning to emerge. Although large-scale sample studies focusing on outcomes and variables may be helpful to clarify issues in the field, they are examples of trickle down research that does not immediately inform practice. The assumptions that basic forms of research inquiry with the development of universally applicable theory will solve socially relevant problems may be misguided (Fishman, 1999; Flyvbjerg, 2001). As has been demonstrated through the rapid advancement of the Culture Change initiatives, practice won't wait for academia to catch up. The contrast between modern positivism and postmodern pragmatism has radical implications for the methods used for seeking and evaluating knowledge to address problems and goals (Fishman, 1999). Future research agendas should attempt to clarify not only the outcomes of new models of practice, but also the assumptions and premises behind the model.

DISCUSSION

As with any research design, the Culture Change Household Model Survey technique has limitations that should be acknowledged. Selection of participants was completed using a snow ball sample and is not suggested to be representative of the entire population of practitioners, regulators, designers, and consultants engaged in long-term care practices. Not all types of stakeholders for long-term care, including older adults who reside in these settings, were a part of the study. Furthermore, the population of participants cannot be identified with how deeply involved, informed, or progressed they are with Culture Change initiatives. Participation across an eligible sample was also limited to those who had accessible e-mail addresses.

Due to the complexities of Culture Change and the numerous variables involved, the survey was lengthy and full participation in the entire survey may have been compromised by survey fatigue or time limitations. The average amount of time spent in a single login completing wave one was 77.4 minutes, with the shortest time being 16 minutes and the longest time being 3.5 hours. Participation rates were also atypically high for the first wave but, as anticipated, dropped off in the last two waves as the Delphi study increasingly attempted to elicit the insight of those who were farther along their Culture Change journey. As with all survey research, participation is biased by those who are willing to participate, but the Delphi embraces its bias because it actively engages those who are invested in a topic in an action-based research agenda. The outcomes could have been much different if practitioners who were not interested in Culture Change were sought to participate.

Despite the limitations, the Delphi process was effective in illuminating the challenges that confront practitioners who are facing changing regulations, policy, and social expectations while embracing Culture Change. The consensus building process clearly demonstrated that although Culture Change strategies may be considered messy and divergent, clear themes can be identified. More specifically, the Delphi study was able to tap into and illuminate the field of practice across a broader segment of Culture Change compared with the previous work of others, which often reports anecdotal stories. It was also effective in identifying where knowledge gaps of practitioners exist. For example, some practitioners argued for the role of the built environment for Culture Change, whereas others indicated that there was no need to change the environment. Such differences and gaps illuminate that there are some limitations in the practice-based knowledge in which the field of environmental gerontology can provide a key role. For the field of environmental gerontology, it is important to ask, "Is it the role of the practitioner to link or bridge gaps? Is it the role of academics, or does the real promise lie in the combined role of practitioners and academics to come together and use their knowledge in a complimentary solution-building way?"

An opportunity exists for environmental gerontology to use a theoretical base to interpret the criticisms of the existing practices that will demand a new way of thinking. Practical assessment instruments are needed that will validate normative approaches and identify where they fail to achieve their states goals and outcomes (Weisman, Chaudhury, & Diaz Moore, 2000). Practice-based research is inherently valuable to inform the field but may result in a loss of objective criticism from practitioners who may have a conflict of interest in questioning the effectiveness of their practice or use of resources. When practitioners are within the confines of their own practice, an inherent bias exists. The role of the academy should be to provide the objective critique and to identify and validate those variables that contribute to experiences.

CONCLUSIONS

The nursing home industry is facing pressure by society, policy makers, regulators, the government, and consumers to change. For environmental gerontology to be relevant for informing the creation of environments for elders, the field must return to Lawton's original desire for the field to focus on solving problems by enabling those who are a part of this complex system. The development of theory for the satisfaction of the research community may be of limited use. A pragmatic focus is aided by research that is informed by the field of practice (Fishman, 1999; Flyvbjerg, 2001). The field of practice for long-term care is severely hampered by the actual and perceived limitation of resources. Therefore, the traditional view of environmental gerontology of solely looking at the environment and the elderly must be expanded to consider the organization, its entire population, and its resources. Although we may be able to create socially desirable models, if these models do not work operationally they will be difficult to sustain and may result in the creation of housing and care options that are not widely available across socioeconomic groups. Thus, a need exists to look across fields of practice, as well as within fields of practice.

Services provided through nursing homes are critical components in the long-term care continuum. If we are to understand how these dynamics effect the quality of the experience for older adults, we must be willing to consider the system in its totality. This expanded outlook requires a broad and systemic view (e.g., Weisman's Model of Place). As the nursing home is reconceptualized from a hospital to a home, the familiarity of home provides a guiding force for practice, which, for the most part, has been missing in the past. The idea of home provides clarity for not only the physical environment, but also the organizational structure that supports and nurtures daily routines and spontaneous activity. Transformative nursing homes may be posited to achieve quality of care and life for the resident, as well as positive financial outcomes for the home. However, little research supports operational linkages between quality of care, operations, financing, and environment. Accordingly, to achieve advancements in policy that provide further insight into practice, it is essential to study Culture Change homes that are attempting to alter the current state of the industry first-hand. This calls for a pragmatic and applied environmental gerontology that will inform the creation of more appropriate settings and programs for older adults.

NOTES

1. Weisman's (1981) Environment-Behavior Systems Model contends that we must consider the influence of individuals, the organization, and the environment to understand place experience. Weisman (1981) stated that the objectives of the organization may be in conflict with individually oriented goals (p. 37). Organizations often have goals and objectives for their environments that are monetarily based (Markus et al., 1972). If one accepts the organization's effect on our place experience, it is also possible to ask the question: how do place experiences for the individual impact the organization? The organization's influence on place experience should be viewed as dialectic of both impacting and receiving (Weisman, 1981).

2. A white paper summarizing all waves of the Culture Change and Household Model Delphi study is available at http://www.ageandcommunity.org/products.attachment/culture-change-and-the-household-model-9408/Culture%20Change%20and%20the%20Household%20Model%20-%20Delphi%20Survey.pdf.

REFERENCES

Abushousheh, A. M., Proffitt, M. A., & Kaup, M. L. (2011). *2010 Stakeholder survey: Culture change and the household model (white paper)*. Retrieved from http://www.ageandcommunity.org/products.html

Adler, M., & Ziglio, E. (1996). *Gazing into the oracle: The Delphi method and its application to social policy and public health*. Philadelphia, PA: Jessica Kingsley.

Angelelli, J. (2006). Promising models for transforming long-term care. *The Gerontologist, 46*, 428–430.

Barry, T., Brannon, D., & Mor, V. (2005). Nurse aide empowerment strategies and staff stability: Effects on nursing home resident outcomes. *The Gerontologist, 45*, 309–317.

Bowman, C. S., & Schoeneman, K. (2006). *Development of the artifacts of culture change tool* (Centers for Medicare & Medicaid Services, Trans.). Baltimore, MD: Centers for Medicare & Medicaid Services.

Braithwaite, J. (1993). The nursing home industry. *Crime and Justice, 18*, 11–54. Retrieved from http://www.jstor.org/stable/1147653.

Brand, S. (1994). *How buildings learn: What happens after they're built?* New York, NY: Viking.

Brannon, D., Zinn, J. S., Mor, V., & Davis, J. (2002). An exploration of job, organizational, and environmental factors associated with high and low nursing assistant turnover. *The Gerontologist, 42*, 159–168.

Briller, S., & Calkins, M. (2000). Defining place-based models of care: Conceptualizing care settings as home, resort, or hospital. *Alzheimer's Care Quarterly, 1*, 17–23.

Calkins, M. (1988). *Design for dementia: Planning environments for the elderly and the confused.* Owing Mills, MD: National Health.

Calkins, M. P. (1997). Home is more important than carpeting and chintz. *Nursing Homes, 44*(6), 20–25.

Calkins, M. P. (2008, April). *Creating home in a nursing home: Fantasy or reality?* Paper presented at the Creating Home in the Nursing Home: A National Symposium on Culture Change and the Environment Requirements, Washington, DC.

Calkins, M. P., & Brush, J. (2009). Improving quality of life in long-term care. *Perspectives on Gerontology, 14*(2), 37–41.

Capitman, J., Leutz, W., Bishop, C., & Casler, R. (2005). Long-term care quality: Historical overview and current initiatives. *Report for the National Commission for Quality Long-Term Care.* Retrieved from http://www.qualitylongtermcarecommission.org/pdf/txBackground03-10-05FINAL.pdf

Chance, S. (2008). Long-term care housing trends: Past and present. Public Administration and Public Policy New York, 143, 221–240.

Cohen, U., & Day, K. (1993). *Contemporary environments for people with dementia.* Baltimore, MD: John Hopkins University.

Cohen, U., & Weisman, G. (1991). *Holding on home.* Baltimore, MD: John Hopkins University.

Creswell, J. W. (2008a). *Educational research: Planning, conducting, and evaluating quantitative and qualitative research.* Upper Saddle River, NJ: Pearson/Merrill Prentice Hall.

Creswell, J. W. (2008b). *Research design: Qualitative, quantitative, and mixed methods approaches.* Thousand Oaks, CA: Sage.

Cutler, L. J. (2008, April). *Nothing is traditional about environments in a traditional nursing home: Nursing homes as places to live now and In the future.* Paper presented at the Creating Home in the Nursing Home: A National Symposium on Culture Change and the Environment Requirements, Washington, DC. Retrieved from http://www.pioneernetwork.net/Data/Documents/NelsonHousehold-ResidentialPaper.pdf

Dalkey, N., & Helmer, O. (1963). An experimental application of the Delphi method to the use of experts, *Management Science, 9*, 458–467.

Day, K., Carreon, D., & Stump, C. (2000). The therapeutic design of environments for people with dementia: A review of the empirical research. *Gerontologist, 40*, 397–416.

Doty, M. M., Koren, M. J., & Sturla, E. L. (2008). *Culture change in nursing homes: How far have we come? Findings from the Commonwealth Fund 2007 national survey of nursing homes.* Retrieved from http://www.commonwealthfund.org/Content/Surveys/2007/The-Commonwealth-Fund-2007-National-Survey-of-Nursing-Homes.aspx

Eppelheimer, C., & Sheahan, M. (2009, October). *Staff empowerment and accountability: A balancing act.* Presented at the Annual Meeting and Exposition of the American Association of Homes and Services for the Aged, Chicago, IL.

Finkler, S. A., & Ward, D. M. (2003). The case for the use of evidence-based management research for the control of hospital costs. *Health Care Management Review, 28*, 348–365.

Fishman, D. B. (1999). The case for pragmatic psychology. New York, NY: New York University.

Flesner, M. K. (2009). Person-centered care and organizational culture in long-term care. *Journal of Nursing Care Quality, 24*, 273–276.

Flyvbjerg, G. (2001). *Making social science matter: Why social inquiry fails and how it can succeed again.* New York, NY: Cambridge University.

Grant, L., & Norton, L. (2003, November). A stage model of culture change in nursing facilities. Presentation at symposium: Culture change II: Theory and practice, vision and reality, the 56th Scientific Meeting of the Gerontological Society of America, San Diego, CA.

Grisham, T. (2008). The Delphi technique: A method for testing complex and multifaceted topics. *International Journal on Managing Projects in Business, 2*, 112–130.

Hagy, A. (2003). Apple health care: Culture change in a privately owned nursing home chain. In A. S. Weiner, & J. L. Ronch (Eds.), Culture change in long-term care (pp. 295–305). New York, NY: Haworth Social Work Practice Press.

Johnson, C. L., & Grant, L. A. (1985). *The nursing home in American society.* Baltimore, MD: Johns Hopkins University Press.

Kane, R. L. (2005) Changing the face of long-term care. *Journal of Aging and Social Policy, 17*, 1–18.

Kane, R. A., & Cutler, L. J. (2008). *Sustainabilty and expansion of small-house nursing homes: Lessons from the Green Houses in Tupelo, MS, Report to the Commonwealth Fund.* Retrieved from http://www.sph.umn.edu/hpm/LTCResource-Center/research/greenhouse/attachments/GreenHouseSustainabilityandExpansionSeptember2008.pdf

Kane, R. A., Lum, T. Y., Cutler, L. J., Degenholtz, H. B., & Yu, T. C. (2007). Resident outcomes in small-house nursing homes: A longitudinal evaluation of the initial Green House® program. *Journal of the American Geriatrics Society, 55*, 832–839.

Kehoe, M. A., & Van Heesch, B. (2003). Culture change in long term care: The Wellspring Model. In A.S. Weiner, & J. L. Ronch (Eds.), Culture change in long-term care (pp. 159–173). New York, NY: Haworth Social Work Practice Press.

Koncelik, J. A. (1976). *Designing the open nursing home.* Stroudsburg, PA: Dowden, Hutchinson & Ross.

Lawton, M. P. (1980) *Environment and aging.* Belmont, CA: Brooks/Cole.

Lawton, M. P. (1998). Environment and aging theory revisited: A focus on housing. In R. J. Scheidt & P. G. Windley (Eds.), *Environment and aging theory* (pp. 1–31). Westport, CT: Greenwood.

Lawton, M. P., & Nahemow, L. (1973). Ecology and the aging process. In C. Eisdorfer & M. P. Lawton (Eds.), *Psychology of adult development and aging* (pp. 619–674). Washington, DC: American Psychological Association.

Linstone, H. A., & Turoff, M. (2002). *The Delphi method: Techniques and applications.* [Adobe Digital Editions version]. ISBN 0-201-04294-0. Retrieved from http://is.njit.edu/pubs/delphibook/

Lustbader, W. (2001). The pioneer challenge: A radical change in the culture of nursing homes. In L. Noelker & Z. Harel (Eds.), *Qualities of caring: Impact on quality of life* (pp. 185–203). Rochester, NY: Springer.

McNiff, J. (2002). Action research principles and practice. New York, NY: Routledge.

McNiff, J., & Whitehead, J. (2002). *Action research for professional development: Concise advice for new action researchers*. Retrieved from http://jeanmcniff.com/Copy%20booklet%20for%20web%20site.doc

Miller, E. A., Mor, V., & Clark, M. (2009). Reforming long-term care in the United States: Findings from a national survey of specialists. *The Gerontologist, 50*, 238–252.

Mitchell, V. W. (1991). The Delphi technique: An exposition and application. *Technology Analysis and Strategic Management, 3*, 333–358.

Namazi, K. H., & Johnson, B. D. (1991). Physical environmental cues to reduce the problems of incontinence in Alzheimer's disease units. *American Journal of Alzheimer's Disease and Other Dementias, 6*(6), 22–28.

Namazi, K. H., Rosner, T. T., & Rechlin, L. (1991). Long-term memory cuing to reduce visuo-spatial disorientation in Alzheimer's disease patients in a special care unit. *American Journal of Alzheimer's Disease and Other Dementias, 6*(6), 10–15

Nelson, G. G. (2008, April). Household models for nursing home environments, *Creating Home in the Nursing Home: A National Symposium on Culture Change and the Environment Requirements*, Washington, DC.

Nolan, B. A. D., Mathews, R. M., Truesdell-Todd, G., & VanDorp, A. (2002). Evaluation of the Effect of Orientation Cues on Wayfinding in Persons with Dementia. *Alzheimer's Care Today, 3*(1), 46–49.

O'Brien, R. (2001). Um exame da abordagem metodológica da pesquisa ação [An Overview of the Methodological Approach of Action Research]. In R. Richardson (Ed.), *Teoria e Prática da Pesquisa Ação [Theory and Practice of Action Research]*. João Pessoa, Brazil: Universidade Federal da Paraíba (English version). Retrieved from http://www.web.ca/~robrien/papers/arfinal.html

Perkins, B., Hoglund, J. D., King, D., & Cohen, E. (2004). *Building type basics for senior living*. Hoboken, NJ: John Wiley.

Rabig, J., Thomas, W., Kane, R. A., Cutler, L. J., & McAlilly, S. (2006). Radical redesign of nursing homes: Applying the Green House concept in Tupelo, Mississippi. *The Gerontologist, 46*, 533–539.

Rahman, A. N., & Schnelle, J. F. (2008). The nursing home culture-change movement: Recent past, present, and future directions for research. *The Gerontologist, 48*, 142–148.

Rantz, M. J., Hicks, L., Grando, V., Petroski, G. F., Madsen, R. W., Mehr, D. R., ... & Mass, M. (2004). Nursing home quality, cost, staffing, and staff mix. *The Gerontologist, 44*, 24–38.

Rogers, E., Singhal, A., & Quinlan, M. (2009). Diffusion of innovations. In D. Stacks & M. Salwon. *An integrated approach to communication theory and research* (2nd ed., pp. 418–434). New York, NY: Routledge.

Rowles, G. D., Oswald, F., & Hunter, E. G. (2004). Interior living environment in old age. In H.W. Wahl, R. J. Scheidt, P.G. Windley, & K. W. Schaie (Eds), *Annual review of gerontology and geriatrics* (pp. 167–194). New York, NY: Springer.

Schneekloth, L. (1987). Advances in practice in environment, behavior and design. In E. H. Zube & G. T. Moore (Eds.), *Advances in environment, behavior and design* (vol. 1, pp. 307–334). New York, NY: Plenum.

Schwartz, B. (1996). *Nursing home design: Consequences for employing the medical model.* New York, NY: Garland.

Siegel, E.O., Young, H. M., Mitchell, P. H., & Shannon, S. E. (2008). Nurse preparation and organizational support for supervision of unlicensed assistive personnel in nursing homes: A qualitative exploration. *The Gerontologist, 48*, 453–463.

Shields, S., & Norton, L. (2006). *In pursuit of the sunbeam: A practical guide to transformation from institution to household.* Milwaukee, WI: ActionPact.

Sommer, R. (1997). Advances in environment, behavior, and design. In G. T. Moore & R. W. Marans (Eds.), *Utilization issues in environment-behavior research* (vol. 4, pp. 347–368). New York, NY: Plenum.

Talerico, K. A., O'Brien, J. A., & Swafford, K. L. (2003). Person-centered care: An important approach in 21st century health care. *Journal of Psychological Nursing, 41*(11), 12–16.

Tellis-Nayak, M. (2009, October). From satisfaction data to action. Presented at the Annual Meeting and Exposition of the American Association of Homes and Services for Aging, Chicago, IL.

Unruh, L., & Wan, T. T. H. (2004). A systems framework for evaluating nursing care quality in nursing homes. *Journal of Medical Systems, 28*, 197–214.

Vitaliano, D. F., & Toren, M. (1994). Cost and efficiency in nursing homes: A stochastic frontier approach. *Journal of Health Economics, 13*, 281–300.

Vladeck, B. C. (1980). *Unloving care: the nursing home tragedy.* New York, NY: Basic Books.

Vladeck, B. C. (2003). Unloving care revisited: The persistence of culture. In A.S. Weiner & J. L. Ronch (Eds.), *Culture change in long-term care* (pp 1–10). New YORK, NY: Haworth Social Work Practice.

Wahl, H.-W., & Weisman, G.D. (2003). Environmental gerontology at the beginning of the new millennium: Reflections on its historical, empirical, and theoretical development. *The Gerontologist, 43*, 616–627.

Walshe, K. (2001). Regulating U.S. nursing homes: Are we learning from experience? *Health Affairs, 20*, 128–144.

Weiner, A. S., & Ronch, J. L. (2003). *Culture change in long-term care.* New York, NY: The Haworth.

Weisman, G. (2001). The place of people in architectural design. In A. Pressman (Ed.), *The architect's portable design handbook: A guide to best practice* (pp. 149–170). New York, NY: McGraw Hill.

Weisman, G. D. (1981). Modeling environment-behavior systems: A brief note. *Journal of Man-Environment Relations, 1*, 32–41.

Weisman, G. D. (1983). Environmental programming and action research. *Environment and Behavior, 15*, 381–408.

Weisman, G. D., Chaudhury, H., & Diaz Moore, K. (2000). Theory and practice of place: Toward and integrative model. In R. L. Rubinstein, M. Moss, & M. H. Kleban (Eds.), *The many dimensions of aging* (pp. 3–21). New York, NY: Springer.

Weisman, G. D., & Diaz Moore, K. (2003). Vision and values: M. Powell Lawton and the philosophical foundations of environment-aging studies. In R. J. Scheidt & P. G. Windley (Eds.), *Physical environments and aging: Critical contributions of M. Powell Lawton to theory and practice* (pp. 23–37). Binghamton, New York, NY: The Haworth Press.

White, D. L., Newton-Curtis, L., & Lyons, K. S. (2008) Development and initial testing of a measure of person-directed care. *The Gerontologist, 48*, 114–123.

White-Chu, E. F., Graves, W. J., Godfrey, S. M., Bonner, A., & Sloane, P. (2009). Beyond the medical model: The Culture Change revolution in long-term care. *Journal of the American Medical Directors Association, 10*, 370–378.

Windley, P. G., & Weisman, G. R. (2004). Environmental gerontology research and practice: The challenge of application. In H.W. Wahl, R.J. Scheidt, P. G. Windley, & K. W. Schaie (Eds). *Annual review of gerontology and geriatrics* (pp. 334–365). New York, NY: Springer.

Winzelberg, G. S. (2003). The quest for nursing home quality: Learning history's lessons. *Archives of Internal Medicine, 163*, 2552–2556.

Zhang, X., & Grabowski, D. C. (2004). Nursing home staffing and quality under the nursing home reform act. *The Gerontologist, 44*, 13–23.

Zimmerman, S., & Cohen, L. W. (2010). Evidence behind the Green House and similar models of nursing home care. *Aging Health, 6*, 717–737.

127

PART III: TRANSFORMING ENVIRONMENTS: HOME AND COMMUNITY CONTEXTS

Age-friendly Philadelphia: Bringing Diverse Networks Together around Aging Issues

KATE CLARK and ALLEN GLICKSMAN

Planning Department, Philadelphia Corporation for Aging, Philadelphia, Pennsylvania, USA

Age-friendly communities are committed to improving the physical and social environments that surround older adults to facilitate independence and neighborhood cohesion. The movement to create these places is being facilitated by policy makers, planners, and researchers from a variety of disciplines who are collaborating under the premise that traditional aging services must be seen within the context of the wider community. Although not a panacea for all the challenges faced by community dwelling elders, this approach will be an important component of the future of environmental gerontology because it rests on acknowledging the effect of the environment on health outcomes.

OVERVIEW

Since January 2009, a new effort in Philadelphia, Pennsylvania, has transformed the city's traditional approach to serving older adults. Called Age-friendly Philadelphia (AfP), the new initiative is being administered by the Area Agency on Aging, Philadelphia Corporation for Aging (PCA). AfP is an integrated policy, planning, and research effort focused on the wider social and physical environments in which seniors live. The purpose of this article is to introduce this new strategy and to identify the

The authors would like to thank the staff at PCA as well as all of the many Age-friendly Philadelphia stakeholders for their efforts to make this agenda a success.

131

ways in which it can augment current and future efforts in environmental gerontology.

THE AGE-FRIENDLY MOVEMENT

Traditionally, most service provision and research in the field of aging have focused on interventions that affect the individual rather than the wider community in which that individual resides. Studies on the effect of factors that influence social interaction and independence, such as sidewalk conditions, accessible public transportation, and the policies that determine the scope of these environmental features (i.e., zoning codes and city planning documents) have been left in large part to policymakers and researchers outside of aging. This is especially true in regard to how multiple environmental factors interact with one another to affect health outcomes. As the population lives increasingly longer and becomes more diverse with respect to a variety of personal preferences, a multi-sector, cross-disciplinary approach must be initiated to support the older adult population. Therefore, professionals in the field of aging must reach out and collaborate with colleagues in other disciplines.

One prime opportunity for professionals to initiate this new approach is through the popular age-friendly efforts. Today, many communities are beginning to recognize the importance of thinking about traditional aging services in the context of the wider communities in which they operate. These new initiatives focus on improving both the physical and social environments that surround elders to facilitate independence and neighborhood cohesion. A survey by the University of California at Berkeley identified approximately 300 such efforts in the country. Many of these initiatives use guidelines established by organizations such as the United States Environmental Protection Agency (2011), American Association for Retired Persons (AARP), the Visiting Nurses Service of New York, or the World Health Organization, which provide a framework for individual efforts.

THE PHILADELPHIA EXPERIENCE: AGE-FRIENDLY PHILADELPHIA (AFP)

Philadelphia's age-friendly effort was created in response to the fact that Philadelphia has the highest proportion of older adults of any of the 10 largest cities in the United States (Hetzel & Smith, 2001). In addition, in 2009, 55% of all older adults (age 60 and older) in the city were minority, foreign born, or both and 45% were low income (American Community Survey, 2009). PCA's award-winning initiative, which has been lead by a Planner

(K.C.) and supported by the agency's Research Program (A.G.), aims to help these older adults remain healthy, active, and engaged in their communities for as long as possible. The agenda has received awards from two national bodies, the United States Environmental Protection Agency and the National Association of Area Agencies on Aging. It also received a grant from the National Institutes of Health's National Institute of Nursing Research and has been written about in national and local publications (Neergaard, 2011).

Four aspects of the agenda set it apart from other national age-friendly efforts:

1. The creation of a formal model called Supportive Age-friendly Environments (SAFE) based on the Environmental Protection Agency's Aging Initiative's framework.
2. A focus on catalyzing the effort rather than building another program with its own budget, staff, and services.
3. Special emphasis on working with emerging leaders in their 20's and 30's to build support for seniors.
4. Ongoing integration of research with policy and planning.

Each of these four aspects of AfP is described below.

Creating a Model: Supportive Age-friendly Environments

AfP is based on the understanding that supportive physical and social environments create more opportunities for healthy living, vibrant neighborhoods, and community engagement. Acknowledging this intimate connection, PCA selected the Environmental Protection Agency's Aging Initiative framework as the basis for a new model called SAFE.

The original Environmental Protection Agency framework is grounded in uniting active aging and smart growth. *Active aging* is a term that signifies both the opportunity for and the willingness of older people to be involved in maintaining their own health and well-being. Smart growth is based on a set of principles that guide urban planners and designers to make communities healthier, more economically vibrant, socially connected, and environmentally safe (Smart Growth America, 2011). The framework breaks down barriers between professions, such as social work and city planning, by embracing terms and concepts that are usually discipline specific. It features four principles that integrate active aging and smart growth, each of which will be reflected in the projects that are outlined in the following section. These principles are:

1. Staying Active, Connected, and Engaged: Where and how we choose to live can affect our health and well-being.

2. Development and Housing: Healthy neighborhoods offer diverse housing choices, gathering places, and ways to connect.
3. Transportation and Mobility: We can build choice back into our transportation system—and make it easier for people of all ages to get around.
4. Staying Healthy: Finding healthy food, keeping active, and getting healthy when you need it can be easier in an age-friendly community (United States Environmental Protection Agency, 2009).

PCA adapted each of the four principles to create the SAFE model, and each revised principle fits well within the context of current city-wide and regional efforts. The new principles can be operationalized using data on older Philadelphians that PCA currently possesses.

1. Social Capital: Being active and connected in one's neighborhood.
2. Flexible and Accessible Housing: Having the option to remain in one's home and/or community.
3. Mobility: Having access to public transportation and a walkable environment.
4. Eating Healthy: Having fresh fruits, vegetables, and other nutritious foods available.

By transforming the original four principles into the SAFE model, PCA has been able to identify new partners whose goals parallel these principles, catalyze specific initiatives for AfP, create champions for the effort, and use research to consider the interaction among these four principles.

Catalyzing the Effort: New Partners & Projects

Unlike many age-friendly efforts that administer programming, PCA primarily functions as a catalyst that identifies partners and innovative ways to collaborate, serves as a matchmaker between the aging network (organizations that serve older adults) and other networks, and provides technical information. In certain cases, the agency has taken the lead in identifying new policies that would move the agenda forward, and in others it has assisted organizations to incorporate older adults into their policies, plans, and programs. PCA defines AfP's success when current collaborators independently take the initiative to promote age-friendly practices and when new collaborators are identified for future projects.[1]

AfP's goals are achieved by bringing together a wide array of organizations to affect the environment in which older Philadelphians live and alter the way in which aging is perceived within the wider network of planners, advocates, and researchers. To do this, PCA's cross-disciplinary approach promotes the importance of government policies that provide a high quality of life for individuals of all ages; a built environment that facilitates healthy lifestyles, safety, and social connectedness; an aging network that considers the effect of the environment on the well-being of consumers; universities that partner with the community to create cutting-edge research; and emerging leaders from all fields who incorporate older adults into their work. Over the past three years, PCA has conducted more than 150 face-to-face meetings to introduce aging issues to organizations that do not traditionally work with older adults. It was discovered that although organizations have significant interest in considering the needs of the older population, there is often a lack of knowledge about networks to connect to for pursuing those interests, such as the aging network; innovative models to support seniors in the community; and research and data about the city's older adults.

PCA aims to provide this type of information and technical support and connect organizations to new networking opportunities so partners do not have to reinvent the wheel. PCA staff serves on numerous committees at a variety of organizations, which has helped to develop new collaborative projects and shows commitment to working with organizations outside of the aging network. It innovatively uses research data, maps, and evaluation expertise to support its practice partners' projects and grant applications, which will be described in detail below. Through these experiences, PCA has identified the motivations behind new interest and commitment to aging:

- AfP projects benefit everyone served by many of these organizations, not just older adults; the phrase "What is good for seniors is good for people of all ages" has been helpful making this point
- Some organizations rely heavily on older adults as donors and volunteers, and participating in AfP illustrates their commitment to this demographic.
- Older adults vote, so knowing where senior centers are located and where the highest proportion of seniors live can be key to a successful campaign.
- Health outcomes are the newest trend in funding; the health of seniors and the willingness of PCA to provide information is key to securing future funds.
- Evaluating projects that affect health outcomes is integral to most grant proposals; PCA's Research Program assists in this process.
- Seniors are often the caregivers of children in Philadelphia, so if the seniors stay in the community, the children receive more supervision.
- Staff at many of these organizations is caring for elder relatives; therefore, AfP appeals to them on a personal level.
- Integrating older adults into policies, plans, and programs helps organizations broaden their scope to look at the entire community rather than at just certain age segments; this contributes to the sustainability and continuity of their efforts.

AfP has facilitated various collaborative practice initiatives based on the SAFE model, four of which are discussed below.

Social Connectedness: The "Age-friendly Parks" Checklist

City parks can provide seniors with the opportunity for social interaction, relaxation, and passive and active exercise. They can also serve as venues to build intergenerational cohesion within neighborhoods. Despite Philadelphia's wealth of open space, seniors are underutilizing parks. In 2010, 72% of older adults in the city reported not attending a public recreation facility (including a park) within the past year, whereas just 1% said that there was no public recreation facility near their home (Public Health Management Corporation, 2010). Mobility issues, transportation to and from parks, perception of safety, lack of shade, and other factors play into this.

In the summer of 2010, PCA and the Fairmount Park Conservancy, a nonprofit organization that fundraises for Philadelphia Parks & Recreation (the Parks Department), partnered to examine these issues and to reach out to other organizations for help in encouraging seniors to use the parks. The organizations jointly created an Age-friendly Parks Checklist, which details the features in a park that would encourage use by seniors. Examples include creating more shaded areas, adding railings along stairways, and ensuring that sidewalks are both wide enough for a wheelchair and firm enough so that it does not sink into the dirt. Philadelphia Parks and Recreation and two environmental advocacy groups, the Next Great City Coalition and the Philadelphia Parks Alliance, provided feedback on the checklist. The list was intended to be used as a tool by seniors, park designers, volunteers, and administrators to evaluate and enhance local green spaces and identify progressive ways to design parks. In December 2010, *The Philadelphia Inquirer* wrote an article about the checklist; in March and April 2011, AARP noted the initiative in its news bulletin; and in July 2011 the Associate Press discussed the initiative in an article that was picked up by over 300 news outlets nation-wide.

In April and May 2011, the working group approached the Philadelphia Association of Senior Service Administrators (PASSA) to assist with its effort to conduct focus groups at three senior centers and one senior housing complex to evaluate and adjust the checklist. It is anticipated that this information will be used along with the checklist for future capital improvement projects and to high-light Philadelphia's signature age-friendly parks.

Flexible and Accessible Housing: The City's New Zoning Code

Many of Philadelphia's elders are active community members, serving as the eyes and ears of their blocks and caring for their grandchildren. Therefore, enabling seniors to age in the community benefits the individual and the neighborhood as a whole. A total of 208,429 Philadelphians aged 60 years and older are homeowners, and 66% of them wish to remain in their current homes for at least 10 more years. Of these older homeowners, 23% report using a cane and 22% report using a railing. In addition, 38% report that it is difficult to cover housing costs (PHMC, 2010). If seniors cannot use their homes to the full extent due to mobility restrictions or they cannot maintain their homes financially, both their homes and their streets can be negatively affected. For example, seniors who cannot use their homes' second and third floors will not be aware of leaks or broken windows, which can affect the structure's integrity and increase housing and maintenance costs. Unfortunately for many elders, moving into a senior subsidized housing facility is not an option because there are long waiting lists for such apartments and for many, these facilities are not located in the community in which they have built their social contacts.

In 2008, Philadelphia began the process of modernizing its zoning code for the first time in 40 years. According to the City of Philadelphia Zoning Code Commission, zoning "seeks to protect public health, safety and welfare by regulating the use of land and controlling the type, size and height of buildings" (Zoning Matters, 2012). Prior to the rewrite, the words "aging," "elders," and "senior citizens" were not mentioned in the code. However, for the past 2 years, PCA has worked with the Zoning Code Commission, the Philadelphia Association of Community Development Corporations, Temple University's Department of Community and Regional Planning, and various aging network and environmental organizations to integrate aging-in-community features into the code.

Accessory dwelling units are one such feature that allows for an alternative way to remain in one's home and are now mentioned in the new zoning code. Accessory dwelling units are subordinate, additional residences that are constructed within a residential property or garage. They can benefit seniors by providing the opportunity to downsize and to live in the same building as caregivers without having to leave the community or go to an institution. Some Philadelphians have built accessory dwelling units illegally, which poses a great challenge for emergency personnel who cannot identify the units. PCA also worked with the Zoning Code Commission to include requirements for at least some new private housing developments to be "visitable." When a home is visitable, it is a place where people of all ages and abilities can enter, circulate, and enjoy; it features three key requirements:

- One entrance to the home at grade-level (i.e., zero steps). This is a critical matter because the majority of Philadelphia's homes are row houses that feature front steps.
- One half-bathroom on the first floor.

- All hallways and doorways on the first floor should be wide enough to accommodate a wheelchair.

These features are important to people of all ages, including older people who have difficulties with stairs, disabled persons who use wheelchairs, parents with children, bicyclists, and those with temporary disabilities, such as a broken leg.

MOBILITY: AGE-FRIENDLY BUS STOPS

In Philadelphia and the surrounding suburbs, seniors have the benefit of riding South Eastern Pennsylvania Transportation Authority (SEPTA) bus, subway, and trolley lines for free. Since the discount began in 2000, more than 200,000 seniors have signed up. Programs like these are extremely important to older adults and to low-income seniors in particular, 50% of whom do not live in a household with an automobile (Ruggles, Alexander, Genadek et al., 2010). The use of public transit by older persons has many benefits, including:

- Providing easy access to senior centers, libraries, shopping, the homes of friends and family members, doctors, and other amenities to help older persons maintain their health and social well-being.
- Walking to and from transit stops increases physical activity and benefits health.
- Interaction with others while taking public transit can reduce isolation and increase a sense of community.
- Public service advertisements available at transit stops and on bus, trolley, and subway cars can provide valuable information and access to needed services.
- Public transport gives independence to older adults who might not feel comfortable driving a car.

All bus stops in Philadelphia are the responsibility of the City of Philadelphia, and their maintenance and upkeep are contracted out to a private vendor. In 2010, PCA collaborated with the Next Great City Coalition to promote the need for more bus stops that are age-friendly, meaning they provide shelter, seating, and lighting. These features benefit people of all ages, yet they can make the most difference to people with mobility problems who may not be able to stand for long periods of time and who can be especially vulnerable to foul weather. In fact, the presence of age-friendly bus stops could be the deciding factor in a senior's decision to use public transportation, get behind the wheel, spend money on a taxi cab, or go to a doctor's appointment.

In March 2010, the City of Philadelphia, through the Mayor's Office of Transportation and Utilities, released a Request for Proposals for a street

furniture program, which would require the redesign, expansion, and installation of new, age-friendly bus stops. However, because of the state of the
economy, the City did not get an adequate response and will rerelease the
Request for Proposals in the near future.

EATING HEALTHY: COMMUNITY GARDENS AT SENIOR CENTERS
AND HOUSING COMPLEXES

An alarming 65% of older Philadelphians report being obese or overweight.
Approximately 91% eat five or less of the Harvard School of Public Health's
recommended nine servings of fruits and vegetables per day, and 56% eat
two or fewer servings per day. Seniors who want to make healthy dietary
choices may find that factors outside of their control prevent them from doing
so. Low-income elderly are more likely to be overweight or obese than those
with higher incomes, and report eating out often at fast food restaurants and
having to travel outside of their neighborhood to a supermarket. They also
report needing a meal program, which indicates having problems shopping
and preparing meals (PHMC, 2010).

In a new effort, PCA is now encouraging community vegetable gardens
at senior centers and senior housing complexes. Being active with a community garden can help promote socialization, physical activity, and better
eating habits. Gardens run by organizations that serve as a resource for
reliable information can also be a way of sharing knowledge about social
services and programs. In February 2011, GenPhilly (a PCA supported, and
subsequently adopted, program discussed more in the next section) held
a groundbreaking event at City Hall called *Germinating Partnerships: Connecting Seniors to Community Gardens,* which fostered new collaborations
around the topic and resulted in an online toolkit to promote more such
gardens (GenPhilly, 2011). PCA is now giving technical support to many
gardens city-wide that are either involved with a senior center or a senior
housing complex.

One example is the Nationalities Senior Center garden, which won a
Nutrition Services Grant (with the support of PCA) through the Pennsylvania
Department of Aging in 2009 to build three gardens at Our Lady of Hope
Catholic Church. Volunteers of all ages donated more than 1,000 hours of
labor to build the gardens, which feature raised beds that allow people of
all ages and abilities to participate. Today, the seniors at the center plant,
harvest, and cook the produce, both at the center and at home, and will
soon be selling it at a nearby farmers' market. Many new partnerships and
increased exposure have resulted from this effort. For example, through
AfP, the Environmental Protection Agency, decided to use the project as
a case study for creating senior-friendly gardens on Brownfield sites (U.S.
EPA, 2011). In addition, the garden director has spoken at PCA's M. Powell
Lawton Conference on Urban Aging, PCA's panel on age-friendly cities

at the 2010 American Society on Aging East Coast Conference, and at the GenPhilly event *Germinating Partnerships.*

Emerging Leaders as Champions of Age-friendly Philadelphia

The success of AfP rests on professionals in the field of aging reaching out to and connecting with professionals whose disciplines have not traditionally addressed the needs of seniors. These disciplines, such as city planning, environmental advocacy, and transportation policy, significantly affect the lives of elders (Lawler, 2009). PCA has approached this challenge by supporting a grassroots effort called GenPhilly (GenPhilly, 2010).

GenPhilly is a peer-led network of emerging leaders who are taking a personal and professional interest in aging issues. Started in 2009, GenPhilly is an award-winning group of professionals in their 20s and 30s who work in a wide range of disciplines, such as urban planning, the arts, social work, government, philanthropy, and marketing. Together, they create professional development opportunities related to aging that tap into popular culture. Unlike traditional "young friends of" groups designed to create a new leadership cadre for an existing organization or conventional intergenerational programming that aims to bring young and old together, the GenPhilly model is organized and run by members who are asking themselves and their peers—"In what kind of city do I want to grow old?" and "How can I get there while helping the current population of seniors?"

Through social media, bimonthly meetings, and public events, GenPhilly shows emerging leaders that there is a competitive professional advantage that results from incorporating knowledge about older adults into their skill set. GenPhilly also serves as a support network for younger individuals whose work relates to the later stages in life. Events break down existing stereotypes about working with seniors and make this topic appealing and cool. Themes have included popular issues such as community gardening, pets, urban planning, contemporary music, women's studies, and environmental sustainability. Events bring different professional networks together to catalyze innovative partnerships that will assist people of all ages and, in most cases, they have sparked new initiatives that other organizations are now are spearheading.

GenPhilly has taken off in popularity in ways unimagined since its inception, boasting more than 250 members, 18 public events, 14 bimonthly networking meetings, and an event listserv of roughly 450 people. It was mentioned in the AARP March Bulletin (Abrahms, 2011), an Associated Press article (which was featured in the *New York Times, Huffinton Post*, and other widely read Web sites), won a 2011 National Associations of Area Agencies on Aging Aging Achievement Award, has been written about in the *Philadelphia Social Innovations Journal* (Groves, 2010), received a local award for its local advocacy regarding pets, and is being recognized by other peer-led young professional groups as a unique, relevant, and valuable resource.

GenPhilly plays an important role in the sustainability of AfP and served as an essential component in its national awards. At the same time, emerging leaders benefit from being a part of AfP because they become the champions and catalysts of programs and policies for their own organization. For example, at PCA's 2010 M. Powell Lawton Conference on Urban Aging entitled *Laying the Foundation for an Age-friendly Philadelphia*, nearly three-fourths of all speakers were GenPhilly members representing their organizations' new interests in aging. In addition, the new collaborations mentioned previously in this article relating to age-friendly parks and bus stops, housing, and community gardens are all being led by GenPhilly members.

In summary, GenPhilly benefits AfP by:

- Building support for and awareness of policy, plans, and programs that relate to aging services in the wider community.
- Facilitating cross-disciplinary learning around issues that relate to older people.
- Creating opportunities for professional development that stress the competitive advantage to know about aging issues.
- Strengthening the workforce in the field of aging.
- Breaking down stereotypes about working with older adults.
- Introducing expertise from outside the aging network to benefit older adults.

The Collaboration of Research, Planning, and Policy

The close cooperation of the Research Program at PCA with the AfP initiative may be unique among age-friendly efforts. The Research Program was created in 2001 to focus on the effect of the urban environment on the experience of aging Philadelphians; its support for AfP is an extension of this agenda. The program has contributed to the AfP effort in four ways, outlined below.

Selecting and Testing the Framework

First, it has worked closely with the policy and planning portion of AfP to develop a Philadelphia-specific framework for collaboration. The process of creating the SAFE model illustrates how the partnership between the AfP effort and the Research Program works. The original framework, developed by the Environmental Protection Agency, was selected based on criteria set by the Planner taking the lead on the AfP agenda. Once selected, the Research Program was asked if it was possible to determine whether the elements in the framework were related to positive health outcomes and other AfP goals. The Research Program was able to operationalize the four principles of the Environmental Protection Agency framework and test the relationship of those four principles to measures of health outcomes, health behaviors, and the desire of older adults to remain in their current homes (PHMC, 2008). The analyses demonstrated that the four operationalized principles are related to positive health outcomes, even when accounting for the effects of minority status and income. This is especially important for illustrating the importance of this approach in Philadelphia, where there are a significant number of low income and minority elders.

PROVIDING INFORMATION

Second, the Research Program's support for AfP extends to the stakeholders in the effort by providing information that can be used in their planning, policy development, grant writing, and advocacy. This information is often shared in the form of geographic information system maps that show the distribution of various characteristics of the city's population (such as functional impairment) in relation to some aspect of the physical environment (such as parks). The Research Program has also assisted with the development of new initiatives by providing technical support. For example, it facilitated the four age-friendly parks focus groups previously discussed. The Research Program has also supported GenPhilly through participation in its programs, conducting surveys on its behalf and providing information and resources as requested.

The Research Program also brings stakeholders together. In 2003, it developed the first M. Powell Lawton Conference on Urban Aging to connect professionals in research, policy, practice, and related fields to examine topics related to older adults who live in large metropolitan areas. The conference has since evolved into a platform to highlight achievements of AfP and to move that agenda forward.

CONNECTING AfP WITH UNIVERSITIES

Third, the Research Program has involved both students and faculty from local academic institutions in the work of AfP as in the case of inviting a university-based researcher to evaluate the community gardens effect on the health of older adults.

PCA RESEARCH PROJECTS

Finally, the Research Program has initiated its own research projects to further the goals of AfP. A grant was recently awarded to PCA by the National Institute of Nursing Research entitled Walkability's Impact on Senior Health (WISH). This project, which involves a local university and a community development corporation, will test hypotheses regarding the effect of walkable neighborhoods on the health and health behaviors of older adults. One of the goals of the WISH grant is to create tools that are constructed based on identifying environmental factors that are related to positive health outcomes, which will be used by AfP to further the goals of the initiative.

IS REPLICATION POSSIBLE?

In considering which aspects of this initiative are unique to Philadelphia and which can be transferred to other urban contexts, it is important to understand the opportunities and barriers that PCA has identified in trying to actualize age-friendly projects and to enlist and maintain partners.

In general, each city's age-friendly effort has a similar goal in mind, regardless of geography. PCA's strategy can be applied in other cities because the SAFE model and its principles are based on popular urban trends: social capital, flexible and accessible housing, improving mobility, and healthy eating. Although cities will vary in using this approach, the objectives—meaning the individual projects—will be catalyzed with partners. Projects should be based on the priorities of cities (their citizens, municipal government, and funders) and should be current initiatives that have multiple stakeholders. Therefore, these projects represent the opportunities that arise due to the unique circumstances that each urban area possesses.

Barriers that have interfered with project and partnership continuity can be attributed to a variety of factors. The first has to do with challenges created by trying to align institutional priorities among PCA, members of the aging network, and organizations outside of the field of aging. In Philadelphia, aging network organizations have legitimately questioned whether it is appropriate for both the Area Agency on Aging and the aging network agencies to provide resources to AfP activities while budgets are strained to the limit. The response has been two-fold: minimal resources (as measured by dollars) are allotted to AfP and staff time is the only true cost. In fact, AfP creates new resources for the aging network via access to technical and alternative financial resources and support for aging issues from the wider community. The majority of these organizations are now supporters of the initiative; however, not all are actively involved with the effort in the form of serving as advocates, project initiators, or ambassadors for AfP to other organizations. This is simply because agencies do not have the staff time to dedicate to projects outside of the primary scope of their funding. In these cases, PCA has assisted the organizations with projects by expending their own staff time to further the goals.

Outside of the aging network, there have not been a lot of friction points about being involved with aging issues (except the occasional case in which an individual appears to have a personal anxiety about growing older). AfP has primarily experienced conflicts when aging issues intersect with other organization's priorities, such as construction costs (i.e., building a "visitable" home on a slope or installing a bathroom in every park can be prohibitive). In these cases, alliance building and public education have been the keys to helping organizations understand the AfP perspective. It is also important that these stakeholder understand that PCA is considerate of their priorities and that one of the agency's long-term goals is to ensure that aging is always a variable in their decision-making process.

Although AfP is a fairly young initiative, the agency has not been able to maintain each partnership at the same level over the period of the effort, which is another barrier that PCA has faced. People leave their jobs; organizations rethink priorities; funding gets cut; political administrations change; and life happens. How catalysts of these efforts can maintain momentum given these constant changes is something to always keep in mind. PCA has realized that working with organizations so that AfP becomes integrated into their institutions missions can help create continuity. At the same time, AfP staff must continue to remain involved with these organizations current trends, projects, and staff.

MEASURING THE EFFECT OF AFP

One of PCA's roles in AfP is to measure its effects, and there are two primary questions that must be answered to do this. First, have the various efforts of AfP met the desired goals? Have they had other, unplanned effects that benefit or damage the goals of AfP? Second, even if the goals are being met (such as more older adults using public parks), how can the role that the AfP effort played in that change be determined?

The first part of this question will be answered by looking for indications of change over time, such as greater ridership of public transportation by older adults or a growth in the proportion of older Philadelphians who report being physically active. Although it may be difficult to determine exactly how much of this change is due to AfP, the change itself is the goal of the project. Furthermore, identifying changes in policies, procedures, and programs to include seniors, especially when these are initiated without AfP staff encouraging the change, are measures of the success of the effort.

The second question will be answered through the formal evaluation of specific projects designed to move the AfP agenda forward. One such project has to do with getting seniors more involved with community gardening. PCA's research arm is now evaluating individual efforts that other organizations (including senior residential facilities, senior centers, and greening organizations) are taking the lead on via building gardens and educating and recruiting volunteers.

MOVING FORWARD

Transforming physical and social environments to improve health outcomes for older indiviuals is becoming an important public health priority nation-wide, as seen through the popular age-friendly efforts. Involvement with these initiatives is an excellent opportunity for professionals in the field of environmental gerontology to expand their networks and collaborate with new disciplines. It is also a chance for those involved with research to become involved with studies of specific communities to determine which types of interventions will have the maximum benefit for seniors. Such studies will also expand the understanding of the relationship between the individual and the environment, which is core to the field's foundation. In Philadelphia, AfP has helped to increase citizens public discourse around aging issues, expose funders and policymakers to AfP projects, and show elected officials why this demographic matters; it has also opened new possibilities for researchers to collaborate around aging issues. The age-friendly movement is one that deserves continuing attention from environmental gerontologists because its effect on the future of every discipline is just beginning.

NOTE

1. Much of the description that follows is adapted from "Laying the Foundation for an Age-friendly Philadelphia: A Progress Report" which was published by PCA (Clark, 2011).

REFERENCES

Abrahms, S. (2011). *Towns and cities prepare for aging populations, older Americans want to age in place.* Retrieved from http://www.aarp.org/home-garden/housing/info-03-2011/towns-cities-prepare-for-aging-populations.html

American Community Survey. (2009). American Community Survey 2009 sample file. Retrieved from http://usa.ipums.org/usa/

Clark, K. (2011). *Laying the foundation for an age-friendly Philadelphia.* Philadelphia Corporation for Aging. Philadelphia, PA: United Staes. Retrieved from http://www.pcacares.org/pca_learn_AgeFriendly_Philadelphia.aspx

GenPhilly. (2010). *GenPhilly.* Retrieved from www.genphilly.org

GenPhilly. (2011). Toolkit for community gardens and seniors. Retrieved from http://genphilly.wordpress.com/resources/tool-kit-for-community-gardens-and-seniors/

Groves, R. (2010). GenPhilly steps up. *Philadelphia Social Innovations Journal.* Retrieved from http://www.philasocialinnovations.org/site/index.php?option=com_myblog&show=genphilly-steps-up.html&Itemid=22

Hetzel, L., & Smith, A. (2001). *The 65 years and over population: 2000.* Washington, DC: U.S. Bureau of the Census, U.S. Department of Commerce Economics and Statistics Administration.

Lawler, K. (2009). Admitting that even Peter Pan grows old. *The Gerontologist, 49,* 859–863.

Neergaard, L. (2011). Aging boomers strain cities built for the young. *The New York Times.* Retrieved from http://www.nytimes.com/aponline/2011/07/09/us/AP-US-Aging-America-Age-Friendly-Cities-1st-Ld-Writethru.html?hp

Public Health Management Corporation's Community Health Data Base—PHMC. (2008, 2010). Philadelphia, PA: Southeastern Pennsylvania Household Health Survey

Ruggles, S., Alexander, J.T., Genadek, K., Goeken, R., Schroeder, M.B., & Sobek, M. (2010). *Integrated public use microdata series, Version 5.0 [Machine-readable database].* Minneapolis, MN: University of Minnesota.

Smart Growth America. (2011). *"What is "smart growth?"* Retrieved from http://www.smartgrowthamerica.org/what-is-smart-growth

U.S. Environmental Protection Agency. (2009). *Growing smarter, living healthier: A guide to smart growth and active aging.* Washington, DC: Author.

U.S. Environmental Protection Agency. (2011). Elder-accessible gardening: A community building option for Brownfields redevelopment (EPA fact sheet EPA 560-F-11-021). Retrieved from http://www.epa.gov/brownfields/urbanag/pdf/elder_accessible_gardening.pdf

Zoning Matters. (2012). Frequently asked questions (FAQs). Retrieved from http://zoningmatters.org/facts/faqs

Assessing and Adapting the Home Environment to Reduce Falls and Meet the Changing Capacity of Older Adults

JON PYNOOS

Andrus Gerontology Center, University of Southern California, Los Angeles, California, USA

BERNARD A. STEINMAN

Institute for Community Inclusion, University of Massachusetts, Boston, Massachusetts, USA

ANNA QUYEN DO NGUYEN and MATTHEW BRESSETTE

Andrus Gerontology Center, University of Southern California, Los Angeles, California, USA

Falls in older adults are a serious problem for individuals, their families, and the health care system. This article describes research regarding fall risk assessment, risk reduction interventions, and public policy aimed at reducing the risk of falls for older adults in home settings. Assessments for frail older adults should include observations of not only the physical environment, but also the interactions among the environment, behavior, and physical functioning so that interventions are tailored to the specific situation of the individual. Home modification and technology can prove useful when designing interventions aimed at reducing fall risks. Problems such as cost, reluctance to adopt or implement suggestions, and a lack of knowledge may present barriers to effective home modification. Program and policy options for the future include improved training for service personnel who visit the homes of older adults, increased awareness of and coordination between programs or interventions aimed at reducing the risk of falls in older adults, new sources of funding, and building more housing that follows the principles of universal design.

Support by a grant provided by the Archstone Foundation.

147

Falling and injuries associated with falls constitute a major risk to the health, well-being, and independence of older adults. Falls frequently serve as a precursor to or indicator of frailty that may result in increased need for help from others or even nursing home placement. Within the community, falls are a leading cause of injury, hospital admissions, and injury-related deaths. Beyond these human costs, falls among older adults also represent a major health care expense for public and private payers of medical claims. In 2000, the total direct medical costs of fall injuries and fatal falls exceeded $19 billion, or about $28 billion in 2010 dollars (Stevens, Corso, Finkelstein, & Miller, 2006). Due to the aging of the population, costs associated with falls are projected to continue increasing to approximately $55 billion (in 2007 dollars) by 2020 (Englander, Hodson, & Terregrossa, 1996). In addition, these direct expenditures fail to account for the long-term costs associated with later disability, formal and informal caregiving services, and other intangible resources. As a public health issue, older Americans' falls are a growing concern across policy domains, and there is common interest in reducing falls in the realms of public health, aging services, and housing.

Greater awareness among stakeholders in the domains of housing and construction/contracting regarding the consequences of falls and techniques for reducing fall risk has corresponded with important work done by occupational therapists and other professionals who provide home assessments and recommendations. The purpose of this article is to describe research on environmental fall risk factors and the strategies, programs, and policies aimed at addressing the problem of falls among a growing population of older adults.

ENVIRONMENT AS A FALL RISK FACTOR

Although Masud and Morris (2001) identified more than 400 individual fall risk factors, falls are commonly thought to result from interactions among multiple risk factors derived from behavioral, intrinsic, or extrinsic origins (Bath & Morgan, 1999; Bueno-Cavanillas, Padilla-Ruiz, Jiménez-Moleón, Peinado-Alonso, & Gálvez-Vargas, 2000; Cesari et al., 2002; Graafmans et al., 1996; Pynoos, Steinman, & Nguyen, 2010). A sometimes-overlooked category, Pynoos et al. (2010) described behavioral fall risk factors as those that reflect the choices of individuals with respect to how they interact within their environments. Examples of behavioral fall risk factors include performing behaviors that could decrease safety (e.g., standing on unstable objects to reach items that are stored on high shelves), failing to perform behaviors that could reduce fall risk (e.g., not turning on lights when using the bathroom at night or not using grab bars or handrails when they are present), or selecting unsafe clothing, footwear, or inappropriate/outdated eyewear prescriptions.

According to Pynoos et al. (2010), intrinsic factors are individually oriented risks that include health conditions (e.g., chronic diseases), degrees of functional impairment (e.g., poor mobility or cognitive decline), or states of being (e.g., advanced age). Other intrinsic fall risk factors include muscle weakness, gait and balance disorders, negative drug interactions, a history of falls, and sensory loss such as vision (American Geriatrics Society, 2012; Pynoos, Rose, Rubenstein, Choi, & Sabata, 2006). Intrinsic risk factors are often dynamic insofar as they may change over time, resulting in health and disability status that is in constant flux between losses and gains.

Finally, extrinsic fall risk factors are described as environmentally oriented and are shared among individuals who inhabit a common environment (Pynoos et al., 2010). Extrinsic factors that have been identified include slippery surfaces; inadequate lighting; loose, deep pile or worn carpets; staircases without railings; unsupportive or badly arranged furniture; poorly designed tubs, toilets, and fixtures in the bathroom; clutter; and pets being underfoot (Clemson, Cumming, & Roland, 1996; Pynoos et al., 2006; Rogers, Rogers, Takeshima, & Islam, 2004). Trips, slips, or stumbles are often attributed to extrinsic factors and may pose an increased risk for falls, especially for community-dwelling older adults whose homes may contain many hazards. In fact, the prevalence of environmental hazards in the homes of older adults was found to be high, with approximately 80% of homes containing at least one identifiable hazard and 39% containing five or more hazards (Carter, Campbell, Sanson-Fisher, & Gillespie, 2000). The degree to which the environment contributes to fall risk is often operationalized by the number of hazards contained in the environment. Nevertheless, research results have varied with respect to the magnitude of effect and circumstances in which hazards in the environment precede falls. For instance, Clemson et al. (1996) found that the homes of fallers were not generally more hazardous than the homes of non-fallers. However, fallers with cognitive impairments had significantly more hazards in their homes than non-fallers with cognitive impairments. Furthermore, homes of those with recent hip fractures had more hazards than those without hip injuries. Among older adults in general, Northridge, Nevitt, Kelsey, and Link (1995) reported that falls were not strongly associated with the presence of home hazards; however, among vigorous older individuals, those living with more home hazards were more likely to fall compared with those with fewer hazards. Thus, evidence exists that the effects of the environment may vary according to the physical capacity and the degree to which the individual is physically active. Indeed, Fleming and Pendergast (1993) found that although 50% of the falls they observed were precipitated by an environmental factor, a large percentage of these were likely caused by physical limitations that prevented residents from safely interacting with their environment.

A MULTIFACTORIAL MODEL OF FALL RISK

Because falls frequently result from multiple risk factors, including hazards in the environment, general consensus exists among researchers that the most effective prevention programs take an individualized and multifactorial approach to improving safety. Great variability is found in the needs, functional capacity, and environments of older adults, and risks may differ substantially between individuals. Therefore, the general approach has been to assess, identify, and address multiple factors that place the individual at higher risk for falls. The best assessment protocols (some examples are discussed below) are designed to be comprehensive in that they are able to identify health and environmental characteristics specific to individuals and their dwellings that place them at greater risk for falling (Rubenstein, Vivrette, Harker, Stevens, & Kramer, 2011). When behavioral risk factors are identified, they are often addressed through raising awareness and educating older adults about safer strategies for accomplishing everyday tasks and activities. To address intrinsic factors, multifactorial fall prevention programs may use medical risk assessments to identify health and functioning problems that can lead to falls. Whether prescribed or in group-based settings, exercise designed to increase strength, flexibility, and endurance can target and reduce the negative effect of intrinsic fall risk factors (Rose, 2011). In addition, home assessments and modifications designed to reduce or eliminate hazards in the environment would seem to be integral in programs aimed at reducing fall risk, especially because, as extrinsic in origin, they are amenable to control and correction.

The complex relationship between health and the physical environment with respect to fall risk has been acknowledged in theory and research aimed at understanding how multiple risk factors can combine to result in falls. In their efforts to describe interactions between older adults and their environments, researchers (Lawton, 1998; Lawton & Nahemow, 1973; Nahemow, 2000) proposed an ecological model in which the competencies of the individual, whether physical, interpersonal, or social/societal, are pressed by the demands of his or her surroundings. According to Glass and Balfour (2003), beneficial elements in the environment may serve as supports that buoy competence by reducing the discrepancy between the physical capacity of older adults (which may have declined due to age) and the relative press of their environments. Outcomes associated with this interaction determine the degree to which person–environment fit is adequate to support the needs and desired lifestyle of the individual (Iwarsson, 2005; Iwarsson, Horstmann, Carlsson, Oswalk, & Wahl, 2009). Elements in the ecological model are also dynamic in that the abilities of individuals and the challenges presented by environments are continually in flux, as is the interaction or relationship between them. Therefore, even when environments have been adapted to address the specific needs of individuals at a specific point in time, continued appraisal of the person–environment fit is necessary to assure that it remains appropriate over time.

The work of Lawton (1998) has served as a seminal theoretical basis for several studies that have attempted to demonstrate the benefits associated with multifactorial interventions. For instance, many studies have examined the role of the environment alone and with respect to other specific intrinsic and behavioral factors. Clemson, Mackenzie, Ballinger, Close, and Cumming (2008) reported on a meta-analysis of six multifactorial fall intervention studies that included an environmental component within community settings. Across studies, a significant 21% reduction in post-intervention falls was reported. In addition, Clemson et al. (2008) found differences in the efficacy of interventions based on the degree of risk experienced by participants, such that greater effects (39% reduction in falls) were reported for populations that had risks associated with previous falls, vision impairments, and functional decline. Similarly, Feldman and Chaudhury (2008) reviewed 25 empirical articles published from 1985 to 2007 that examined the role of environmental hazards, home modifications, and cognitive factors as they relate to falls in older adults and concluded that modifying the home environment was an effective intervention to prevent falls among this group. Based on such research, a conceptual model of multifactorial fall risk was developed that includes factors related to health and mobility, risk-taking behavior, and the physical environment (Feldman & Chaudhury, 2008). Collectively, these findings support the assertion that multifactorial fall risk is cumulative, such that fall risk increases as a function of factors individually or in combination with other factors (Rubenstein, Robbins, Josephson, Schulman, & Osterweil, 1990).

Another line of study has suggested that differences in the efficacy of multifactorial fall prevention programs may depend on the intensity of the interventions and the specialization of professionals conducting assessments. For example, Clemson et al. (2008) reported on four studies in which interventions with an environmental component were conducted by occupational therapists and found that these programs were more effective than similar interventions that did not include an occupational therapist. Pighills, Torgerson, Sheldon, Drummond, and Bland (2011) reported the results of a randomized controlled trial, which assessed fall outcomes for at-risk older adults following an environmental assessment and home modification intervention by either an occupational therapist or other trained assessor. Results of this study also found a significant reduction in post-intervention falls for the group that received the intervention from an occupational therapist, whereas the group that received the intervention from a trained assessor experienced no significant reduction in falls. In unpublished research reporting outcomes associated with the InSTEP (*Increasing Stability Through Evaluation and Practice*) program, which was funded by the Archstone Foundation, Kramer, Harker, Mitchell, and Rubenstein (2011) evaluated interventions at three intensity levels. The high intensity model included medical assessment by a physician, in-home assessment and follow-up assessment by an occupational therapist, and a focused balance and gait program taught by a trained, certified exercise professional. The medium intensity model used social workers for the medical risk and home assessment components, and a physical activity instructor to lead exercise classes. The low intensity model challenged older participants to be more proactive with their fall prevention efforts, with senior center staff or volunteers to follow-up and provide support. Although self-reported falls per year were reduced significantly for participants with previous falls, in this study program intensity level did not have a major effect on rates of falling. With respect to different types of assessors, Steinman and Nguyen (2011) analyzed the environmental assessment component of InSTEP, and the number of hazards found by various types of professionals who administered the Falls Home Assessment tool (described below). Occupational therapists identified more hazards than social workers, although this difference was not statistically significant. Statistical differences were reported regarding the location of hazards, with occupational therapists reporting more hazards than social workers in pathways and entrances leading to homes, on steps and stairs, and in a nonspecific "other" category that included the garage and the backyard. Thus, mixed evidence was found regarding to what extent the qualifications of the assessor, as well as the intensity of the assessment, influence the effectiveness of environmental fall-prevention interventions.

ASSESSMENTS FOR FALL RISK

For environmental modification to be effective, assessment tools are needed for identifying problems and offering solutions to hazardous areas in homes. Several home assessment tools have been developed that differ with respect to their complexity and the amount of time, training, and resources needed to administer them. The simplest and least expensive environmental assessment tools are self-administered checklists that help identify common hazards or solutions to hazards that exist in the homes of many older adults. In addition to their relative low cost and ease of administration, checklists usually require little or no training to conduct and may be disseminated directly to older adults via facilities where older adults may congregate to receive services (such as senior centers and health clinics) or through Internet sites that target older adults in need of services. Checklists can also be used or distributed by professionals such as builders and remodelers to engage clients and residents in the process of creating safe homes and in defining and prioritizing unsafe areas for improvement of the home environment.

An example of a home assessment checklist is "Check for Safety: A Home Fall Prevention Checklist for Older Adults," disseminated by the Centers for Disease Control (CDC) (2005) and attainable in large print from the CDC's website (http://www.cdc.gov). Another resource produced by the CDC is a self-administered fall-risk checklist, Stay Independent, adapted from a checklist developed by the Greater Los Angeles VA Geriatric Research Educational Clinical Center (Rubenstein et al., 2011). In addition to tips for making homes safer, items in this tool connect intrinsic fall risks to interactions with the environment (e.g., "I steady myself by holding onto furniture when walking at home" and "I need to push with my hands to stand up from a chair") and encourage individuals to discuss their fall risk factors with health care providers. Similarly, the Rebuilding Together Home Safety Checklist, created in partnership with the U.S. Administration on Aging (http://www.rebuildingtogether.org) covers not only the identification of fall hazards, but also accessibility and safety considerations.

Despite their convenience, it should be noted that checklists vary greatly with respect to their comprehensiveness and suggested solutions may be generic or may not apply in all cases (especially in the case of older adults who have impairments that require specific types of modification) (Pynoos et al., 2010). For example, checklists that are designed for older adults in general may overlook some problems that are especially important for individuals who are blind or visually impaired (Steinman, Nguyen, Pynoos, & Leland, 2011). The adoption of recommendations presented by checklist assessments may also vary according to the willingness of older adults to change aspects of their homes and their confidence about the extent to which making changes will influence their likelihood of falling (Cumming et al., 1999). Therefore, checklists may be more effective if they are accompanied by other educational materials that inform older adults in appropriate terms about research-validated findings emphasizing the correct use of home modifications and the efficacy of making specific changes to reduce fall risk.

In contrast to checklists, some assessment instruments, designed for use by health care or social service professionals, identify fall risk factors in the environment and explore the interactions of the individual with their surroundings (functional assessments). Environmental fall risk assessments use a more comprehensive approach that requires greater expenditure of time and resources to administer. In addition to items present on the assessment tool, assessors may call on their past experiences to provide an array of possible solutions to address hazards. Some examples of assessment instruments include the Falls Home Assessment, which has been developed and tested as part of the InSTEP program at the Fall Prevention Center of Excellence (http://www.stopfalls.org), and the more broadly based Comprehensive Assessment and Solution Process for Aging Residents (http://www.ehls.com) (Sanford, 2010; Sanford, Pynoos, Tejral, & Browne, 2002). These assessments incorporate a decision-making process that directly involves older adults in identifying their greatest needs or problems. Input from older adults may be helpful in selecting solutions among a variety of alternatives and setting priorities about what aspects of the home environment to change. It may also be important to include caregivers and family members in the process of identifying problems and setting priorities (especially in the case of individuals with Alzheimer's disease) to determine the best solutions given the individual's current state of health, projected changes to health, affordability of alternatives, as well as the attractiveness, safety, and ease of use of the solutions (Gitlin, Corcoran, Winter, Boyce, & Hauck, 2001).

Several other fall home assessment tools exist that differ with respect to their structures and key areas of focus. The Housing Enabler (http://www.enabler.nu/) uses a multi-step procedure to make predictive, objective, and norm-based assessments and analyses of accessibility problems in the physical environment. "Safety Assessment of Function and the Environment for Rehabilitation–Health Outcome Measurement and Evaluation" is an occupational therapy assessment developed for use with the elderly and adults with disabilities living in the community. It consists of an easy-to-use checklist grouped into 12 areas of concern: living situation; mobility; environmental hazards; kitchen; household; eating; bathroom and toilet; medication, addiction and abuse; leisure; communication and scheduling; personal care and wandering. The 100-page manual provides administrative instructions, detailed guidelines and seven case studies (Chiu, Oliver, Tamaki, Faibish, & Sisson, 2001). Finally, In-Home Occupational Performance Evaluation is a performance-based measure that evaluates 44 activities in the home with four subscales including activity participation; client's rating of performance; client's satisfaction with performance; and severity of environmental barriers (Stark, Somerville, & Morris, 2010). Although this is by no means an all-inclusive list of fall prevention checklists and assessments, they provide some insight into the types of tools that are currently available.

UNIVERSAL DESIGN, HOME MODIFICATIONS AND TECHNOLOGY

Over the past 20 years, greater emphasis has focused on designing and building dwellings that are sensitive to the needs of individuals with disabilities or those who may acquire disabilities at some point in the future. Public policies including the Americans with Disabilities Act of 1991 and the Fair Housing Amendments Act of 1988 have required that public and private environments be accessible and promote inclusion of people with disabilities. Similarly, activism by disability and aging groups has raised awareness about issues of accessibility and visitability (discussed later) of new and existing structures (Alley, Liebig, Pynoos, Banerjee, & Choi, 2007). A greater promotion of design that is accessible and supportive along with home modifications and assistive technology aims to accommodate individuals with physical and mental impairment in both new dwellings and housing that is older or poorly designed.

The concept of universal design has been used to create products, buildings, and exterior spaces that reduce environmental demands for people of all ages, sizes, and abilities to the greatest extent possible without the need for adaptation. Effective universal design minimizes barriers and increases supportive features to facilitate participation in activities of daily living and leisure activities (Mace, Hardie, & Place, 1996). Among many other possibilities, universal design features that can reduce the number of falls at home include a zero-step entrance with flush or low-profile threshold; high-contrast trim and glare-free floor surfaces; a curbless or roll-in shower in bathrooms; short, wide hallways that can accommodate a person using a wheelchair or walker, as well as caregivers providing assistance; and motion-sensor lighting that automatically turns on and off when individuals enter or exit the room (Pynoos, 1992; Pynoos et al., 2010; Young, 2006).

In homes that are older or poorly designed, the process of home modification refers to the converting or adapting of environments to make everyday tasks easier, reduce accidents, and support independent living (Pynoos, Sabata, & Choi, 2005). The dynamic nature of health and functioning among older adults, especially those with chronic diseases, mandates the continued monitoring of home safety even after homes have been assessed and features such as grab bars and handrails are in place. Even though in some circumstances, a single event might precipitate the need for home modifications, the process is better viewed as one that occurs over time. Follow-up visits or telephone calls by health professionals can help determine whether more training should be offered or if additional modifications are needed to respond to the changing needs of the older person.

According to Steinman and Nguyen (2011), home modification recommendations made by a home assessor (e.g., an occupational therapist or social worker) to individuals about their environments can be grouped into at least four categories: additive, subtractive, transformative, and behavioral modifications. The most common recommendations are for additive modifications in which supports or structures are added to the environment to facilitate access and functioning of the user. Additive modifications may include major additions (e.g., installing ramps for wheelchair users) or relatively minor additions (e.g., adding an automatic nightlight in the hallway). Because additive modifications commonly require professional installation of new features by hired contractors or other professionals, they may be relatively expensive compared with other types of modifications.

By contrast, subtractive modifications involve the removal of items or hazards to improve safety and access to the environment. Subtractive modifications include changes such as removing unsecured floor mats or clearing clutter from the floor. Subtractive modifications tend to be less expensive and may be easier for individuals to implement on their own without professional assistance because they do not involve installing new features.

Transformative modifications involve restructuring existing characteristics to better facilitate the use of environmental features. Widening doorways to improve accessibility for individuals who use wheelchairs is an example of a major transformative modification. Transformative modifications may also include relatively minor changes, such as rearranging furniture to clear pathways or relocating frequently used objects such as cooking utensils, so that they are within easy reach.

Finally, behavioral modifications include avoidance or adoption of specific behaviors to improve safety. Behavioral modifications involve altering how individuals interact with their environments. For example, when stairs are identified as a hazard, individuals may modify their behavior by sleeping on the first floor instead of the second. In accordance with Lawton and Nahemow's (1973) ecological model of person–environment fit, behavioral modifications are unique because they acknowledge the potential of behavior change as a means to reestablish equilibrium between the capabilities of individuals, and the environments in which they function. Thus, when suggesting behavioral interventions, providers should explore how personal attributes of the individual and their environment interact as they perform daily activities.

Advances in mainstream technology (marketed to the public at large) and assistive technology (designed to promote independence for individuals with disabilities) also promote the ability of older adults to continue to live in their own communities as they age (Vasunilashorn, Steinman, Liebig, & Pynoos, 2012). Smith and Small (1983) described the major benefits of applying technological advances for increasing the safety of older individuals living in their own homes, especially those living alone. Since that early period, innumerable advances in technology have been made that promise to improve the capacity of individuals to remain at home. As is true with universal design and home modifications, technology may be useful in fall prevention interventions as potential buoys to problems that are either created or exacerbated by interactions between physical capacity and the environment. For example, several low-tech assistive devices (e.g., that assist with reaching and gripping) and mobility devices (e.g., canes, walkers) are on the market that can substantially reduce fall risk. In addition, a growing number of high-tech devices are being developed that gather biological and kinesthetic data to detect when falls have occurred or are imminent (Yu, 2008). In very frail older adults, sensors embedded in garments can be used to detect suspicious movements that often precede falls and may be able to alert caregivers to a potentially hazardous movement or balance-related situation. Cameras and ambiance devices that detect movement or vibrations have been equipped with sophisticated software programs that connect to personal emergency response systems. The improved ability of technology to interpret high-risk movement patterns has facilitated the process of alerting caregivers when risky behaviors are undertaken. Older adults who are less frail have also benefited from the explosive growth in technological devices that range from motion-activated lighting to phone applications (apps) that help monitor and send reminders to take medications. In the spirit of universal design, many technological devices used by people of all ages are now designed to also accommodate the changing physical needs and capacities of individuals as they age. Whereas research has shown that older adults are often willing to adopt technologies that would help them remain independent (Brownsell, Bradley, Bragg, Catlin, & Carlier, 2000), it is important that technology is designed to facilitate access and avoid barriers to use. Simple-to-use, unobtrusive technology, as it continues to develop, will be integral in promoting safety by accommodating disability associated with cognitive, sensory, and mobility impairment.

BARRIERS TO SAFE HOME ENVIRONMENTS

Despite great improvements, much of the current built environment, including the homes of older adults, still contain hazards that increase the risk of falls and lacks features to prevent or reduce falls. The mismatch between the needs of older adults and their environments exists for sundry reasons that relate to scarcity of resources and limited support and information available to older adults about alternatives that address environmental risks. Older adults may be unaware that environments contain hazards or may be unable to make the changes themselves or get a friend, neighbor, or relative to do it. In addition, a lack of trained assessors exists, and it is often difficult to locate a skilled installer. Older adults may even reject home modifications due to their often non-residential appearance or the costs associated with making changes. Indeed, costs are often a major barrier to implementing home modifications. Those who have low incomes and live in substandard housing with problems such as broken stairs or crumbling bathroom walls may need structural repairs before adding such home modifications as handrails, stair glides, or grab bars. Likewise, many low- and high-tech assistive devices may be beyond the financial means of individuals with low incomes. Moreover, because many home modification programs are often lodged in housing agencies, there can be difficulties in coordinating with health and human services because they target different population groups, vary in the qualifications for eligibility, and operate under different time frames.

PROGRAMS AND POLICIES

Several policies and programs have been developed to address barriers that have stood in the way of reducing environmental fall risks. Among the multi-faceted programs included in the CDC's Compendium of Effective Fall Interventions (Stevens, 2010), many include a component that focuses on home assessment and modification. In addition, recent efforts have been made to upgrade the skills of individuals who conduct home assessments and modification and to address the problem of inaccurate or cursory assessments. Educational and skill-building programs include a series of multi-session online certificate programs in home modifications that are available from the University of Southern California's Davis School of Gerontology; the American Occupational Therapy Association; I.D.E.A.S., Inc. has a set of online education modules that pertain to home modifications and the environment, including one on falls; the University of Buffalo has several online courses on universal design and home modification; and The National Association of Home Builders offers remodelers a 2-day program on aging in place and accessibility.

In addition to the growing focus on training programs, efforts have also been made to increase the absolute number of assessors who are available by enlisting new groups to participate in the assessment and referral process. Other professionals who could do a quick assessment of the home include firefighters and emergency medical services (EMS) responders. In addition to responding to fires, firefighters and EMS personnel frequently address medical emergencies, such as cardiac arrests and falls. As trusted personnel, firefighters and EMS responders have the opportunity to capitalize on these teachable moments by administering a quick in-home environmental screen to identify common fall risks within the environment and referring individuals to programs and services in the community. FP Connect, a project at University of Southern California's Andrus Gerontology Center, is working with local firefighters and EMS personnel to determine the best way to provide fall prevention and reduction training so they can use the short period of time they are in the individual's home to effectively conduct a home assessment, leave recommendations for changes, and refer them to individuals or organizations that can make changes.

At the federal level, the National Affordable Care Act's "Independence at Home Demonstration" (Centers for Medicare and Medicaid Services, 2012) is testing the efficacy of house call visits for frail older individuals by doctors. Once common in the United States and still a practice in countries such as England, physician house calls provide a potentially effective avenue for identifying fall risks. Although the demonstration does not provide designated funds for home modifications, it offers the opportunity for physicians to observe how older individuals function in their own settings overtime and, if needed, make appropriate referrals to other services, such as occupational therapy and handy workers. Similarly, other health care or social service professionals (e.g., nurses, case managers, and in-home workers) who have access to older adults in their homes can be trained in assessing environments for fall risks. It is expected that these types of visits will increase as health care moves more into home settings (National Research Council, 2011).

With respect to funding for home modifications, several housing programs exist in the United States, such as Community Development Block Grants and Veterans Administration grants (targeted to wounded and disabled veterans), that can pay for home repairs and modification. Health-related programs such as Medicaid Waivers may also allow funds to be used in modifying homes. Still, expenditures for home modification programs are optional, and they are often at a high risk for elimination or retrenchment when government budgets are cut. Newer programs, such as PACE (Program of All Inclusive Care for the Elderly) and Cash and Counseling, which have greater flexibility in how funds are used, may institute home modifications as a strategy to keep frail older adults in the community. They have the advantage of caring for frail older individuals over an extended time, the opportunity to conduct home assessments as part of care plans, and the ability to integrate fall prevention (including home modifications) as part of on-going services that they provide. Even though they are increasing in number, due to their limited resources such programs are able to serve only a relatively small percentage of older individuals who could benefit from their services and are restricted to those with a very low income. Depending on their particular policy, middle- and upper-income individuals who have purchased private long-term care insurance and who meet the threshold for services may be able to use funds for home modifications. Likewise, older homeowners who take out a reverse mortgage can use funds from it to make repairs and modifications.

FUTURE DIRECTIONS

Many policy and research challenges lie ahead in the realm of falls prevention via hazard reduction and environmental assessment. To adequately address the role of the home environment in falls—a problem that is only likely to grow over time—new strategies and interventions must be developed, and new resources must be committed to ameliorating fall hazards in homes of older adults. In addition to material resources, greater advocacy is needed to assure that policymakers are well-informed about what works, what resources are needed to improve environments, and what is at stake in terms of human and economic costs. Moving forward, the combined efforts of professionals in the domains of public health, aging services, and housing will likely continue to focus on the development of environmental solutions that accommodate and support the greater physical and cognitive demands that often accompany aging. For example, improved integration of universal design principles into housing designs will benefit older adults by improving home access and safety for all people. Activists and advocates in the disability movement have also served to raise awareness of the role of environment in activity participation and safety of older adults. The concept of visitability, originally conceived by Eleanor Smith of Concrete Change, has promoted housing codes in the United States that would require a small set of essential features on the first floors of visitable houses to allow for access by individuals with mobility concerns, including a level entrance, an accessible bathroom on the first floor, and wide doorways and hallways that allow for the passage of a wheelchair. Although visitability has not yet had the large effect that its advocates hope to eventually achieve, as of 2008 approximately 30,000 homes were built according to its requirements (Pynoos, Nishita, Cicerso, & Caraviello, 2008; Rehabilitation Engineering Research Center on Universal Design, 2008).

In addition to improved advocacy, programs that serve older adults should have access to research results by way of wider dissemination of information translated into clear, easy-to-understand formats available to professionals outside of academic and scholarly journals. Stronger ties and relationships between researchers and service providers will help to ensure that interventions related to the environment are efficacious and based on a wide body of scientific evidence.

With respect to research, new data sources aimed at understanding the causes of falls and methods of intervention need to be developed. Many of the data regarding environmental fall risk factors are cross-sectional, and better national longitudinal data could include well-formulated questions about falls experienced by older adults, and home modifications implemented to address falls (Beasley, Jason, & Miller, 2011). New sources of data could be derived from different types of providers that have contact with older adults who have fallen. For example, when older adults who experience serious falls are transported by EMS personnel to hospital emergency departments, this negative scenario has potential to result in more positive outcomes if EMS personnel used the opportunity to collect more detailed and uniform information about contributing factors leading up to falls, including medical precursors and the role of the environment. Similarly, states could improve access of researchers to emergency room discharge data that pertain to falls (Wallace, Molina, & Jhawar, 2007). Health Maintenance Organizations and programs such as PACE that operate using a comparatively holistic approach to providing health care for older adults would seem to have a strong interest in collecting improved falls-related data and testing interventions to reduce falls. Since passage of the Deficit Reduction Act of 2005, hospitals and nursing homes in particular now have a greater incentive to understand and prevent falls through collection of better data. As a result of Deficit Reduction Act, the Centers for Medicare and Medicaid Services no longer reimburse hospitals for the treatment of fall-related injuries that occur within their facilities.

Finally, more research is needed that clearly explains the role of the environment in the complex mosaic of fall risk. Much of the falls research to date has focused on identifying risk factors for falls, demographic analysis of adults who fall, and interventions designed to prevent falls. This work has demonstrated, and it is now generally agreed, that falls are a result of complex interactions between factors that are intrinsic and extrinsic to the individual. As a result, many programs have begun to include assessment and modification of the environment as a central component of multifactorial fall-reduction interventions. Even so, additional research is needed to ascertain the effectiveness of different types of assessors (e.g., occupational therapists, social workers, family members, and older adults themselves) and various methods of assessment (e.g., self-administered checklists, functional assessments). In addition, expanded research will lead to better understanding the extent to which costs, ease of making modifications, appearance of modifications, tenure of residents (renter vs. owner), living arrangements, and the perceived usefulness of home modifications influence the decisions of older adults to implement changes in their homes.

Successful efforts to improve the environments of older adults and to reduce their risk for falls and fall-related injuries are complex and transdisciplinary undertakings. As such, future efforts to improve home safety will require that policymakers, practitioners, and other stakeholders in the medical, public health, housing, transportation, and social service sectors each acknowledge the role of physical and behavioral characteristics of older adults in context with their environment in falls risk, while embracing policies and practices designed to improve the home environments of older adults. Although many challenges and barriers remain, environmental gerontology continues to develop new opportunities and advancements to address these pressing problems. Indeed, future efforts to reduce fall risk that is attributable to a mismatch between functional health and the environment should focus on assessments, technology, and public policy aimed at reducing the environmental press in homes where older adults live.

REFERENCES

Alley, D., Liebig, P., Pynoos, J., Banerjee, T., & Choi, I. H. (2007). Creating elder-friendly communities: Preparations for an aging society. *Journal of Gerontological Social Work, 49*, 1–18.

American Geriatrics Society. (2012). *AGS/BGS clinical practice guideline: prevention of falls in older persons.* Retrieved from http://www.americangeriatrics. org/health_care_professionals/clinical_practice/clinical_guidelines_recommenda tions/prevention_of_falls_summary_of_recommendations/

Bath, P. A., & Morgan, K. (1999). Differential risk factor profiles for indoor and outdoor falls in older people living at home in Nottingham, UK. *European Journal of Epidemiology, 15*, 65–73.

Beasley, C. R., Jason, L. A., & Miller, S. A. (2011). The general environment fit scale: A factor analysis and test of convergent construct validity. *American Journal of Community Psychology.* doi: 10.1007/s10464-001-9480-8.

Brownsell, S. J., Bradley, D. A., Bragg, R., Catlin, P., & Carlier, J. (2000). Do community alarm users want telecare? *Journal of Telemedicine and Telecare, 6*, 199–204.

Bueno-Cavanillas, A., Padilla-Ruiz, F., Jiménez-Moleón, J. J., Peinado-Alonso, C. A., & Gálvez-Vargas, R. (2000). Risk factors in falls among the elderly according to extrinsic and intrinsic precipitating causes. *European Journal of Epidemiology, 16*, 849–859.

Carter, S. E., Campbell, E. M., Sanson-Fisher, R. W., & Gillespie, W. J. (2000). Accidents in older people living at home: A community-based study assessing prevalence, type, location and injuries. *Australia New Zealand Journal of Public Health, 24*, 633–636.

Centers for Disease Control. (2005). *Check for safety: A home fall prevention checklist for older adults.* Retrieved from http://www.cdc.gov/ncipc/pubres/toolkit/Falls_ToolKit/DesktopPDF/English/booklet_Eng_desktop.pdf

Centers for Medicare and Medicaid Services. (2012). Medicare demonstrations. Retrieved from https://www.cms.gov/demoprojectsevalrpts/md/itemdetail.asp?itemid = CMS1240082

Cesari, M., Landi, F., Torre, S., Onder, G., Lattanzio, F., & Bernabei, R. (2002). Prevalence and risk factors for falls in an older community-dwelling population. *Journals of Gerontology Series A: Biological Sciences and Medical Sciences, 57*, M722–726.

Chiu, T., Oliver, R., Tamaki, T., Faibish, S., & Sisson, A. (2001). *The Safety Assessment of Function and the Environment for Rehabilitation–Health Outcome Measurement and Evaluation (SAFER-HOME).* Unpublished manuscript.

Clemson, L., Cumming, R. G., & Roland, M. (1996). Case-control study of hazards in the home and risk of falls and hip fractures. *Age and Ageing, 25*, 97–101.

Clemson, L., Mackenzie, L., Ballinger, C., Close, J. C. T., & Cumming, R. G. (2008). Environmental interventions to prevent falls in community-dwelling older people: A meta-analysis of randomized trials. *Journal of Aging and Health, 20*, 954–971.

Cumming, R. G., Thomas, M., Szonyi, G., Salkeld, G., O'Neill, E., Westbury, C., & Frampton, G. (1999). Home visits by an occupational therapist for assessment and modification of environmental hazards: A randomized trial of falls prevention. *Journal of the American Geriatrics Society, 47*, 1397–1402.

Deficit Reduction Act of 2005, Pub. L. No. 109-171. (2006).

Englander, F., Hodson, T. J., & Terregrossa, R. A. (1996). Economic dimensions of slip and fall injuries. *Journal of Forensic Sciences, 41*, 733–746.

Feldman, F., & Chaudhury, H. (2008). Falls and the physical environment: A review and a new multifactorial falls-risk conceptual framework. *Canadian Journal of Occupational Therapy, 75*, 82–95.

Fleming, B. E., & Pendergast, D. R. (1993). Physical condition, activity pattern, and environment as factors in falls by adult care facility residents. *Archives of Physical Medicine and Rehabilitation, 74*, 627–630.

Gitlin, L. N., Corcoran, M., Winter, L., Boyce, A., & Hauck, W. W. (2001). A randomized, controlled trial of a home environmental intervention: Effect on efficacy and upset in caregivers and on daily function of persons with dementia. *The Gerontologist, 41*, 4–14.

Glass, T., & Balfour, J. L. (2003). Neighborhoods, aging, and functional limitations. In I. Kawachi & L. F. Berkman (Eds.), *Neighborhoods and health* (pp. 303–334). New York, NY: Oxford University Press.

Graafmans, W. C., Ooms, M. E., Hofstee, H. M. A., Bezemer, P. D., Bouter, L. M., & Lips, P. (1996). Falls in the elderly: A prospective study of risk factors and risk profiles. *American Journal of Epidemiology, 143*, 1129–1136.

Iwarsson, S. (2005). A long-term perspective on person-environment fit and ADL dependence among older Swedish adults. *The Gerontologist, 45*, 327–336.

Iwarsson, S., Horstmann, V., Carlsson, G., Oswalk, F., & Wahl, H. W. (2009). Person-environment fit predicts falls in older adults better than the consideration of environmental hazards only. *Clinical Rehabilitation, 23*, 558–567.

Kramer J., Harker, J., Mitchell, M., & Rubenstein, L. (2011, November). *InSTEP: Major research questions.* Symposium, Gerontological Society of America, Boston, MA.

Lawton, M. P. (1998). Environment and aging: Theory revisited. In R. J. Scheidt & P. G. Windley (Eds.), *Environment and aging theory: A focus on housing* (pp. 1–31). Westport, CT: Greenwood Press.

Lawton, M. P., & Nahemow, L. (1973). Ecology and the aging process. In C. Eisdorfer & M. P. Lawton (Eds.), *Psychology of adult development and aging* (pp. 619–674). Washington, DC: American Psychological Association.

Mace, R. L., Hardie, G. J., & Place, J. P. (1996). *Accessible environments: Toward universal design.* Raleig, NC: North Carolina State University, The Center for Universal Design.

Masud, T., & Morris, R. O. (2001). Epidemiology of falls. *Age and Ageing, 30*(S4), 3–7.

Nahemow, L. (2000). The ecological theory of aging: Powell Lawton's legacy. In R. L. Rubinstein, M. Moss, & M. H. Kleban (Eds.), *The many dimensions of aging* (pp. 22–40). New York, NY: Springer.

National Research Council. (2011). *Health care comes home: The human factors.* Washington, DC: The National Academies Press.

Northridge, M. E., Nevitt, M. C., Kelsey, J. L., & Link, B. (1995). Home hazards and falls in the elderly: The role of health and functional status. *American Journal of Public Health, 85*, 509–515.

Pighills, A. C., Torgerson, D. J., Sheldon, T. A., Drummond, A. E., & Bland, J. M. (2011). Environmental assessment and modification to prevent falls in older people. *Journal of the American Geriatrics Society, 59*, 26–33.

Pynoos, J. (1992). Strategies for home modification and repair. *Generations, 16*(2), 21–25.

Pynoos, J., Nishita, C., Cicero, C., & Caraviello, R. (2008). Aging in place, housing, and the law. *The Elder Law Journal, 16*, 77–105.

Pynoos, J., Rose, D., Rubenstein, L., Choi, I. H., & Sabata, D. (2006). Evidence-based interventions in fall prevention. In S. M. Enguidanos (Ed.), *Evidence-based interventions for community dwelling older adults* (pp. 55–73). New York, NY: Hawthorn.

Pynoos, J., Sabata, D., & Choi, I. H. (2005). The role of the environment in fall prevention at home and in the community. In *Falls free: Promoting a national falls prevention action plan* (pp. 41–54). Washington, DC: National Council on the Aging.

Pynoos, J., Steinman, B. A., & Nguyen, A. Q. D. (2010). Environmental assessment and modification as fall-prevention strategies for older adults. *Clinics in Geriatric Medicine, 26,* 633–644.

Rehabilitation Engineering Research Center on Universal Design. (2008). *Existing local visitability laws.* Retrieved from http://www.ap.buffalo.edu/idea/visitability/reports/existingcitylaws.htm

Rogers, M. E., Rogers, N. L., Takeshima, N., & Islam, M. M. (2004). Reducing the risk for falls in the homes of older adults. *Journal of Housing for the Elderly, 18,* 29–39.

Rose, D. J. (2011). Reducing the risk of falls among older adults: The Fallproof balance and mobility program. *Current Sports Medicine Reports, 10,* 151–156.

Rubenstein, L. Z., Robbins, A. S., Josephson, K. R., Schulman, B. L., & Osterweil, D. (1990). The value of assessing falls in an elderly population. *Annals of Internal Medicine, 113,* 308–316.

Rubenstein, L. Z., Vivrette, R., Harker, J. O., Stevens, J. A., & Kramer, B. J. (2011). Validating an evidence-based, self-rated fall risk questionnaire (FRQ) for older adults. *Journal of Safety Research, 42,* 493–499.

Sanford, J. (2010). The physical environment and home health care in national research council: The role of human factors in home health care—Workshop summary (pp. 201–245). Washington, DC: National Academies of Sciences.

Sanford, J. A., Pynoos, J., Tejral, A., & Browne, A. (2002). Development of a comprehensive assessment for delivery of home modifications. *Physical and Occupational Therapy in Geriatrics, 20*(2), 43–55.

Smith, D. B. D., & Small, A. M. (1983). Aging and technological advances: Human factors. In P. K. Robinson, J. Livingston, & J. E. Birren (Eds.), *Symposium on aging and technological advances: NATO conference series* (pp. 363–368). New York, NY: Plenum Press.

Stark, S. L., Somerville, E. K., & Morris, J. C. (2010). In-home occupational performance evaluation (I–HOPE). *The American Journal of Occupational Therapy, 64,* 580–589.

Steinman, B. A., & Nguyen, A. Q. D. (2011, November). *Outcome analysis of the InSTEP home modification component.* Symposium, Gerontological Society of America. Boston, MA.

Steinman, B. A., Nguyen, A. Q. D., Pynoos, J., & Leland, N. E. (2011). Falls-prevention interventions for persons who are blind or visually impaired. *InSight, 4,* 83–91.

Stevens, J. A. (2010). *A CDC compendium of effective fall interventions: What works for community-dwelling older adults* (2nd ed). Atlanta, CA: Center for Disease Control and Prevention, National Center for Injury Prevention and Control.

Stevens, J. A., Corso, P. S., Finkelstein, E. A., & Miller, T. R. (2006). The costs of fatal and non-fatal falls among older adults. *Injury Prevention, 12,* 290–295.

Vasunilashorn, S., Steinman, B. A., Liebig, P. S., & Pynoos, J. (2012). Aging in place: Evolution of a research topic whose time has come. *Journal of Aging Research.* doi:10.1155/2012/120952

Wallace, S. P., Molina, L. C., & Jhawar, M. (2007). *Falls, disability and food insecurity present challenges to healthy aging.* Policy Brief (UCLA Center for Health Policy Research), (PB2007-5), 1–12.

Young, L. C. (2006). *Residential rehabilitation, remodeling and universal design.* Raleigh, NC: North Carolina State University, The Center for Universal Design.

Yu, X. (2008). Approaches and principles of fall detection for elderly and patient. *2008 10th IEEE Intl. Conf. on e-Health Networking, Applications and Service,* Singapore. 42–47.

Aging and Dying in Place: A Personal Journey

RUTH BRENT TOFLE

Department of Architectural Studies, University of Missouri, Columbia, Missouri, USA

A phenomenological case study of a 93-year-old woman is a discussion of her transitions during a short two and a half week period of morbidity from living independently, to hospital, to nursing home, to grave. Her daughter, an environmental gerontologist, provides intimate conversations and reflections chronicled as she keeps vigil by her side 24 hours a day, 7 days a week. The phenomenological approach captures the emotional dying process and amplifies major issues of aging and dying in place for future study.

This is a case study of a 93 year old woman who transitions during a short two and a half week period of morbidity from living independently, to hospital, to nursing home, to grave. She lived in a small town along the Missouri River. This journal began as a way to inform family and friends of the shocking, sad news: "Your mother has acute leukemia, and she can live up to three weeks." It evolved as I tried to remember mother's last experiences, thoughts, and words. Staying by her side in constant vigil, I witnessed her decline as her lifespan shortened from the emergency room diagnosis to her death in my arms. From the emergency room to hospital rooms, intensive care, her nursing room deathbed, and grave, writing to describe this journey was cathartic. This text may be seen as a personal case study in environmental gerontology. The story begins with an alerting email to family members:

BACKGROUND—1/4/12 UPDATE ON MOTHER'S HEALTH

This note is to let you know what's going on with mother's health. Mother has been in a lot of pain recently with her back to the point that she couldn't lift her legs, [is] not sleeping, and [is] in this tremendous pain. I just called to check on mother and she is now resting at home and feeling some better.

Last week after we talked through things, mother put her name on the list at an Assisted Living Facility in her home town. We visited the place and had lunch there a while ago. After visits to several places, it is the one we both like the best. There were six ahead of her on the wait list and we said that is fine since she is not yet ready. I suggested we try to get through another gardening season which is so important to her—and then we can see how things are in October. Mother and I considered having her move out of town to be with me which would be easier for me—but we both think staying in her home community is a better solution since she would be near her friends. I will continue to make the regular road trips once every other week or more often as needed. While I tell mother I won't make her do anything she doesn't want to do, we both see her frailty and the need to have more and more care on a daily basis.

DAY ONE: 1/8/2012 THE NEWS

My 2-hour road trip every week or two to assist mother with personal hygiene, shopping, and business matters were routine until the morning of January 8, 2012. When I enter her bedroom, she is in a fetal position feeling excruciating pain. Complaining of a sore on her hip, she asks what it looks like. I take a photo on my iphone to show her and then call her doctor. I describe her situation, and hear the doctor say "bring her to the emergency room." During the slow, painful walk from her bed, out the back door, and to the car, I hide my worst suspicion. I know this is the last time she will walk out of her own home.

At the emergency room, while waiting for results of multiple blood tests, we are informed she will spend the night in the hospital. With my own interests in the environment and gerontology, mother has always enjoyed being my point of reference. My mother is an academic case study. I wrote about her in a manuscript to describe how she was successfully aging in place and have the pages in my brief case to read to her now:

> Dorothy-from-Kansas owns and manages five rental properties despite her 93 years. Her relative affluence makes her ineligible for low income senior housing. Remembering the Great Depression during her formative years, being frugal with living sustainable practices characterize her chosen way of life. She lives alone in the same house she entered as a bride

nearly 70 years ago. Above doorways of wide varnished oak moldings she displays collections of antique ironstone tea-leaf dishes.

Five walkers assist her in maneuvering her three-story house and yard. Staying active, she climbs stairs by tightly gripping handrails and slowly transferring to another walker at each level. The conveniently placed indoor walkers have yellow tennis ball tips muffling the scooting floor noises while giving her control to safely ambulate. One walker is reserved to the back porch and garden. She transfers to a metal chair where she sits between rows of tomato plants to weed. To lift her spirits, she goes to her garden on a sunny day.

While showing frays, she loves her home. The vermillion draped kitchen table is the social epicenter, and her modest bedroom is the private domain's heart. Alpha and omega, her bedroom is where her two children were conceived and where she would like to breathe her last breath. The bed is pushed to the wall, making room for a small desk with a lamp, sewing supplies, and magazines. Perched in the arm chair she reupholstered, she admires hand stitched patchwork quilts of her dresses. A small duct tape square marks the spot where her kitchen chair glides have worn through the linoleum floor. A lamp's pull chain has a heavy plumbing washer to improve grasp and the 1950's sturdy oak kitchen table and chairs serve to stabilize her gait.

Dorothy's facial wrinkles and stooped arthritic carriage suggest her years. Defying her years, however, she avidly reads *The New Yorker* and stimulates intriguing conversation as she ambitiously tackles her sewing crafts. She takes minimal medication of a daily baby aspirin—suggesting the health of a much younger woman. Called a "white tornado" when young, she was manic in household cleaning and robust in pulling weeds. Now with diminished strength, she limits travel to be close to the bathroom, recognizes vision problems, and becomes fatigued every couple of hours. If living independently would be too difficult, she says she will go to an assisted living facility . . . as long as she could take her sewing machine.

After the death of her 60 year old son, she accepted her own mortality and decided to streamline and simplify accumulations with an auction. Preparing for the concurrent two-ring public sale, she and her daughter sorted memorabilia in stuffed closets, jammed chests, and overflowing shelves to trade procurement stories and determine the fate of items. The piles were labeled "keep," "pitch," "sell," or "donate" to one of three museums. The auction sold tools, furniture, and household treasures accumulated from her deceased husband and her own mother who lived to be 98. A "keeper" is the framed heirloom stitched sampler with colorful wool thread made by her grandmother Emma Jane and hung in her childhood home reads "What's Home Without a Mother." The carefully centered jewelry box atop the bureau was somewhat of a shrine, revealing the greatest legacy stories as necklaces and pins were untangled and admired.

Dorothy's museum-like dwelling is nearly a 1940's period room— without a television, dish washer, or computer. The interior's modern advancements are minimal: microwave, life-line call service, cordless phone with answering machine, and digital clock radio. She is asked if she ever considered remodeling, and her response reflects what she considers remodeling to be. She says she once imaged the house without the decorative iron radiators ... "but got used to the way things were."

As time passes in the Emergency Department, I am anticipating a temporary move to a nursing home for rehabilitation. I ask to talk to a social worker to understand how Medicare works. If she stays in the hospital for 3 nights, she qualifies for skilled nursing home stay, and Medicare will pick up expenses.

A large man wearing a physician's white coat enters the room. He doesn't mince words: "Your mother has acute leukemia, and she can live up to 3 weeks." Thinking the word "acute" means the opposite of chronic and surely an acute ailment could be treated, I was in disbelief hearing the second part of the sentence: "Do you mean 3 weeks of a lifespan?" He answers clearly, "Yes. Lifespan." I immediately turn and lean down to talk to mother while holding back tears. "Mother, the doctor says you have acute leukemia and have 3 weeks to live." Her reaction is silence.

"Can't we give her any medicine?" I ask. The doctor explains, "The normal white blood count is less than 10,000 and your mother's is over 200,000. We will use a medicine called Hydrea, trying to control the white blood count. I am also contacting an oncologist."

Dizzy with the news and feeling the urgency of getting word to family and friends, we begin a new journey as chronicled in emails:

LATER THIS DAY: EMAIL READS "MOTHER'S LIFESPAN"

Today the doctor said my mother has up to about 3 [weeks] to live. Mother knows everything—no secrets. They are controlling pain, but she is very frail. I'm spending the night at hospital and will know more tomorrow after the oncologist comes. ... I feel blessed to have this time to be with mom to talk about things and help her say goodbye to family and friends. The minister has been here and a steady stream of company. I'm so glad we are in her home town.

For years I have carried a notebook with all mother's legal papers in the trunk of my car to have whenever I visited her—Living Will, Power of Attorney, etc. I easily hand over the necessary documentation to the hospital. And, a purple "Do Not Resuscitate" [DNR] bracelet is secured on mother's wrist. Trying unsuccessfully to hold back emotions, I explain to mother the meaning of the DNR purple bracelet. She understands but is silent.

DAY TWO: 1/9/12 COMMUNITY SUPPORT

We've had a parade of ladies from church, family, neighbors, and friends. We are chatting to help realize the love created, and I'm acting as mother's social secretary. The leukemia came so very fast, and I'm here to help her say goodbyes. At the end of each visit with friends, there is not a "see you later" statement, but a matter of fact, "good bye." Mother says she is comfortable and at peace. We talk about how happy she was to have lived in her own home independently, and we both feel blessed by her really long, good life. I'll know more today after more tests. The doctors and staff have been wonderful. Mom is on morphine and comfortable and cogent.

DAY THREE: 1/10/12 MEDICAL UPDATE

Today we heard pretty much what we learned yesterday—with a few more specifics. Mother has AML. Acute myloid leukemia. With the large white blood cells, they could stick to her heart or brain (heart attack or stroke), and death would be very fast. We are beginning a regime of Hydrea to get the blood count down. They are now saying the median expected life expectancy is 4 weeks. Eventually, she will transfer to a private room with hospice care in a local nursing home. We are trying to extend life now. With hospice care she won't be in pain. She will take oral pain meds now and move to morphine as hospice determines—to orchestrate a good death as much as possible. I will stay by mother's side. I told mother I would not leave her. Grandchildren want to come to visit now instead of attending memorial service.

LATER THIS DAY:

The doctor just told us her blood work with new medicine seems to be helping to buy more time but still only up to a month. And after scans, we just learned mother does not have any cancer mass or bone cancer—it is all in her blood. The doctor wants mom to try to get out of bed today. She is really excited about seeing her grandchildren and trying to think of stories to tell.

DAY FOUR: 1/11/2012 BUYING TIME

We are moved to the ICU [Intensive Care Unit] at the hospital trying out a rather new drug for leukemia. It is a pill, but there may be complications so that's why she is in ICU for monitoring. The doctor said he would give it to his own mother if she were in this situation. Last night, her white blood cells continued to climb, but she is stable with all vital signs before the drug begins to do its work. Her very caring doctor called mother's nurse three times between 11:00 last night and 7:00 this morning. It may take 2-21 days to see if it will work, and they will be monitoring clinical health to see how long she will continue on drug. We just need to take things one day at a time—as you've noticed things change in her treatment regime.

LATER THIS DAY

Mother is still "holding court" in the ICU with visitors. For the first few hours in the ICU, when we are both scared about a possible drug reaction as the medicine drips in her veins, we hold hands. I pull a chair near her bedside and lean over to share pillows as we try to sleep.

After a while, I move to the recliner chair by her bedside. We are in a semiprivate room without a nearby shower. There is a unisex bathroom (with smelly urinal) that I use and must do my best to freshen up with crunchy paper towels. Friends are doing my laundry. I'm not even leaving her to eat—but living on granola bars. It is nice to see so many friends from my childhood. No news yet on mother's white blood cells. They draw blood every morning to check progress. So far no bad drug reaction.

DAY FIVE: 1/12/12 NIGHT TIME REFLECTIONS

Mother took a Percocet (Endo Pharmaceuticals Inc., Chadds Ford, Pennsylvania) at about 2:00 p.m. today for pain, and we are trying to get on a schedule so pain doesn't get ahead of her. This is a rather low level pain med[ication]. She is also getting steroids and insulin to counteract affects. I watch monitors and worry when her blood pressure drops much too low—which may mean the need for a central line. I decide to start asking questions about the extent of what is too invasive. Talking to friends, I learn about "DNR plus" and have my notes to discuss with doctors tomorrow. I feel less frightened now understanding this better.

She got out of bed to sit in a chair and she is exhausted. While in the ICU, I am limiting visiting to help mother get more sleep. Non-family visitors may stay 10 minutes to protect her strength. And I'm trying to help visitors lead conversation rather than mother (this is hard for her).

At 4:00 a.m. they draw blood, and by 6:00 a.m. her doctor will have results to tell us. We are all eager to learn her white blood count. We are taking things day by day. So far she is tolerating this new medicine for the hope of a longer lifespan—knowing it is still terminal. Again, vitals are good, no cancerous mass, no cancer in the bones, and this is so rapid. She was living alone up until recently, so we are encouraged to try.

Mother is in good spirits, bedridden, too chatty for her own good sometimes, bright, and at peace with her terminal condition. We are talking about her memorial and cremation calmly. I remind her we will use the small antique iron safe we cleaned up together a couple of years ago for her remains to be buried, and that I think I will put my remains in her tea-leaf casserole dish when I die. Mother speaks up instantly, "I want the tea-leaf casserole!" Laughing and appreciating her spunk, "Okay, mom, you can have the casserole."

Mother is looking forward to seeing our out-of-state family members beginning tomorrow. Thanks to wonderful friends, I showered, washed my hair, put on clean clothes, was able to read a chapter of the Steve Jobs biography to her, and eat above my normal calories.

DAY SIX: 1/13/12 LIVING IN THE INTENSIVE CARE UNIT

Mom's white blood count this morning is now 138,000. ... Remember, less than 10,000 is normal. The drop is good, but her red blood cells are also dropping, so today she will get platelets. Her veins are problematic, which causes concern. She has two bad infections—leukemia and a general one. The side with the red spot continues to be enflamed, hot, swollen. They are going to change her antibiotic today.

Mother is classified as DNR. She is weak, very weak. She tried sitting up on the side of the bed by herself with the physical therapy but got too dizzy. Her blood pressure and lungs are good. She eats some food slowly, as it is difficult to swallow. She likes hot water and ice water. She is still getting her IV. And her pee went from tea colored to now being red blood colored. She needs platelets. She hasn't had a BM [bowel movement] for a couple of days, so she will get a laxative today.

Coming from out of state and driving through snow, all grandchildren and a new great grandchild arrive to visit in the cramped and sterile ICU. Mother and I really enjoy these visits. Mom is relieved that her grandchildren are smart and grasp the family business. When the night is quiet, a grandson uses my iPad and Pandora to help mother select four songs for her memorial service as I doze.

Being in this ICU semi-private room for days is unpleasant. Ironically, we go to such lengths with HIPAA regulations for health information privacy, and yet in a semi-private room we are bludgeoned with the most intimate information I don't want to know. On a busy night when all ICU beds are occupied, emergency surgery was performed at 3:30 a.m. to insert a central line in a lady's neck—just 4 feet from my mother's bed and every word is heard. On another night when the bed pan from another patient on the other side of the "privacy curtain" was particularly noxious, mother woke up and screamed, "Something is burning!" I had to whisper in her ear to calmly explain it was not a fire but the bowel movement of the lady in the other bed.

A friend/genealogist/and former funeral director stopped by and gave us contact information as we also plan the cremation and burial. Our Pastor has been here several times as we all held hands and prayed.

Special thanks go to cousins for helping with showers and sheets for our out of town family members. One cousin arrives each morning to visit and is truthful in telling me what I look like after sleeping every night in a chair ... which brings humor.

I rarely leave mothers side—unless to go to the bathroom, bring back food from cafeteria, or [run] quick errands. Mother wants me to feed her, and I help with giving fluids, changing bed position, being advocate with staff, asking for nursing help, holding hands during painful blood sticks, and sometimes with bathing, hair washing, and bedpan work. Mother bragged about me working so hard to the doctor and the doctor's retort was, "Dorothy, you are making us ALL work hard!"

DAY SEVEN: 1/15/12 ONE WEEK AND SINGING

Today's blood report comes with good news. We entered the hospital 1 week ago today with the white blood count of over 200,000. That jumped as high as 230,000 when the normal is 4,000 to 9,800. Today, her count was 11,200, which is in the high normal range. Apparently, she was able to pee out the bad stuff without hurting her kidneys. Her red blood count has been low however. Yesterday, she got platelets, and today she got 2 units of blood because this count was 8.1 when the normal was 11.8–14.8.

We are buying time, not a cure for her terminal leukemia. She still has leukemia but the two drugs they used for her—the Hydrea and Accutane (also used for acne) drug—seem to be making a difference. You may remember how frightened we were in trying the risky Accutane derivative drug because of the potential side effects—which is why we were so closely monitored in the ICU and had to confront the DNR Plus issues.

She has been bedridden all week, and as a result she is very weak. The doctors are tapering down pain medication as well so she may be sleeping less. Her appetite is pretty good and her mind continues to be sharp.

Finally, we are moved to a small private room with a sink, toilet, and shower that I can use. Mother is now SINGING to herself—really. She memorized the lyrics to songs in a couple of pioneer song book years ago. Living alone, her routine is to sing these songs or recite poetry to herself—out loud. In her words, this "gets me going for the day."

> "The pedigree of honey
> Does not concern the bee;
> A clover, any time, to him
> Is aristocracy." Emily Dickinson
> "Oh, mairzy doats and dozy doats and little lambsy divey
> A kiddle divey, too. Wouldn't you?"

While here, I'm trying to take care of some of mother's household and business details as she has been managing several rental units while living alone. I'm still sleeping next to my mother at the hospital and get away for only short tasks. I've turned off her telephone, paid bills, and am making appointments to keep rental houses going. I am so happy to be here near my mother. We are doing important work together in this end-of-life phase of her magnificent life.

DAY EIGHT: 1/16/2012 AWARE OF PLACE

Mother had a hard night last night. During the night she describes seeing things through a long silk scarf with scales. Sometimes during sleep she calls out to me to ask, "Am I okay?" She also talks about turnstiles—"there is only one way through." And, more than once she says, "I can see myself going right out the window." At night, I close the draperies.

With a large window with a low sill running the length of the private room, she asks about the red balls marking power lines near the helicopter pad and flags whipping in the wind. The ever-flowing Missouri River is only visible for a small stretch between tree branches. Lighting in our room offers different levels of illumination for functional purposes and multiple outlets allow for computer and iPhone recharging to connect with the outside world. A pastel sage-green wallpaper border of vines defines the edge where the ceiling meets the walls and I wonder if patients who spend most of their days looking up will notice this detail. Mom is flanked with hospital bed linens and a soft green snow-flake plush lap blanket drawing many compliments. Her head is cradled by her own feather pillow encased in her hand-made patchwork pillowcase. She knows she is becoming weaker, and it is hard to adjust to her total incontinence. A catheter is now in place. She is sleeping more, and when she is awake in a slow, low pitch voice recites another poem or gruffly sings lyrics. Pandora iPad music was rejected because she "would rather sing to herself." Her hearing is getting worse—I have to speak distinctly near her right ear. Talking less, she points to what she wants. She wants me to read from the Steve Jobs biography and appreciates me reading the missing lyrics from my computer to the song, "Don't Fence Me In."

Her blistered bottom and purple-bruised left arm from veins that blew during IV/blood work [are] now swollen and blistering too. Nurses were finally able to remove her gold ring, and today a nurse switches her Christmas "Happy bracelet" and watch to the right arm. During a visit by a buff Physical Therapist, he stretches to remove the "Livestrong" yellow bracelet my brother wore during his last days with cancer. The yellow rubber bracelet is now around my wrist until I return it my brother's family.

We continue to get company from friends, but she is now more detached from conversation. Tomorrow, the last of out-of-state family will be here. Mother directs me to be sure and call them if she dies before they arrive—so they can turn around and go home and just come back for the memorial.

Our private room is small and compact with seating for five—and still some visitors stand. There are cut flowers in water becoming murkier as leaves become brittle. An antique 1800-something Valentine is nearby—something she reminded me about and therefore retrieved. I read "Be my Valentine" as I know how unlikely it will be to make it to February 14. Her photo album is nearby, and I show off the July feature story with mother on the cover and brag that she is also the featured center-fold story because of her 4-H acclaim in being the first woman to win the American Royal for the Grand Champion steer. During the Depression, she bought a gold watch and a college education. I want all the nurses and staff to know my mother is a celebrity. Discovering her identity might make a difference in connecting on a caring, personal level.

I'm in the reclining chair where I sleep facing my bedfast mother (Figure 1). Her soft vanilla skin loosely laps over deep wrinkles and sunken cheeks. I tell her often that I love her as I stroke her hair and kiss her

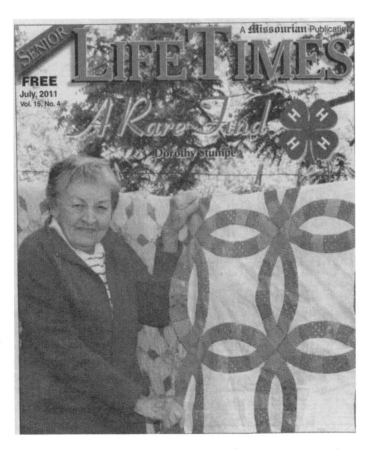

FIGURE 1 Feature story of mother in local magazine 6 months earlier is shown to health care providers.

cheeks. With barely opened eyelids, she raises her hands from her bed to make the OK sign with thumb and index finger. I reminded her how she told me throughout my life how she wore out a rocking chair comforting me when I was a baby ... and now it was my turn to comfort her. Also, I never missed a Christmas away from her—and I was going to be near her for her good death too.

Like the first night I slept by her side, I wonder if this is reality or a dream. I don't think about my normal life—but know the hospital hourly clocked routine. Barely leaving her sight, I report to the nurse's station if leaving for scant minutes to bring up cafeteria food. I've lost sense of time and check the patient orientation board for the day of the week and date. When the nurse quizzes mother today however, she correctly says, "It's Martin Luther King's Birthday."

We talk about who to ask to speak at her memorial service. I have an idea of what I will say, and mother approves with a smile. She tells me she wants to sleep tonight. I smooth her blankets and calculate the next hour she will receive pain medicine. Good night mother, I'm right here for you.

DAY NINE: 1/17/2012 WHEN?

"Pain medication as needed" means it is MY responsibility to calculate hours between meds and request they be administered. When left up to mother, she doesn't get them in time to handle the minutes between doses kicking into action. Last night, her medication was good and this morning she asks, "Am I going to die?" I tell her "Yes, you have cancer all over your body and you are getting weaker all the time." She then asks, "Well, why do I feel so good?" I reiterate my promise that I won't let her suffer. She asks, "When?" Responding, "I don't know, only God knows. Would you like to say the Lord's Prayer with me that has that line 'Thy will be done'?" She nods, we hold hands, and we recite the words.

DAY TEN: 1/18/12 MOVING TO A NURSING HOME

Arriving by ambulance, mother's next residence is a local nursing home—just down the street from the hospital. Tomorrow I'll become immersed in Medicare reimbursement procedures. I have 62 legal pages awaiting to read and sign. It is delayed from this first day of admittance. I'm an interior designer, so I have the challenge of making this room more homelike. Challenged indeed. I was surprised by the stark emptiness of this institutional room—a bed, small chest, and cubicle curtains—that's it.

How can I stay with my mother in this room? Can I bring in my air mattress? It was agreed they would bring in another twin bed. Mom and I now have matching twin beds in this "semi-private" room offered as a single room. We can be together 24/7, and I can actually sleep horizontally instead of snoozing contorted in a chair as I've done in the past week and a half. I rearrange the beds for her to look directly out the window and also see a small shelf of photos and six of her requested small, home-made prairie dolls. The bed is also positioned so her face is in my direct line of sight when I'm in my bed.

The western-facing window gives light from the street. The room has a sink and toilet but no shower. The heater/air conditioner unit is controllable. Wi-Fi is available, albeit remote in another part of the facility. Visitors from town continue to come on a regular basis, and I am also brought a meal tray to eat the same food as mom. The privilege of eating nursing home food is not thrilling, but I'm happy to have it.

It is too early to assess staffing—we're just getting acquainted. When given the choice of a newer facility with poor staffing or an older facility with better staffing as described by mother's doctor, I chose the older facility with better staffing. The cost, one way or another, wasn't considered. It was an easy decision to make but curious given my professional background that I put staffing above importance of environment. Staff takes the time to introduce themselves, and we try to make family connections. Mother says, "You should write a book about my experience here."

Here's the down side of this place—it's a 1960s nursing home. I was in high school when I attended its Sunday afternoon open house. In that era, nursing homes were designed with double*loaded long corridors, a large dining room, and showers were not included in rooms. I'm in a time warp with mint green walls (I love to hate) and scalloped trim on furnishings popular in the 1960s or before. Showing signs of age and heavy wear, the beds need to be hand-cranked and furniture and walls are marred, scuffed, or chipped. I'm told the community shower room would not be a good place to shower. It's smelly. Should I try showering late in the evening when no one else is around?

This is likely to be the room where my mother will die. Even though she has other things on her mind and she thinks it is okay, is this death bed good enough for my mother? Because we are not going to be here very long, I'm wondering what and how much to haul into this place to make it more homelike. In the first hour, I personalized the place with photos, [a] quilt of patches from childhood dresses, mother's hand-crafted dolls, and mother's pillow. If I knew I had to be here for a long time, I'd begin painting the entire room, change out the light fixtures, bring in our own furniture and more accessories, and rid the place of institutional features. The structure of the interior room reads institution. Cubicle curtains are only used in medical institutions. Let's get cubicle curtains outlawed! Even the ceiling is scarred with its tracks. Then there is the institutional intercom with buzzes, rings, and announcements—installed before cell phones were conceived.

Important family stories are retold and clarified. She reveals voting for FDR [Franklin D. Roosevelt] and how she "fell" for my dad fast—at 25 she was at the right age and they saw each other every weekend. "We just fit." Mother asked me to tell the family story of the wild horse that bucked the son of a Kaiser military man—an ancestor. She would listen to how I told the story to make sure I told it correctly. ... Despite warnings, the son rode the stallion and then felt ashamed to tell his parents when crippled and therefore didn't get medical attention. Limiting his career options to follow his father in the military, the family left Germany to come to the U.S.

"I've tried to beat this long enough" she grumbles. And, being in the nursing home, things are taking its course. The doctor says the white blood cells will rise again—just keep her comfortable and let her do what she wants to do. Mother has no IV's. She uses a catheter and bed pan. Still on Percocet, she sleeps a lot with her head back and her mouth open. The inside of her mouth and esophagus is sore as a result of the leukemia medicine, so she is eating tiny little bites of soft food—canned pears, overcooked meat, Jell-O, and liquids.

Mom's 81-year-old Kansas brother is with us today—the last of the out-of-state family. In the long good-bye, we know this will be the last time they'll see one another and words spoken cannot express the deeper feelings. Mother's German heritage of not saying the words "I love you" also make the heavy moments linger and hurt. I say the three words for her. She adds, "that's right." To which I conclude, "And, mother, I love you."

DAY ELEVEN: 1/19/2012 PLACE MAKES A DIFFERENCE

After grandchildren visited mother this past week, they were invited to select items from mom's house to remember her. Using their iPhones, they photographed their selections so they could come back and show mother what they thought was most precious and learn more stories.

While the house is torn up and picked over, I am able to transport a nice collection of possessions to personalize her nursing home room. Within about 24 hours, mother's nursing home room is rearranged and decorated to be functional and provide delight for both mother and me. Most of the framed pieces have their own story, and it feels good to see mother light up as the pictures were hung. This act of love is for me too—that I can do something positive for her to appreciate and also feel personal comfort. I believe place makes a difference—for both of us. I have my own workstation (card table) where I can work at a table by her bedside. The process is not unlike preparing a dorm room—only I have no idea how long we will be set up. The photos show the before and the after. I will be glad I went to this effort for however long she is able to appreciate this place (Figures 2 and 3).

She is sleeping a lot—during the day and in the night with medication. In the middle of the night, I heard her talking about "handsome Jonathan" and "pretty Jessica"—my children. Later in the morning, I asked what

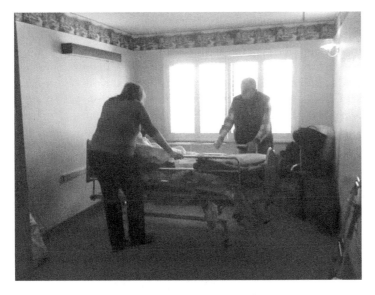

FIGURE 2 The empty nursing home.

she dreamed about last night and she remembered exactly what she said. Throughout the day, however, she talks during sleep about things that don't connect. Within a short period of time she talked about a "policeman making this bed," "Is Kathy still eating?" "Take it through the bottom drawer," and "Blueberry, my God Almighty!"

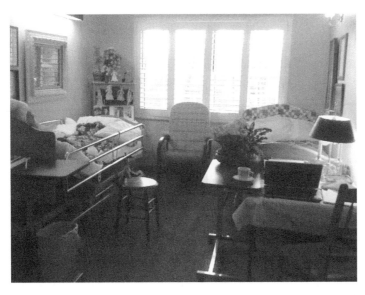

FIGURE 3 The same room accommodating patient and caregiver with personal possessions 24 hours later.

I've filled out all the Medicare papers. We are at a private for-profit nursing home. The cost of our private room is $152/day, calculated to be $4,561/month. Having transferred from acute illness, Medicare Part A pays for the cost of a semi-private room in the nursing home (we pay the $23/day difference for a private room and [it's] worth every cent) and rehab for 100 days. At the recommendation of her physician, she came as a nursing home patient. We all know the transfer to hospice, however, is imminent. Medicare will pay for either hospice or the nursing home. I'm eager to talk to her doctor tomorrow for him to advise if we should go to hospice.

I have a list of questions for mother's doctor tomorrow. While she tells me she is not in pain, there is a new problem. Tonight, my mother's temperature went from 99.6∞ to 100.5∞ between 8:00 a.m. and 4:00 p.m., and I admit I'm worried. My friend Sally has been with me tonight, and we are putting a cool wash cloth on her forehead and wiping the back of her neck to cool her off. It appears she has an infection somewhere, and her body can't handle it. Her immune system can't handle an infection. Perhaps she may become septic, and this will be what takes my mother.

DAY TWELVE: 1/20/2012 HOSPICE BEGINS

Days begin thinking nothing new will happen. ... Then, the journey becomes more arduous. Mother's long-time regular family doctor returned from knee surgery recovery to assume his normal duties, and we were finally able to meet. Limping into the room, he hugs mom and says, "Dorothy, Dorothy, Dorothy, how did this happen?" Sitting on my low antique stool near her pillow, our geriatric physician is attentive to mother's slow speech. After mom's best shot to speak, I blurted out the chronology of events, recorded details, and my specific bottled-up questions.

Bottoming the list was "timing of hospice." With tears streaming from both eyes simultaneously and nose dripping, I confessed, "Sometimes I want her to go faster ... and sometimes I want to hold on to her just so I have my mother." The doctor turns to me and gives me a hug as if I'm now the patient. He comforts and consoles me. The words are soft and clear, "Your mother is dying, and it's time for hospice." Me: "Do you think I did the right thing to agree to that Accutane drug?" Doctor: "Absolutely, it was a low-risk good try, and you would really be feeling guilty if you wouldn't have tried." Doctor: "Do you want to stop the antibiotics too?" Me: "I think we should let mother go." Doctor: "I agree. That's what I would recommend." I feel a sense of relief when he agrees. Rationalizing, I am following professional advisement.

He writes the prescriptions: Ativan, 1 mg every 4 hours as needed for anxiety/nausea, and Roxanol (morphine), 10 mg every hour as needed for pain or shortness of breath. Expressing my frustrations, "I don't know when she needs more pain medication." Again his reassurance, "You won't have to make this decision." Me: "How will it happen?" Doctor:

"Commonly, it is from pneumonia, 'the old man's friend', but we don't know." Me: "When will it happen?" Doctor: "Days ... not longer than a month." Me: "Tell mother. Be honest. We have no secrets." Doctor: "Dorothy, you are dying. There is no cure."

The notebook carried in my car trunk for so many years containing copies of signed documents is finally needed: Living Will and Durable Power of Attorney for Health Care Decisions and Living Will and Durable Power of Attorney for Health Care. Now, I am presenting them to a hospice nurse. White paper forms are flashed in front of me at a dizzying pace requiring signature consent as mom's "legally authorized representative": requesting hospice admission, the Missouri's hospice election statement, authorization for release of medical information, Medicare secondary payer screening form. ... Then, a purple card stock paper is presented: "Outside the Hospital Do-Not-Resuscitate Order."

It's 3:00 in the afternoon, and I haven't had lunch. I sign all without reading and grab a granola bar so I don't faint. The hospice nurse examines mother as she looks for cardinal markers. I know to look for bluish color under nails and from the feet as it travels up. In the exam, the nurse checks vitals and turns mom's stiff body from side to side as we hear loud groans. She has a temperature of 101. Continuing the exam, mother is in and out of sleep and answers calls from nowhere. The hospice nurse questions, "Who do you see?" Mother: "They are calling me." Nurse: "Who is calling you, do you know their names?" Mother: "I don't know. I just see their initials." Nurse: "Where are they?" Mother pointing to the air above her, "Hovering."

Sitting on the edge of my bedside, the nurse says this is common in the last days. "You could call the crematorium or our social worker can call ... and you can talk to our Chaplin or he can call your own minister." We cover a few more details. ... And, as if a miracle in timing occurs, there is a knock at the door. Our Pastor walks in with his black communion satchel.

My mother was raised Methodist and then converted to Lutheran when she married my dad. She is somewhat of an agnostic, although both my brother and I attended parochial Lutheran grade school. Earlier in this ordeal, we talked about how "it doesn't hurt to believe." Now, I feel a new burden of responsibility to help my mother have a stronger faith in the everlasting during her last hours. I speak clearly in mom's right ear: "Pastor has come to give us communion." Mother nods in agreement. The nurse's aide interrupts to empty the urinal bag, Pastor prepares the communion, and I shut the door.

Removing us from this earthly location, Pastor begins the Holy Communion ritual by belting out a loud and committed voice as is heard from the pulpit. Scripture I memorized when in grade school is recited. As I hold both of mother's hands, he asks mother questions about her faith in Christ and tells her she can agree by nodding. Three questions are asked, three nods given. He gives her the wafer to eat and she coughs, not able

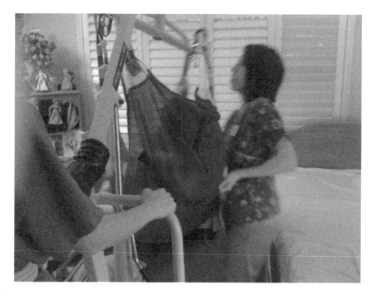

FIGURE 4 Hoisted in hammock, mother is temporarily moved so her own bed can be switched to a low air-loss mattress.

to eat the entire wafer as instructed, but nibbles a small morsel. With my eyes closed, a wafer melts in my mouth. The wine is then offered and received by mother and also by me. Mother chokes again and asks for more wine. Instead of offering more wine, the minister stands up and says he will get water—but grabs the clear glass of 7-Up. When I clarify the difference (does 7-Up nullify the power of the wine?), he says it is okay, and also removes the wafer from her fingers. We say the Lord's Prayer slowly together. Concluding the ritual, he gives me a 29-page brochure entitled "Heaven" and suggests I read it to mother.

Thanking him for his service, I reveal I'd never had Communion outside of a church. He talks to me as he pitches mom's remaining wafer in the trash can. I suddenly recall discussions in religious instruction about the sanctity of the blessed wafer and ask if it was "okay" to pitch. "I guess I should have eaten it myself ... but God forgives me," he says. What a relief to know he allows slippage.

The excitement for the day concludes with hospice services arriving with a low air-loss mattress—like a Sleep Number Bed. To switch out the mattress, mother must be hoisted into a hammock in a power lift and temporarily placed in the bed where I sleep for 30 minutes while inflation is completes. Mother is not liking this—but she rallies to show her spirit as she sings with the nurses' aides and me, "Rockabye baby in the tree top" (Figure 4).

When released in my bed for her mattress to complete its inflation, the first thing she does is reach up to the ledge of the picture frame of a favorite Grant Wood print nearby to check for dust. Giggling, I quickly

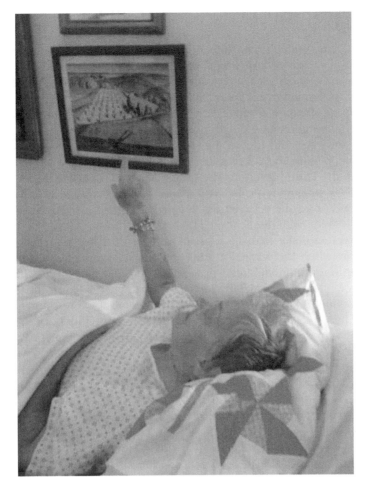

FIGURE 5 Mother checks for dust on a frame of a favorite Grant Wood picture.

respond: "I caught you checking! You didn't believe me when I told you I dusted the pictures before I hung them up!" I cannot believe she is so attuned to her pictures. She still wants to make sure they are clean and presentable! (Figure 5)

Mother is talking more to herself. She talks out loud to no one about my role as an interior designer who fixed up this room so nicely ... and how much she likes the prairie dolls she made. I hand her a doll to hold—with its dress matching the quilted patches on her pillow. She also says things that make no sense. Then, being absolutely cogent she calls me over to say, "Get a nurse to be with you." Me: "Do you mean you don't want me to be alone when you die?" She nods in agreement, "Get a nurse to be with you. And, don't cry unless you have to." A true mother, she is worrying about her daughter.

DAY FIFTEEN: 1/23/12 SLIDING

"Am I getting enough nourishment to stay alive?" "How long will it take to die?" "It's hard work staying alive." Then, "It's hard work to die." "Am I being abandoned?" "What do you want me to do?" These are the slowly spoken, penetrating, and poignant thoughts.

A recurring dream/nightmare is with someone knocking angrily at the door. In the middle of the night, she was actually knocking on the wall by her own bed and frightening me. It was real, and her eyes showed fear. I jumped up and talked to her and then started reading the religious material the Pastor gave me. The only other reading material I had was Steve Jobs' biography or the New Yorker. I pulled up the lyrics on my iPad for a song she selected for her memorial and she lip synced the refrain, "Abide with me."

Two days ago, she told me to make a flash card that said "water" so I'd know when she wanted a drink. Mother has made "flash cards" all her life in teaching children—now she is the one who needs this aid. She even attempted to write words on a card when I didn't understand her. Communication is now more with nods, facial expressions, slowly raising her hands to point, making the OK sign, raising up both palms as if to say "I'm doing what I can," and saying few words. I guess and she confirms—or I keep trying.

Now, well-constructed, reflective sentences are over for this former English teacher. Struggling this morning, she barely gets out the agitated words associated with scary thoughts: "They give me the lie first!" "They are tricked!" "Did you tell them the secret?" Her eyes and expressions tell me she is afraid. I do the best I can to repeat what she is saying and keep trying to get an affirmative nod and then try to comfort. In the middle of the night for the past two mornings, I awake startled by her restlessness and fright. I stroke her hair, hold her hands and calmly say, "Don't worry, mamma, I'll take care of everything, I promise. It's okay. You had a wonderful life. We love you. I'm here for you."

Meanwhile, I ask for morphine. As the liquid is being squirted and absorbed in her mouth, I pulled up the iPad words to "Abide with Me" and sang. She nods to confirm I should continue singing, but mother is no longer able to sing the refrain. I learn these scary ideas are the result of her drugs.

Once she is asleep, I am dreary in walking to the nurse's station to inquire about the timing of her pain medication. The nurse tells me she had a pain pill in the evening. Pressing harder, I learned the last Percocet pill was at 5:00 p.m., and it becomes apparent that the 11:00 p.m. pill was not given. I continue to press, "Did you try to give the pill to mother and she refused?" Not answering my question, the nurse responds: "She has the right to refuse medication." Me: "I want my mother to have her Percocet on schedule even if she says she doesn't need it. When she does not get her medication on schedule, the pain is too hard on her between doses." I don't hear the words or the compassion I expect.

At a more civilized hour of 8:00 a.m., after breakfast, a CMT (Certified Med Tech) makes it a point to tell me she overheard our conversation and will report it to the Director of Nursing and will also try to get a request to mom's doctor to make sure this medication occurs on schedule along with the morphine as needed. She can't directly make the request with the doctor because she is not a nurse. She comes back later to say the doctor agreed.

Walking down the hall, I occasionally hear a patient calling out for help, "Nurse?!?" The call light gives out a noise that sounds like a loud annoying swarm of mosquitoes on microphones. It's an alarming sound . . . and yet, after a while, I too am able to ignore the noise. I'm glad I'm here to be my mother's advocate. I don't even bother with the call light, I hunt down the staff.

I don't see another person bunking with their loved one as I am doing in end-of-life care. Apparently, it is occasionally done for a family member who stays for a day or two to "settle someone." In one other case I know about, an attendant is paid by the family. She is a former High School classmate who graciously greets me and tells me about fellow classmates. She is hired to help a 94-year-old patient/resident from 5:00 a.m. to 11:00 a.m. each morning.

What do staff members think about me being here? They are glad I can help interpret needs, feed meals, and make the patient/resident comfortable. Not just that I do some of their work, they see the tenacity of love I have for my mom. They tell me they "admire" me and how they have been in my shoes seeing a parent or husband die. One staff member says she feels sorry for those who don't have a soul to be their advocate. She resents family members who ignore their loved one or only make visits on holidays a couple times a year.

Many rooms have no personalization whatsoever—just the standard bed, chest, and chair. Who are these anonymous people? I want to see the quilts and dolls they make, their wedding pictures, the trophies of their life's triumphs. I can't blame the patient/residents who have health problems, and I'm not blaming the nursing home staff. If I can blame anyone, it is the family of these resident/patients. If I can scrounge around to find meaningful pictures and memorabilia for a 2-week stay, surely any other family could also expend the effort to honor the past lives of their loved ones (Figure 6).

Most rooms have a television running incessantly. And, the majority of rooms are what I believe would be intolerable—double occupancy. I shudder thinking about giving my mother a bed in a semi-private room with cubical curtains cutting off natural light of windows and hearing other people's grief when we have our hands full with our own. When death is knocking at the door, I want to sing to my mother to comfort her in the darkness of night. And, I want my mother to see her joyous young granddaughter romping around her room drawing pictures and playing with dolls.

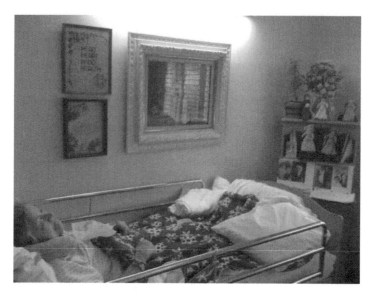

FIGURE 6 Closest to mother's eye-sight is a framed letter a 4-H member wrote to her and the 4-H sampler she made when she was 13 years old: "Head, Heart, Hands, Health." Prairie dolls she made and photographs are at the foot of her bed.

I used to give nursing homes a bad rap. I am recanting some of my criticisms. With a single room, the flexibility to make it a "home away from home," no qualms about hammering on the walls to hang pictures and adjust lighting, a small-town everybody knows everybody else neighboring, and my advocacy in working with the staff, it is ideal. Wheelchair scrapes on the wall don't bother me, and other marks are covered with our own adornments. The place is clean. I don't smell urine in this wing. Except for the one error noted above, staff members are kind and caring. Being at a nursing home provides needed medication and care around the clock, which I could not administer on my own while giving easy access for local friends to stop by for visits.

Mother's condition is printed in the Sunday church bulletin—a major communication conduit. On weekends, significantly more family visitors are present and the meals are better. Probably intentionally, the Sunday noon meal is like Thanksgiving—timed for families getting out of church to see their loved ones. Otherwise, food is overcooked and mushy, but edible. For my mother's generation, milk gravy is comfort food and Jell-O with canned fruit satisfies a legitimate food group. Every meal time, I'm invited to get my own tray when I feed my mother. I enjoy their breakfasts—hardest to screw up: hard boiled eggs, raison bran and milk, orange juice, and pancakes or wheat toast with butter and jam.

What is mother eating? Itty-bitty tiny bites of meat with gravy and small sips from straws of juice, 7-Up, or water. Her urine bag output shows she is drinking much less. She motions for a stick with a small blue foam rubber tip—an oral care swab—to scrape the yuck from her mouth. This morning, her lips had the black crust of dried blood.

In addition to responding to mother during her moments when awake, I give updates on mother's situation and visit with the steady stream of wonderful friends and family members who love my mom and visit us on a regular basis.

While dramatically sliding, she still recognizes all of her family members and friends. It is so hard to see my mother in this bodily shell when she is not in control—being so "out of it." The toil of the past 2 weeks has ravaged her spirit and body. She doesn't act like herself or look like herself. I tell her doctor, "I hate seeing my mother like this." Doctor: "There is no other way. It won't be long." Mumbling between tears: "This week?" Doctor, reaching out arms to hug and giving a best guess: "Yes."

DAY SEVENTEEN: 1/25/12 WAITING ... AND THEN DEATH

Is this the death date I will remember? Just like we remember birthdates, maybe today, January 25th, will be the death day engrained in my memory. The morning visit of the hospice nurse includes a report. Mother is now in the "active dying stage." A hospice volunteer appears and hangs white feathers on the wall for me to see. She calls them "angel wings." She sits with me as I hold my mother's hand. I'm afraid to let go. I send an email message to family and friends at 9:00 a.m.: "The time of death is close. Death rattle, bleeding internally, pneumonia, gray fingernail beds, unresponsive. ... We're holding hands. I'm comforted by hospice, minister, many of her friends and my cousins. My husband is on his way. Probably sometime today??"

At 11:00 a.m., mom rallies to squeeze my hand. Breathing still hard and gurgling. My cousin and the hospice nurse are with me. More morphine administered. Pastor was here, and we prayed. We are all at peace and waiting with mom. Some apnea where breathing stops for a while with morphine.

By afternoon, word is out. Mother will not last long. Several of her closest friends stop by during the day or after work—including my son. Meanwhile, I constantly hold mother's hand. It is getting late. Mother's vitals show a fever of 102 degrees.

By 8:00 p.m., people leave to go home. I am tired too. At 9:00 p.m., I decide to take a short nap. and when I wake up again I go back to mother's bedside. I adjust the upholstered chair and pillows to get comfortable and convince myself I can sleep the rest of the night like this.

At 10:00 p.m., when a nurse comes to check on mom, I look over at mother and see she has a large glob of foam dripping from the right side of her mouth. I jump up to get a tissue to wipe it away when I see her eyes open. Her unresponsive arms and hands now reach up from her body. They are now stiff and very strong. Responding to her being awake, I repeat: "I love you momma, I love you momma, I love you momma." Moments later, her arms collapse and eyes close. I glance at the nurse in tears, "Is she gone?" The nurse is afraid to answer, but I see it in her eyes. I continue to talk to mother as I now tearfully climb on top of her to hug her in her deathbed, "Momma, you worked so hard, so hard, I love you, I love you, I love you." I know it is over—but her feverish shoulders still give me my mother's comfort. I can't let go.

It is 10:15 at night as I continue to caress her warm shoulders. I try to close her gapping mouth and it springs back open. I know there is a chance she still hears, "Momma, we are going to play your songs now." The iPad plays her memorial songs—Abide with Me; Joyful, Joyful We Adore Thee; Come Thou Almighty King; Oh Shenandoah-Across the Wide Missouri. "Let's pray the Lord's Prayer."

"She is still warm," and I don't want to stop holding her. Finally, I look up and see the nurse is ready to officially declare death, so I let go of mother's warm shoulder. The nurse uses a stethoscope to listen for a heartbeat, checks her eyes, [and asks] "Do you want us to bathe her?" I answer, "Yes, let's bathe her, and you can call the undertaker." As the staff come to wash her naked body, I stare at her from the foot of the bed. This is the woman I know—but she is not moving. She does not have the mottling signs expected. This is definitely my mother—but she is different. Her face is sunken without muscle tone around her skull.

I begin to make tearful phone calls to family and friends. They are expecting it. The calls are all short. I am trying to balance my emotions with being practical. I know it is now time I must send a factual email and write: "Mother passed away in my arms at 10:15 tonight. I will try to arrange a memorial service for next week Saturday. Thanks for your love and support. More later. Love, Ruth."

Mother's good friend calls back, "I'll come and help you move things out." I accept, "Okay." As we wait for the undertaker, I begin packing up a large collection of personal possessions. Framed pictures are taken off the walls, quilts are folded, and papers are shuffled together. While the white daisies are now wilting, I pluck the stem with the most life and lay it on my mother's left shoulder. On the right shoulder, I lay a copy of mother's birth certificate—so there would be no mistake in identity.

11:30 p.m. Within another hour, everything we own is packed up and removed from the room. All that remains is the body of my mother in her bed—the walls are again barren as when we entered just 1 week earlier. The undertaker arrives with a hospice nurse, and he explains, "You are verifying the identity of this body." I sign. He then suggests, "You may not want to stay for the rest of this." My reply: "I want to stay for it all."

He writes my mother's name on a yellow plastic strip and fastens it as an ankle bracelet. They scoot her body to this narrow blue painted board and then to the silver metal gurney on wheels. He covers her face with a white sheet. I interrupt the process to uncover her face and kiss her, "Goodbye momma, I love you." Covering up her face again, the

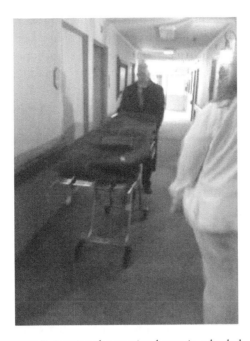

FIGURE 7 Leaving the nursing home in a body bag.

stiff, red-purple body bag is zipped up entirely. Now it's about 1:00 in the morning, and I direct, "You lead the way." The undertaker is first, then mother with her head first, then the hospice nurse. My husband and I slowly and quietly trail behind. We are floating down the empty nursing home hallway and out the back door. A cool misty rain falls as the stretcher smoothly glides into the back of a dark minivan. Before the van's hatch door is closed, I go up to the body bag and squeeze the foot of my now deceased mother, "Good bye momma" (Figure 7).

THE DAY AND DAYS AFTER

After a sleepless night, my husband takes the wheel to drive through the rain to St. Louis. There is no crematorium in my small town. The well-appointed funeral home, while comfortable and attractive, seems alien and brings back morbid, ghoulish memories of people in caskets. I'm so glad mother will be cremated and her visitation will be at her familiar church narthex where we have stood so many times before. Here, the song will play, "Oh Shenandoah, Across the Wide Missouri." I give the undertaker my mother's social security number, middle names of parents for death certificate information, and pay the bill. I don't have the energy to argue about buying a container for the remains I won't use.

The next week is a blur. Two days late, mother posthumously receives her 50-year award for being a 4-H leader. At this 4-H banquet, I give a speech to thank the community—and tell them how mother had her 4-H sampler "Head, Heart, Hands, and Health" near her bed along with a letter a 4-H member had written to thank her. The audience gives a long and emotional standing ovation. My presentation is practice for my eulogy at mother's memorial service.

During the day, I busy myself with arrangements—newspaper for final inspection of the obituary, organist, florist, Ladies Aid President to serve the luncheon, grave digger, and minister. I tell the Missouri Synod Lutheran minister about the Jewish tradition of mourners who see the remains of the body lowered below ground and are invited to shovel dirt in the grave at the gravesite service. Fortunately, he is familiar with the ritual, "We have Jewish roots."

My parents bought four graves in 1955. It is the only piece of land not in mother's Trust because the contract confirms our family ownership "forever." A large red granite tomb stone has been in place for 20 years marking my father's grave. Engraving gives the name and birth and death dates of my father and the name and birth date of my mother—awaiting the date that I will soon direct be chiseled, January 25, 2012.

Over 170 people sign the guest book for my 93-year-old mother. I make it a point to thank the crowd in my eulogy at the Memorial for helping her stay in her own home and live there independently until her last 2.5 weeks of life. I'm so glad I did not uproot her from her friends and community that meant so much to her. At the completion of the Memorial service, I carefully lift the tea-leaf lidded casserole dish of her remains from the encircled fresh flowers. Tucking it in my grandmother's straw sewing basket, I then ceremoniously walk down the church's center aisle escorted by the Pastor to our black car. Thirty cars, with their lights aglow, trail us in the slow drive two miles outside of town to the cemetery (Figure 8).

If you want to know where home is to someone, ask them where they will be buried. It was never questioned in our household; my parents' final home is at this church cemetery. My father's parents, grandparents, cousins, aunts, uncles, and friends are nearby.

Again, the air has a chilly mist. The cemetery ground is saturated. At the gravesite, the floral wreath of Kansas sunflowers is propped up near my father's grave and family tomb stone. The ceremony begins. Ashes to ashes ... "for dust thou art, and unto dust shalt thou return." Mother's remains are in the casserole dish with those of my deceased brother's and the "Happy bracelet" she wore since Christmas. Now encased in a hard plastic shell serving as a vault, they are lowered underground as scripture is read. In silence, the minister provides the first shovel of dirt. I take the shovel next. Out of respect, family and friends take their turn as her burial is in the hands of loved ones instead of strangers. In this last act of shoveling dirt to fill the grave, we have left nothing undone. My mother, at last, finds her permanent earthly place that is her final home.

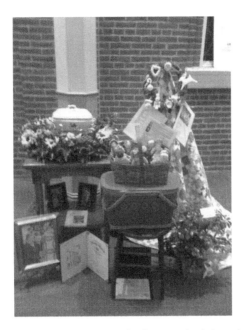

FIGURE 8 Visitation displayed the lidded, tea-leaf casserole dish with her cremated remains encircled with a wreath of Kansas sun-flowers, her hand-made prairie dolls and crafts, photos, sewing basket, and a quilt with her own dresses she had as a child.

EPILOGUE

This humanistic case study contributes to the field of environmental gerontology in two respects. First, it exposes the emotional transition from one's own home to the grave with the depth of intimate experiences and the nuances of reality rarely revealed. A strictly factual and abstract explanation of these transitions would have ignored the wide range of sensitive emotions I felt as a caregiver and my mother felt as patient: anguish, fear, grief, hope, pride, joy, sadness, love, and fright. As human beings, we are moved by emotions and stirred by the search for personal meaning as we approach death. Rather than detached involvement in these transitions, understanding the context and process of being with a loved one during the intense moments of dying and death can be a personally rewarding experience beyond imagination.

Second, the case study amplifies major motifs of aging and dying in place for future study: generational relationships, attitudes toward housing transitions for the elderly, the role of community involvement, attachment to possessions, design making a difference, medical intervention to extend life, the role of religious beliefs and spiritual dimensions to give strength, and the mystery of death. Thomas R. Cole so beautifully writes in *The Journey of Life*, "Mysteries require meaning. Born of moral commitment and spiritual reflection, the experience of meaning helps individuals to understand accept, and imaginatively transform the unmanageable, ambiguous aspects of existence"

(p. xxiii). Although I can no longer feel the comfort and warmth of my mother's shoulder, I can silently play the melody and lyrics of experiences to discover new associations. And, my mother's angel wings abide with me.

REFERENCE

Cole, T R. (1992). *The journey of life: A cultural history of aging in America.* New York, NY: Cambridge University Press.

PART IV: TRANSFORMING ENVIRONMENTS: CARE-BASED SETTINGS

Veterans Health Administration: A Model for Transforming Nursing Home Care

SONNE LEMKE

Center for Health Care Evaluation, VA Palo Alto Health Care System, Menlo Park, California, USA

The Veterans Health Administration nursing homes, now called Community Living Centers (CLCs), are engaged in systematic transformation of their environments and their care and work practices. A brief history of nursing home care for Veterans illustrates the competing values that influence CLCs. Monitoring data show that CLCs have reduced institutional features, improved the personalization of care, and empowered direct care staff. Although CLCs differ in many respects from community nursing homes, their experiences offer valuable lessons for culture change, underline the complementary importance of top-level commitment and grassroots engagement, and offer untapped opportunities for research in environmental gerontology.

This research was supported by the Department of Veterans Affairs, Veterans Health Administration, Office of Research and Development, Health Services Research and Development Service (HSR&D) (IIR 03-243 and PPO 09-279). The findings and conclusions are those of the author and do not necessarily represent the Department of Veterans Affairs or the United States government. The author thanks Dr. Christa Hojlo, Director of VA Community Living Centers, for her continuing and active support for research on culture change, Kathy Fung and Vidhya Balasubramanian for their valuable contributions to data file management and the data analyses reported here, and my colleagues, Penny Brennan and Jeanne Schaefer, for their comments on an earlier draft of this article.

INTRODUCTION

The Veterans Health Administration (VHA) oversees nursing home care in 133 facilities, making it one of the larger providers of long-term care in the United States. Since 2004, these facilities, now called Community Living Centers (CLCs), have been involved in a transformation effort intended to make them more humane environments for residents, staff, and families. This article describes the historical roots of VHA CLCs and the characteristics that distinguish them from community nursing homes (CNHs). It then outlines the culture change effort in CLCs, including practical strategies being used to implement it and the extent and types of culture change achieved. It concludes with consideration of future research directions and the opportunities provided by the ongoing transformation of CLCs.

HISTORICAL BACKGROUND

A historical examination of the development of long-term care for veterans highlights recurrent and critical issues that are likely to confront any reform effort. These issues include the models of care that have currency in society and the value systems they embody. The articulation and clarification of these values are important to the success of culture change.

In the colonial period and early days of the United States, support for needy citizens mirrored conditions in England. There was an intentional effort to discourage dependence on government-funded institutions, known as almshouses, by ensuring that living conditions and the stigma attached to residence would ensure that no one would willingly choose to live there. Within this framework, questions were inevitably raised about some categories of needy. Exceptional classes, such as orphans and virtuous widows, were gradually defined and made the focus of philanthropic efforts.

Care for Veterans

Men who had served in the armed forces were among those viewed as specifically entitled to humane government support. This social obligation initially took the form of pension payments to veterans of the Revolutionary War, French and Indian War, and the War of 1812. When the family was unable to provide needed services, the veteran could use this pension to board in someone else's home.

The Civil War had a massive effect on the number of military veterans and on their needs. More than 1.9 million Union Soldiers survived the war (U. S. Department of Veterans Affairs, n.d., p. 4), and these individuals represented all strata of society, not just professional soldiers as in most previous conflicts. New weaponry, improved medical treatment, and the conditions of battle and in prisoner-of-war camps meant that veterans of this war often survived with chronic diseases or horrific wounds, both physical and mental. Initially, Civil War veterans were expected to return to their home communities and resume their lives, with some financial support from the government in the case of those with combat-related injury or disease. (This and the following historical information regarding the National Home is derived from a report to the National Park Service by Julin [n.d.].)

Roots of CLCs

Such reintegration was not always successful, as indicated by the movement to establish the National Asylum for Disabled Volunteer Soldiers (later the National Home for Disabled Volunteer Soldiers), an outgrowth of charitable efforts begun during the war. The branches of the National Home, which eventually numbered 11, received government support and served veterans of U.S. military service with combat-related disabilities. (Confederate veterans were not eligible, although some separate philanthropic homes were developed in the South.) In the beginning, veterans moved in and out of these homes as the need arose. Vocational training was an important part of the program, and the National Home largely depended on resident labor.

As the century progressed, the characteristics of residents changed substantially. In 1884, criteria were relaxed to permit the admission of veterans who did not have any direct combat-related disability or illness but who had aging-related needs. Residents were no longer able to provide most of the labor, and many older residents entered the National Home and remained there for the rest of their lives. Medical services and care provision were in greater demand, and hospitals within the National Home grew increasingly overcrowded.

The population of the National Home peaked in 1906 with 21,000 residents, most of whom were aging Civil War veterans (Julin, n.d.). With the influx of young, severely injured veterans of World War I, the emphasis on provision of medical care, including extended nursing care, increased during the 1920s. By this time, several agencies had developed to serve veterans' needs, and both the Public Health Service and the Department of Treasury became involved in aspects of the National Home operation. These separate agencies became increasingly unwieldy, and in 1930 they were consolidated into a single federal agency, the Veterans Administration, which became the Department of Veterans Affairs in 1989 (both abbreviated as VA). Over the next 40 years, the major emphasis within the VA was on providing hospital care for both acute and chronic conditions.

By mid-century, the aging of the large World War I cohort meant that VA wards were increasingly serving an older population with chronic conditions that prevented discharge back to the community. The need for a less medically intensive and less expensive alternative became apparent, and in

1963 the VA nursing home care program was formally recognized, with the first units being established in modified hospital wards. Subsequently, stand-alone nursing homes were constructed, but the hospital ward continued to serve as a model, both in terms of architecture and in terms of staffing and care routines. In 1971, VA nursing homes had a census of about 4,600 residents; by 1995, the census had increased to 13,600 residents (National Center for Veterans Analysis and Statistics, n.d.), and by 2010 it had decreased to approximately 10,500 residents as new options for home- and community-based care became available and veterans' demographics changed.

CLC CHARACTERISTICS

In part because of their history and in part because of the population they are designed to serve, CLCs currently differ from their community counter-parts in many respects. Table 1 summarizes some of these differences; data for this table were drawn from analysis of VA administrative databases con-taining September 2004 census records for CLCs and from the 2004 National Nursing Home Survey (Jones, Dwyer, Bercovitz, & Strahan, 2009). The most obvious difference between CLCs and CNHs is that nearly all CLC residents are men (97% vs. 29%, respectively). Another major difference is that CLC residents are, on average, much younger than CNH residents; in 2004 the median age was 76 years for CLC residents versus about 83 years for CNH residents. The marital status of CLC residents differs from that of CNH resi-dents, reflecting the gender and age differences of their populations, as well as other influences (e.g., higher rates of substance use disorders and mental illness). Compared with CNH residents, CLC residents were much less likely to be widowed (17% vs. 53%, respectively) and more likely to be married (38% vs. 20%, respectively) or separated, divorced, or single (45% vs. 26%, respectively).

Beyond average age, the age distribution of CLC residents is different from that of CNH residents. Although CNHs will experience some shifts in their age distribution as the Baby Boomer generation ages, CLCs are subject to much greater fluctuations because the veteran population is concentrated in particular age cohorts coinciding with the military-age population dur-ing periods of major conflict. For example, analysis of VA administrative databases reflects that the large Vietnam Era cohort has begun using CLCs, increasing the proportion of residents under age 65 from 18% in 1998 to 26% in 2004 and 31% in 2010. Meanwhile, the massive World War II age cohort increased the proportion of residents who were 85 years and older from 9% in 1998 to 14% in 2006 and 23% in 2010. Together, these shifts have radically altered the age distribution of CLC residents but left the average age relatively unchanged (Lemke & Schaefer, 2010). The increase in size of the youngest and oldest age groups will begin to reverse itself over the next

TABLE 1 Resident Characteristics in Community Living Centers (CLCs) and Community Nursing Homes (CNHs)

Characteristics	CLCs[a]	CNHs[b]
Resident Demographics		
Men (%)	97	29
Marital status (%)		
Married	38	20
Widowed	17	54
Separated, divorced, single	45	26
Age (%)		
Under 65 years	26	12
65-74 years	21	12
75-84 years	39	31
85 years and older	14	45
Nursing Home Stay		
Median length of stay (days)	259	463
Selected primary diagnoses (%)		
Malignant neoplasm	5.4	1.8
Diabetes mellitus	2.1	3.9
Mental disorders	22.6	14.2
Alzheimer's disease	8.6	8.5
Other nervous system/sense organ disease	6.9	5.5
Heart disease	3.4	8.3
Acute cerebrovascular disease	.3	5.8
Other circulatory system disease	8.0	9.6
Respiratory system disease	3.5	6.7
Digestive system disease	1.1	3.1
Skin, subcutaneous tissue disease	2.7	1.4
Musculoskeletal/connective tissue disease	2.6	4.5
Symptoms and signs	2.5	5.6
Injury and poisoning	2.0	1.3
Post-hospital aftercare	21.0	8.8

[a]Based on $n = 12,466$ CLC residents in census records for September 30, 2004.
[b]Based on National Nursing Home Survey, completed for a cross-section of residents in 2004 (Jones et al., 2009).

decade as the Vietnam Era cohort moves into the 65- to 75-year age range and as World War II veterans die.

Given these differences in the demographics of their populations, as well as in the policies under which they operate, CLCs and CNHs differ in their use patterns and in resident medical and mental health status (Table 1). In 2004, the median length of stay for a cross-section of CLC residents was 259 days, and the mean was 681. Comparable data for the National Nursing Home Survey show a median stay of 463 days and a mean of 835 days.

For both CLCs and CNHs, the broad category of mental disorders (which excludes mental retardation and organic brain syndrome) was a common primary diagnosis, but this diagnostic category was much more frequent for CLC residents (23% vs. 14%). For CLCs, this category comprises primary diagnoses of schizophrenia (9%), delirium (9%), and smaller numbers with depression, substance use disorders, and manic disorders. CLCs thus play a more substantial role than do CNHs in care of the chronically mentally ill. In fact, some CLCs have developed specialized psychogeriatric units.

Hospital aftercare was frequently listed as the primary diagnostic code for both CLCs and CNHs, but it was more common in CLCs (21% vs. 9%, respectively). As part of an integrated care system, CLCs often function as a transition from hospital to community. The heavy use of CLCs for hospital aftercare helps to explain the shorter length of stay of their residents. CLCs also provided care to more residents with cancer (5.4% vs. 1.8%, respectively), likely reflecting the fact that many CLCs have developed formal hospice or palliative care units, another factor that probably contributes to shorter resident stays. As a primary diagnosis, Alzheimer's disease had similar frequency in both settings (9%). Primary diagnoses of heart disease, respiratory disease, acute cerebrovascular disease, and diabetes mellitus were more common in CNHs than in CLCs.

CLCs and CNHs also differ substantially in their staffing. CLCs have more nursing staff and more licensed personnel among their nursing staff. Data from a sample of 50 CLC units, selected for their high substance use disorder prevalence rates and evaluated in 2006 (Lemke & Schaefer, 2012), indicate that the overall ratio of full-time equivalent (FTE) nursing staff per resident was .99 and that nursing assistants constituted 37% of the nursing staff (Table 2). This contrasts with the situation in CNHs, where the nursing staff FTEs per resident ratio was .63 in 2004 and where nursing assistants and aides were 66% of the nursing staff. This pattern of high staffing, particularly by licensed personnel, also holds for non-nursing staff. In contrast with CNHs, each CLC has an assigned, VA-employed physician, and new VA guidelines require one FTE psychologist for every 100 CLC residents. In the sample of 50 CLC units, units provided almost one FTE of mental health staffing and one FTE of rehabilitation staffing for their average census of 34 residents. In general, these staff members are assigned to the CLCs rather than accessed on a consultative basis, facilitating their integration into care teams.

Another contrast between CLCs and CNHs is the relatively low turnover rate among CLC nursing staff. In the survey of 50 CLC units, 83% of the nursing staff had worked in the unit for more than a year. Even if some positions had been filled more than once during the year, we can assume that the turnover rate was most likely less than 25%. In contrast, a 2007 survey of U.S. nursing facilities found that the yearly turnover rate for nursing assistants was 66%, indicating two terminations for every three nursing assistant positions. The turnover was somewhat lower for registered nurses (RNs) and licensed vocational nurses (LVNs) (41% and 50%, respectively) (American Health Care Association, 2008).

TABLE 2 Staffing Characteristics in Community Living Centers (CLCs) and Community Nursing Homes (CNHs)

Characteristics	CLCs[a]	CNHs[b]
Staffing		
Nursing staff/patient ratio	.99	.63
Nursing staff type (%)		
RN	35	13
LVN	28	20
Nursing assistant	37	66

[a]Based on survey of 50 CLC units in 2006.
[b]Based on National Nursing Home Survey in 2004 (Jones et al., 2009).

Although systematic information is limited, the environments of VA nursing homes and CNHs have historically differed in emphasis. For example, assessments of elder care facilities performed in the late 1970s and early 1980s were used to compare proprietary community and veteran facilities of similar size that served residents with comparable functioning (Lemke & Moos, 1989; Moos & Lemke, 1994). The facilities serving veterans were housed in older buildings that provided a higher level of comfort (amenities and social-recreational features) and a similar level of security (accessibility, supportive architectural features, safety features). The veterans facilities scored lower on autonomy (less privacy and less flexibility for residents to structure their own daily lives), although this difference was not reflected in residents' and staff members' assessments of resident control, which was relatively low in both community and veterans facilities. Finally, both residents and staff reported a lower level of rapport or warmth of interpersonal relationships in veterans than in community facilities.

MODELS AND VALUES FOR LONG TERM CARE

One issue addressed in the development and management of the National Home for Disabled Volunteer Soldiers was determining which veterans merited access to these resources and how these individuals should be viewed by society. Several decisions, including the name change from asylum to home and the emphasis on architectural quality and attractive grounds, reveal a concern for the protecting residents' dignity. In 1890, the National Home Board explicitly stated that "the Home is neither an hospital nor alms-house, but a home, where subsistence, quarters, clothing, religious instruction, employment when possible, and amusements are provided by the Government of the United States. The provision is not a charity, but is a reward to the brave and deserving" (Julin, n.d., p. 26).

Another issue relates to the appropriate model on which the National Home should be run. Founders and early directors vigorously debated these issues, and different branches embodied different conceptions. In general, as implied by the original name, they were viewed as a temporary refuge and had the goal of returning residents to society as well-functioning and productive citizens (Julin, n.d.). Some branches of the National Home were structured along military lines, with residents living in barracks, authority exercised in a hierarchical structure, and a fixed schedule and limited resident autonomy. The rationale for this model was that this lifestyle was familiar to veterans and that those who failed to function well in the outside community did so because they lacked self-discipline and were in need of external constraints. The health spa or rest home served as another model. There, the emphasis was on protecting the resident from the stresses of city life by providing an idyllic physical environment isolated from its surroundings, with a self-contained, "healthful" community life provided within the Home.

Whatever the model, the National Home was generally viewed as operating *in loco parentis*. For example, consumption of alcohol was initially barred, reflecting awareness that many of the residents had problems resulting from alcohol use and that these problems often explained their failure to manage in the wider community. Drinking establishments inevitably grew up around these homes and created ongoing problems for their administration (Julin, n.d.), leading to relaxation of alcohol use policies from the late 1870s until 1906.

Paralleling the development of facilities for veterans, the wider society wrestled with how to care for its needy older citizens. Skepticism about the capacity of institutions to provide adequate care, expressed when the National Home was first developed, have regularly reappeared, such as in the Social Security Act of 1935, which barred funds being paid to individuals residing in public institutions. Describing the history of care, Levine (1979) noted that "Advocates of 'indoor relief' (care in institutions) and 'outdoor relief' (cash payments to maintain people in their own homes or communities) vied with each other over the centuries. The popularity of policies seesawed back and forth as each approach produced its own welfare scandals, or as politicians pointed with alarm to rising welfare costs" (p. 3).

As medicine became increasingly effective, specialized, and professionalized during the latter half of the 20th century, a new model for nursing home care entered the mix. This model drew from the production line and scientific management and envisioned improved efficiency and quality of care in centralized, large-scale institutions. Ideally, these settings could classify and sort residents into homogeneous populations with uniform needs, cared for in a hygienic, hazard-free environment. Bathing, meals, sleeping, and provision of medications were organized for narrowly defined efficiency and staff convenience, and the relationships between residents and staff and among staff were increasingly depersonalized.

Throughout the 20th century, attention was repeatedly drawn to the inhumane conditions of care for older, chronically ill, and needy individuals. These included old, poorly maintained buildings, fire hazards, lack of privacy, limited and unpalatable food, lack of sufficient medically trained staff, corruption, and inefficiency. More recently, criticisms have focused on the sterility, loss of autonomy, and dehumanization of the newer model nursing homes. Over the years, books and reports on conditions in nursing homes appeared regularly, with titles such as "Buried Alive," "Hell's Vestibule," "A Home is not a Home," and "Unloving Care."

The social response to such exposés has often been to shift the venue of care or to specify new standards of care. However, as critics have remarked, these standards generally take the providers' perspective (Levine, 1979) and have ignored critical issues related to residents' quality of life (Kane, 2001).

> Not facing up to our ambivalence and not accepting the realities of the problem of chronically dependent groups, we have not really tried to describe in detail what we mean by good care for them, nor have we thought seriously about more than the financial issues. ... Of course legislative draftsmen and behaviorally oriented social scientists have in common the difficulty of dealing with "fuzzy" concepts such as decency and dignity. It is much easier to specify square feet of space per person, ratios of patients to employees, or the way tranquilizers should be locked up, than it is to specify a psychological atmosphere. (Levine, 1979, p. 15)

CLCs (and nursing homes in general) represent tensions between the impulse toward the humane care of older individuals and concerns about the cost of such care and society's responsibility for its provision, between the desire to make these settings safe and secure and to provide a true home for the older person, between neglect and paternalism, between the efficiency of large institutions and the personalization of small ones, and between an idealized home (or Eden) and the realities of illness, debility, and loss.

THE CULTURE TRANSFORMATION MOVEMENT

In recent years, the balance between these various forces has shifted, as exemplified by efforts occurring within CLCs and by the reform movements and support networks from which they draw. Several threads have united to strengthen reform efforts, including the disability rights movement, consumer-centered care, and separation of housing and services in the form of assisted living (Kane, 2001). Groups supporting nursing home reform include the Pioneer Network, an organization formed in 1997 to promote person-directed long-term care, and the initiatives promoted by Advancing Excellence in America's Nursing Homes, a coalition of organizations representing nursing home providers and practitioners, quality improvement experts, consumers, government agencies, and foundations and focusing on improving the quality of care and of life in nursing homes. Various models of culture change have been developed in recent decades (e.g., Eden Alternative, Green House project, PlaneTree Continuing Care Model, and the Wellspring model) (Rahman & Schnelle, 2008).

Key elements of humane, person-centered care include knowledge of and responsiveness to individual characteristics, values, and preferences; a holistic view of the individual; choice and reasonable risk taking based on the individual's needs and preferences; and involvement of the family and broader social network. Kane (2001) detailed 11 quality of life domains: sense of safety, security, and order; physical comfort; enjoyment; meaningful activity; relationships; functional competence; dignity; privacy; individuality; autonomy and choice; and spiritual well-being. However, despite increasing awareness of the culture change movement among nursing home staff, a 2007 survey of community nursing homes found that the adoption of culture change principles is limited (Doty, Koren, & Sturla, 2008).

Transformative Efforts in VA

In 2005, the VHA Office of Geriatrics and Extended Care hosted a national summit of VA nursing home staff, with the goal of initiating nursing home culture change designed to provide cost effective, competitive and compassionate care to veterans.

VHA Handbook 1142.01, a field-driven guide to implementing cultural transformation, was issued in August 2008 (Veterans Health Administration, 2008). This handbook authorized the official renaming of VA nursing homes as CLCs and established expectations in the areas of person-centered care (personal preferences in provision of care), the environment of care (home-like environment, de-institutionalized facility space, privacy), nutrition and food services (scheduling, availability of food), activities of daily living (scheduling, encouragement of active participation and independence), life enhancement (customs and rituals, culture, spirituality, community, meaningful activities, and family involvement), and end-of-life issues (Veterans Health Administration, 2008).

The centralized organization of VHA has facilitated culture change in several ways. National Geriatrics and Extended Care leaders have articulated a consistent, committed vision of culture change that reinforces the broader VHA efforts to encourage resident-centered care. Geriatrics and Extended Care leaders have used a variety of tools to provide training and guidance to CLC staff undertaking culture change. These include presentations by outside experts and CLC staff in national conference calls, resource materials and guidelines on a VA intranet web site (vaww.infoshare.va.gov/sites/geriatrics/CLC/default.aspx) accessible to all

CLC staff, and readily available links to other resource sites. Each CLC has designated culture change leaders to plan and guide their efforts. National leaders recognize innovative efforts and celebrate the accomplishments of CLC staff in a variety of ways, and local recognition also is strongly encouraged. Illustrating these various efforts, the National Nursing Assistants Culture Change Collaborative pairs nursing assistants who want to take an active role in culture change with a peer leader and RN coach and provides opportunities for training, leadership, and professional advancement. The Nursing Assistants Olympics provides 8 to 12 weeks of training, culminating in competition among teams for gold, silver, and bronze medals in a variety of resident-centered events. Another example is the Under Secretary for Health Award for Innovation in the VA CLC, given in 2011 to the Lake City, Florida, CLC, which was selected from among 19 CLC submissions.

Where needed, new policy guidelines and memoranda have been developed and broadcast to the field, where they can be used in working with mid-level managers who may be resistant to change or anxious about regulatory compliance. For example, fire codes under which VA medical centers operate have recently been revised to explicitly accommodate kitchens for resident use in CLCs, and VHA policies allow CLCs to develop alcohol-use policies as distinct from the general prohibition of alcohol on VA grounds. Where local regulations may be impeding change, culture change leaders can solicit policy memoranda and documents from other CLCs to serve as examples. CLC culture change participants can post blogs on the website in which they discuss their experience with new initiatives.

Despite this strong central support, discussions of culture change within VHA, such as those occurring at CLC Cultural Transformation Summit Meetings or in monthly national calls, highlight the tension that exists between this model of nursing care and the infrastructure in place in VA Medical Centers. Among numerous issues, concerns center on infection control, fire safety, patient safety and security, efficiencies of scale, ethics regulations, suitability of the model to varying patient populations, and staff workload and burnout. For example, ethics regulations prohibit staff members from consuming VA-purchased food, creating a challenge for birthday celebrations or other special events that bring residents and staff together in an informal social atmosphere. Another recent example is offered by bird feeders, which offer CLC residents a pleasurable activity but may raise a concern about attracting unwanted animals (e.g., pigeons, rats) and possible disease transmission.

Documentation of Change

Beginning in 2008, CLC staff used a measure termed Artifacts of Culture Change (ACC) to report the facility's performance in key areas of transformation. This instrument was initially developed for the Centers for Medicare and Medicaid Services to measure the quality of care in long-term care settings (Bowman, 2006) and adapted for use in CLCs. This checklist covers care practices (dining schedule and snack availability, daily schedules), environment (privacy, adaptive features, décor, outdoor areas), family and community (intergenerational program, availability of space for families and community functions), leadership (involvement of nursing assistants, residents and family members), workplace (stable staff assignments, nursing assistants responsible for scheduling, job development), and outcomes (staff turnover, occupancy).

Between 2008 and 2010, facilities reported six aggregate scores to the VHA Office of Geriatrics and Extended Care on a semi-annual basis and were expected to show a 5% improvement from one measurement to the next. Indeed, as shown in Table 3, the total culture change score improved from 51% to 64% over a 1.5-year period, with all scales except Outcomes showing substantial increases. Reflecting the historically low turnover of VA nursing staff, the Outcomes scale was initially at a ceiling for many facilities (average score of 80%). In addition, because this scale measures turnover and bed occupancy, it is subject to other influences not under the control of the culture change planning group, such as the local unemployment rate and the Medical Center occupancy rate. Excluding the Outcomes scale gives a more accurate picture of the environmental and practice changes put into effect by the CLC.

The measure used to monitor culture change in CLCs was updated in January 2011 to include an expanded set of items and more detailed definitions and clearer specification of the conditions required for each item score, as well as data entry and report availability through the Pioneer Network Web

TABLE 3 Average Percentage Scores on Culture Change Monitors in Community Living Centers

	ACC[a]			ACCT[b]		
Culture Change Domain	No. of Items (points)	July '08 Mean (SD)	Jan. '10 Mean (SD)	No. of items (points)	Jan. '11 Mean (SD)	Oct. '11 Mean (SD)
Care practices	9 (45)	57 (18)	77 (14)	14 (70)	54	65
Environment of care	23 (180)	44 (11)	55 (12)	27 (320)	37	42
Family/community	6 (30)	46 (24)	61 (23)	6 (30)	52	59
Leadership practices	5 (25)	52 (23)	72 (24)	5 (25)	49	59
Workplace practices	11 (55)	61 (21)	75 (15)	14 (70)	56	61
Outcomes	4 (20)	80 (16)	86 (14)	13 (65)	81	84
Total score	58 (355)	51 (11)	64 (10)	79 (580)	48	53

[a]Scale scores but not item frequencies were available for the Artifacts of Culture Change (ACC) survey completed by $n = 126$ CLCs in July 2008 and by $n = 134$ CLCs in January 2010. Standard deviations are shown in parentheses.
[b]Overall item scores were available for the Artifacts of Culture Change Tool (ACCT) completed by CLCs in January and October 2011 and were used to calculate item percentage scores and scale scores. Because individual CLC scores were not available, standard deviations could not be calculated.

site. As shown in Table 3, the percentage scores on the January 2011 Artifacts of Culture Change Tool (ACCT) decreased from the scores obtained a year earlier, even for scales with no new items, such as Family/Community Practices and Leadership Practices. It seems unlikely that CLCs actually regressed in their culture change achievements. Rather, the lower scores are likely due to the more explicit scoring standards and, for some scales, to the addition of new items. As with the previously used measure, scores on ACCT scales have generally increased over the 9-month period represented in Table 3. With a target of a 10% yearly improvement, most scales have shown a 5% to 11% improvement over 9 months. However, even with many new items the Outcomes score has remained relatively flat.

Areas of Change

Many of the items showing the most progress in the first 9 months of 2011 reflect systematic efforts by national CLC leadership. For example, the largest percentage change (a 26% increase) has been in CLC adoption of "Bathing without a Battle" (Sloane et al., 2004), a new ACCT item. This approach to bathing has been discussed in national calls, and an instructional video was formally introduced nationwide in October 2011. Direct care staff was asked to enter information on aggressive incidents around bathing, to watch the Bathing without a Battle video, and to practice the demonstrated skills under supervision. Follow-up data are being collected at the national level to measure the effect of this new approach on the incidence of aggression. CLC staff members have blogged about their experiences with this bathing approach and the generally positive outcomes they have observed. Several other new and related ACCT items also showed a marked increase, such as use of warm towels after bathing and availability of massage (each with a 17% improvement).

Another major effort has focused on consistent assignment of nursing assistants as part of the initiative, Advancing Excellence in America's Nursing Homes. This goal was introduced in a February 2011 national call, and CLCs began to use the consistent assignment calculator developed by the Advancing Excellence initiative to monitor their progress. A later national call presented information on the existing empirical support for consistent assignment, as well as the first-person experiences of staff members working on a unit that had adopted this staffing model. Again, the web site has carried some additional staff accounts. On the ACCT, the item tapping consistent assignment of nursing assistants has increased by 8% in the first 9 months of 2011. The current score indicates that the average CLC provides consistent nursing assistant assignment for some but not most residents.

Some items that CLCs have been working on since the beginning of culture change also have increased substantially in 2011, again with strong support from VHA leadership. Learning circles or similar structures designed to give participants an opportunity to share ideas or opinions have been modeled in national CLC meetings and have increased in use from 54% to 71% of CLCs. Nursing assistant involvement in care conferences has increased relatively quickly (a 12% improvement). Approximately 78% of CLCs now offer community meetings at least once a month that include residents, staff, and families, increasing from 68% a year earlier.

Progress has been substantial with regard to food availability and the eating experience. More CLCs now bake or cook food in the resident area, and larger numbers now offer options at mealtimes, such as flexible hours or restaurant, buffet, or family-style service. In addition, 74% have a special dining room for family use or special gatherings, half offer a café or restaurant area on the unit and 46% now provide a common kitchen area in the unit. Each of these items showed an increase of 8% or more in the average score in 2011.

Significant progress is discernible in terms of workplace practices. Staff self-scheduling has increased, as has the inclusion in employee evaluations of support for resident choice and control (71% of possible points), the use of staff awards to recognize commitment to culture change (70% of CLCs), and career ladder positions for nursing assistants (52% of CLCs). Each of these workplace practice items showed a 7% to 10% improvement in 2011. A new item assesses whether uniforms are required; the percentage of CLCs with no requirement for uniforms has increased from 29% to 38%. Another indicator of the move away from a hospital model is the decreased use of overhead paging systems; 58% of CLCs have turned off the overhead paging system, up from 50% a year earlier.

Adoption of Culture Change Practices in CLCs

Aside from looking at recent changes in adoption of specific culture change practices, it is instructive to look at the breadth of adoption across CLCs of different practices and to compare CLCs with CNHs in this respect. Complexity theory offers one possible explanation of the speed and extent of adoption of particular culture change practices. For example, researchers rated the complexity of 16 practices based on the extent of agreement needed to put them into place and the certainty of achieving the intended outcome. Among the low complexity practices were residents' choice about when to go to bed, availability of food, and opportunities for nursing assistants to be involved in care planning. In terms of the physical environment, eliminating nurses' stations and shifting from tray to dining service were rated as low complexity. Involving residents in decisions about who will provide care, inclusion of direct care workers and residents in the management team, and developing self-managed work teams were rated as highly complex practices. The less complex practices tended to be more economical and easier to implement; not surprisingly, these were the first and most frequently adopted practices among nursing homes at various stages in the culture change process (Sterns, Miller, & Allen, 2010).

To some extent, the situation in CLCs mirrors these patterns but also shows other influences. The most recent assessment, completed by CLCs in October 2011, shows that some individual measures have been widely adopted (average scores of 80% or more of the possible points). In the area of care practices, these include "I" care plans, written in the first person and in the resident's voice; resident choice about waking time and the frequency of bathing; snacks and drinks available to residents at all times; individual birthday celebrations; and formal memorial or remembrance services for residents who die.

In terms of the physical environment, CLCs generally provide a high level of adaptive features. Given accessibility regulations, this was likely the case even prior to the culture change initiative. However, in addition to adaptive features, CLCs have been successful in offering some physical features that provide residents greater flexibility and personalization. For example, residents are generally welcome to decorate their rooms, and additional lighting is available on request. Laundry facilities are available to individual residents or their families. Most CLCs now provide a protected outdoor garden, raised gardening beds, and a path for walking or wheelchair use.

Certain workplace practices that strengthen the role of direct care staff also have become common practice in CLCs. These include paid conference attendance for non-managerial staff, formal job development programs (e.g., nursing assistants to become LVNs), and activities planned and performed by staff other than those formally designated, such as nursing staff or housekeeping staff planning an event.

Comparison of Culture Change in CLCs and CNHs

In general, CLCs surpassed non-VA nursing homes that have entered ACCT scores on the Pioneer Network Web site, as illustrated in Table 4. This table compares the scores reported by CLCs in October 2011 with those obtained by non-VA nursing homes recording ACCT scores on the Pioneer Network Web site. The latter scores were calculated by subtracting out the scores reported by the 133 CLCs in January 2011 from all the scores summarized by Pioneer Network for the period ending in March 2011 (http://www.artifactsofculturechange.org/Data/Documents/Tools%20for%20 Change-Artifacts%20v3.pdf). Among the 319 nursing homes covered in this report, 32% (approximately 102) were proprietary, 23% (approximately 73) were nonprofit, and 45% (approximately 144) were government-run, including the 133 CLCs. Thus, the non-VA sample consists of 186 facilities

TABLE 4 Comparison of Community Living Centers (CLCs) and Community Nursing Homes (CNHs) for Scales and for Selected Items on the Artifacts of Culture Change Tool Items (ACCT)

Scale/Item	Possible Points	CLCs (n = 133)	CNHs (n = 186)	Item Difference
Care Practices	70	41	31	
"I" care plans	5	4.1	1.4	2.7
Memorial for resident	5	4.5	2.3	2.2
Baking on unit	5	2.2	.6	1.6
Bathing without a battle	5	3.3	2.7	.6
Residents allowed to bring dog or cat with them	5	.7	1.1	−.4
Expanded dining	5	2.5	2.7	−.2
Environment of Care	320	133	91	
Privacy enhanced rooms	25	9.7	3.8	5.9
No traditional nurses stations	25	8.2	4.0	4.2
Laundry facilities for residents/families	5	4.3	.6	3.7
Computer/internet adaptations	10	6.7	3.1	3.6
Overhead paging turned off	5	2.9	2.2	.7
Residents welcome to decorate rooms	5	4.2	4.3	−.1
Residents can page staff; staff communicate with pager/radio/telephone system	5	.9	1.2	−.3
Refrigerators in residents' rooms	5	2.5	3.3	−.8
Bathing rooms with radiant heat	5	1.5	2.5	−1.0
Family/Community	30	18	14	
Private guestroom	5	2.9	1.0	1.9
Common kitchen area	5	2.3	1.7	.6
Community groups meet in home	5	3.6	3.2	.4
Leadership	25	15	6	
Community meetings	5	3.9	1.0	2.9
Nursing assistants participate in care conferences	5	3.5	1.5	2.0
Learning Circle or similar structures	5	3.6	1.9	1.7
Residents/families on quality committees	5	1.5	.5	1.0
Workplace Practices	70	43	27	
Job development programs	5	4.8	2.4	2.4
Awards to staff for culture change work	5	3.5	1.2	2.3
Activities led by staff in other departments	5	4.4	2.6	1.8
No required staff uniforms	5	1.9	.8	1.1
Nursing assistants consistently work with residents of the same unit/neighborhood	5	3.3	3.6	−.3
% of non-nursing staff with nursing assistant certification	5	.4	1.0	−.6
Outcomes	65	55	44	
Job longevity of RNs	5	4.4	2.5	1.9
Job longevity of nursing assistants	5	4.1	2.7	1.4
Occupancy rate	5	3.8	2.8	1.0
Use of agency nursing assistants	5	4.5	4.6	−.1

in 47 states and Canada (55% proprietary facilities, 39% nonprofit facilities, and 6% non-VA government-run).

Table 4 indicates that CLCs scored higher on all dimensions measured by the ACCT, particularly on measures of leadership and workplace practices. Selected items also are included in Table 4 to illustrate these differences.

Some of the well-established practices noted earlier for CLCs are less well established in CNHs involved in culture change. These include the use of first-person care plans written in the resident's words, memorial services following the death of residents, job development programs to support career advancement of all nursing staff, and the use of staff in various departments to plan and carry out activities.

A few items, such as radiant heat in the bathing areas and refrigerators in residents' rooms, have been more broadly adopted in this sample of CNHs than in CLCs. Perhaps more significantly, CNHs report greater use of consistent nursing assistant assignment than do CLCs, despite the focused effort underway in CLCs. However, it is possible that this is not so much a difference in practices as it is in how consistent assignment is measured. CLCs are asked to answer this item in terms of the criteria established by the Advancing Excellence initiative. These criteria require that 85% or more of residents receive care from a maximum of 8 nursing assistants in a given month. No such directions are given to CNHs completing the ACCT. In fact, a recent study found that in a representative sample of nursing homes, 68% reported that they used consistent assignment of nursing assistants, but only 28% met the criteria used in the Advancing Excellence campaign (Castle, 2011).

Case Examples

For its Innovation Award entry, the Lake City CLC highlighted the continuing and progressive nature of changes in all aspects of the program (Lake City Community Living Center, 2011). Their efforts included forming neighborhoods and changing terminology to give the neighborhood a unique identity and to include staff, family members, and visitors as care partners. The neighborhoods have a fully functioning kitchen, family room, computer laboratory, and new décor. Residents' rooms are personalized, and the shower rooms were remodeled to make them feel spa-like. Buffet-style dining is available to residents, as well as the opportunity to prepare food in the neighborhood kitchen. A trained dog was donated to the unit and is a source of meaningful activity and positive interactions for residents. Other activities focus on exercise, nutrition, healthy living, intergenerational sharing, and gardening. The key to success for this program has been an active interdisciplinary team effort and inclusion of residents in substantive decision making, both in regards to their individual routines and to CLC functioning. Residents participate in weekly Neighborhood Meetings and monthly Resident's Council meetings. (For other examples of CLC efforts, see "Putting the Home into Home," 2009; Scott, 2011; Whipple et al., 2009).

Another innovative effort focuses on the construction of new CLCs along the model of small homes. The VA Illiana (Danville, Illinois) Healthcare System is the first VA medical center to pilot a Green House home, with two homes of 10 residents each opened in October 2011. Each resident has a private living space and bathroom within the home, situated around an open kitchen and dining room. Residents are free to adopt their own daily schedule (Gala to celebrate, 2011; Wicoff, 2011). The VHA is currently working to develop position descriptions for the "universal worker" used in these settings, as well as in more traditional CLCs.

CONCLUSIONS

CLCs differ from CNHs in many important respects, but their commonalities point to the possibility of deriving important lessons for nursing home culture transformation from the CLC experience. As demonstrated here, CLCs have successfully embarked on changing both their physical and social environments. Some of these changes are relatively superficial, such as new furnishings, but others go deeper by explicitly acknowledging the personhood of those receiving and those giving care and the critical role of relationships in quality of life.

CLCs have been systematically monitoring culture change in terms of structure and process measures, which are in turn assumed to be linked to desired outcomes. For example, in the development of the ACCT, empirical support for inclusion of items generally cited purported effects of these structures and processes on desired outcomes. In addition, individual CLCs have measured outcomes as part of some of their change efforts. The monitoring of aggressive incidents associated with bathing is an example of a national effort to monitor the effect of an innovative care process (i.e., "Bathing without a Battle").

Nevertheless, research to evaluate culture change initiatives has been relatively limited, and the empirical support for them remains weak. A 2005 review of research on innovations in long-term care drew the conclusion that many innovations are supported solely by anecdotal evidence or simple pre- and post-comparisons, and that those studies using a control group did not control for non-random selection of facilities or residents (Port, Sloane, & Zimmerman, 2005). Rahman and Schnelle (2008) attributed the absence of empirical research to several factors: reliance on face validity rather than empirical outcomes to support change, indifference or aversion to measuring quality of life among some culture change leaders, and the scope and extended process of change. Given the difficulties of introducing substantial changes into complex organizations within a limited timeframe, it is not surprising that most nursing home intervention studies are undertaken in a small number of nursing homes. As a consequence, limited sample size often results in insufficient statistical power or improperly inflated sample size based on treating individuals within a nursing home as independent observations.

The 2005 Pragmatic Innovations in Long-Term Care Conference set the following as high priority areas for future research: (1) to define, describe, and evaluate culture change, (2) to study how organizational and management structures affect change and innovative practices, and (3) to explore the differential needs, treatment, and outcomes of residents (Sloane & Zimmerman, 2005; see also Feldman & Kane, 2003; Rahman & Schnelle, 2008). As well as being a laboratory for implementing culture change, CLCs offer an opportunity to address these issues. Such research benefits from the availability of linkable VA administrative database, the sustained national support for culture change, and the large numbers of units involved, representing varied resident populations, staffing characteristics, and environmental features.

One research goal would be to describe and catalog the changes that have been achieved in CLCs. For instance, what are the specific solutions CLCs have adopted for transforming meal experiences and providing food preparation opportunities? How has direct care staff been given an increased voice? What procedures are used to manage staff assignments within a consistent assignment approach? How can good staff communication and adequate work areas be ensured when institutional features are removed? Documentation of practical alternatives could provide a rich resource for nursing homes undertaking particular types of change.

Another important research goal is to identify unit characteristics that facilitate or impede change efforts. This could be done for overall culture change scores or for adoption of particular interventions, such as "Bathing without a Battle" or consistent staff assignment. For example, existing research has highlighted the critical role of organizational leaders and less hierarchical organizational structure for effective innovation (Scott-Cawiezell, 2005). In the case of culture change, resistance may be greater when unit resources are limited, such as when staffing levels are low or staff turnover is high (e.g., Castle & Banaszak-Holl, 1997). Characteristics of a resident population may place demands on staff that make it more or less difficult to implement culture change. Better understanding of the factors related to successful culture change can be used to refine and strengthen existing implementation strategies. Results of this research also could serve as the basis for more systematic, randomized interventions or implementation evaluations.

The change achieved by CLCs offers an opportunity to address another critical research area, evaluating the effect of culture change and of particular interventions. Retrospective analysis of the CLC experience is necessarily limited to outcomes captured in existing databases, but these include the resident characteristics tapped by the Minimum Data Set, diagnoses and care history captured in resident treatment records across the spectrum of care offered by VA, staff employment characteristics, and annual assessments of workplace characteristics. For example, these data could be used to explore whether adoption of consistent staff assignment is associated with any change in nursing assistant turnover, improved resident social engagement, better maintenance of resident functional capacities over time, or decreased resident problem behaviors. Similar comparisons could be undertaken for other major culture change initiatives. Findings would strengthen the evidence base for innovative practices that have substantial intuitive appeal. If unintended negative consequences are identified, they can be addressed, and doing so will improve the implementation process and the effectiveness of culture change.

Large numbers of older people will spend at least some time in a nursing home, a dreaded prospect for most older people and their families. As indicated by high turnover, staff members working in these settings also appear to find the work conditions far from ideal. VHA has taken bold steps to transform their nursing home units, offering potent models for change and a wealth of research opportunities.

REFERENCES

American Health Care Association. (2008). *Report of findings, 2007 AHCA survey: Nursing staff vacancy and turnover in nursing facilities.* Retrieved from http://www.ahcancal.org/research_data/staffing/documents/vacancy_turnover_survey2007.pdf

Bowman, C. S. (2006). *Development of the artifacts of culture change tool.* Report of Contract HHSM-500-2005-00076P, submitted to Centers for Medicare & Medicaid Services, April 21, 2006, Edu-Catering, LLP. Retrieved from http://www.culturechangenow.com/pdf/artifacts.pdf

Castle, N. (2011). The influence of consistent assignment on nursing home deficiency citations. *Gerontologist, 51,* 750–760. doi:10.1093/geront/gnr144

Castle, N. G., & Banaszak-Holl, J. (1997). Top management team characteristics and innovation in nursing homes. *Gerontologist, 37,* 572–580. doi:10.1093/geront/37.5.572

Doty, M. M., Koren, M. J., & Sturla, E. L. (2008). *Culture change in nursing homes: How far have we come? Findings from the Commonwealth Fund 2007 National Survey of Nursing Homes.* The Commonwealth Fund, 91. Retrieved from http://www.commonwealthfund.org/Publications

Feldman, P. H., & Kane, R. L. (2003). Strengthening research to improve the practice and management of long-term care. *Milbank Quarterly, 81,* 179–220. doi:10.1111/1468-0009.t01-1-00051

Gala to celebrate VA Illiana Green House Homes. (2011). Retrieved from http://thegreenhouseproject.org/gala-to-celebrate-va-illiana-green-house-homes/

Jones, A. L., Dwyer, L. L., Bercovitz, A. R., & Strahan, G. W. (2009). The National Nursing Home Survey: 2004 Overview. National Center for Health Statistics. *Vital Health Stat, 13*(167). Retrieved from http://www.cdc.gov/nchs/data/series/sr_13/sr13_167.pdf

Julin, S. (n.d.). *National home for disabled volunteer soldiers: Assessment of significance and national historic landmark recommendations.* Retrieved from http://www.nps.gov/history/nhl/Downloads/NHDVS/NHDVS%20Draft%20Two.pdf

Kane, R. A. (2001). Long-term care and a good quality of life: Bringing them closer together. *Gerontologist, 41*, 293–304. doi:10.1093/geront/41.3.293

Lake City Community Living Center wins VA Award for Innovation. (2011). Retrieved from http://northflorida.va.gov/NORTHFLORIDA/features/CLCInnovation Award.asp

Lemke, S., & Moos, R.H. (1989). Ownership and quality of care in residential facilities for the elderly. *Gerontologist, 29*, 209–215. doi:10.1093/geront/29.2.209

Lemke, S., & Schaefer, J. A. (2010). Recent changes in the prevalence of psychiatric disorders among VA nursing home residents. *Psychiatric Services, 61*, 356–363. doi:10.1176/appi.ps.61.4.356

Lemke, S., & Schaefer, J. A. (2012). Addressing substance use disorders in VA nursing homes. *Journal of Social Work Practice in the Addictions, 12*, 89–106. doi: 10.1080/1533256X.2012.646630

Levine, M. (1979). Congress (and evaluators) ought to pay more attention to history. *American Journal of Community Psychology, 7*, 1–17. doi:10.1007/BF00893159

Moos, R. H., & Lemke, S. (1994). *Group residences for older adults: Physical features, policies, and social climate.* New York, NY: Oxford University Press.

National Center for Veteran Analysis and Statistics. (n.d.). *Trend data—1971–1995.* Retrieved from http://www.va.gov/VETDATA/docs/SurveyAndStudies/TREND 1971-1995.pdf

Port, C., Sloane, P. D., & Zimmerman, S. (2005, April 4–5). *Pragmatic innovations in long-term care: Developing a research agenda. Literature review.* Paper prepared for conference Pragmatic Innovations in Long-Term Care. Baltimore, MD. Retrieved from http://www.pragmaticinnovations.unc.edu/Pragmatic%20Innovations%20Literature%20Review.pdf

Putting the home into nursing homes. (2009). *Newletter on Aging, 7*(1), 3–4. Retrieved from http://centeronaging.ucsf.edu/files/UCSF.NOA.Spr09.pdf

Rahman, A. N., & Schnelle, J. F. (2008). The nursing home culture-change movement: Recent past, present, and future directions for research. *Gerontologist, 48*, 142–148. doi:10.1093/geront/48.2.142

Scott, A. (2011). Miami VA long-term care creates bright, homelike environment for residents and staff. *Advances for Nurses.* Retrieved from http://nursing.advanceweb.com/Article/Culture-Change-2.aspx

Scott-Cawiezell, J. (2005). Are nursing homes ready to create sustainable improvement? *Journal of Nursing Care Quality, 20*, 203–207.

Sloane, P. D., Hoeffer, B., Mitchell, C. M., McKenzie, D. A., Barrick, A. L., Rader, J., . . . & Koch, G. G. (2004). Effect of person-centered showering and the towel bath on bathing-associated aggression, agitation, and discomfort in nursing home residents with dementia: A randomized, controlled trial. *Journal of the American Geriatrics Society, 52*, 1795–1804. doi:10.1111/j.1532-5415.2004.52501x

Sloane, P. D., & Zimmerman, S. (2005, April 4–5). *Improvement and innovation in long-term care: A research agenda.* Report from the Pragmatic Innovations in Long-Term Care, Maryland, MD. Retrieved from http://www.pragmaticinnovations.unc.edu/FinalReport/Pragmatic%20Innovation%20Final%20Report%2001-9-05.pdf

Sterns, S., Miller, S. C., & Allen, S. (2010). The complexity of implementing culture change practices in nursing homes. *Journal of the American Medical Directors Association, 11*, 511–518. doi:10.1016/j.jamda.2009.11.002

U. S. Department of Veterans Affairs. (n.d.). *VA history in brief.* Retrieved from http://www1.va.gov/opa/publications/archives/docs/history-in-brief.pdf

Veterans Health Administration. (2008). *VHA Handbook 1142.01: Criteria and standards for VA Community Living Centers (CLC).* Retrieved from http://www.va.gov/vhapublications/ViewPublication.asp?pub_ID=1736

Whipple, Y. Y., Magill, M., Decker, C., Koegel, DA, Keen, D., & Wooten, M. (2009). Culture transformation in action: The experience of one VA Community Living Center. *Practitioner Forum.* Retrieved from http://www.fedprac.com/PDF/026100040.pdf

Wicoff, M. (2011). Pilot housing project moving ahead. *Commercial-News.* Retrieved from http://commercial-news.com/local/x564244732/Pilot-housing-project-moving-ahead

European Long-Term Care Models:
An Interview with Victor Regnier

RICK J. SCHEIDT

School of Human Development and Family Studies, Kansas State University, Manhattan, Kansas, USA

My first meeting with Victor Regnier occurred at the Andrus Gerontology Center at the University of Southern California in 1975. I was a Postdoctoral Fellow in Lifespan Human Development, working with K. Warner Schaie. Victor held a joint-faculty appointment in the Environment-Aging Lab in the Andrus Gerontology Center and the University of Southern California School of Architecture. At that time, he was just emerging as an influential and respected leader in environmental gerontology. It is not quite correct to say that Victor first *introduced* me to the environment–aging paradigm; rather, he *infected* me with the wisdom and usefulness of the perspective for understanding the role that environments play in moderating and directly affecting the quality of life experienced by elders living within community-based and long-term care residential settings. As his professional biography below shows, a special issue dedicated to exploring the current status of environmental gerontology would be remiss if it did not tap into the experiences and views of this outstanding architect and scholar. Our invitation to him to join our group of authors in this special issue found Victor in a constant cycle of travel as a consultant in the United States and Europe. We asked if he would consent to a telephone interview and he graciously agreed. Despite exceeding 2 hours in length, our discussion covered but a few of the several questions we had intended to ask. The heart of the interview deals with Victor's views of both mentors and models within environmental gerontology that have most influenced his thinking, of people and directions that continue to excite his work. In addition to being expedient, the interview format flows with an ease and informality that shows his mind

---

Supplementary material is available for this article. Go to the publisher's online edition of Journal of Housing for the Elderly for the following free supplemental resource(s): The Academic Work of Victor Regnier.

at work, as well as his continuing excitement and dedication to improving the well-being of older adults in so many venues around the world.

BIOGRAPHICAL SKETCH

Victor Regnier is a teacher, researcher, and architect who has focused his academic and professional life on the design of housing and community settings for older people. He holds a joint professorship between the University of Southern California School of Architecture and the Leonard Davis School of Gerontology, which is the only joint appointment of this type in the United States. He also serves as the Vice Dean for Administration and External Affairs of the School of Architecture at University of Southern California. He is the only person to have achieved fellowship status in both the American Institute of Architects and the Gerontological Society of America. From 1992 until 1996, he served as the University of Southern California's Dean of the School of Architecture.

He has published 6 books and 60 articles and book chapters dealing with various aspects of housing and community planning for the elderly. He has received awards for his scholarship from the American Society of Landscape Architects, the American Planning Association and Phi Kappa Phi, as well as two Progressive Architecture Research Awards. He has also received a traveling Fulbright Research Award and the Thord-Grey Award from the American-Scandinavian Foundation.

Victor's interest in balancing theory with practice has led to many different and distinct honors. For example, he is the only architect to receive the Gerontological Society of America's M. Powell Lawton award for applied research. On the practice side, he was named by the National Association of Home Builders as an "Icon of the Industry" for his educational and teaching activities in senior housing. University of Southern California Architecture named him as their "2007 Distinguished Alumnus." In 2008, in recognition of his teaching and research, the American Collegiate Schools of Architecture named him one of three Distinguished Professors that year. (Since its inception in 1985, only 100 professors have been given this designation from the 125 schools of Architecture in North America.)

As an academic, he has directed over 20 research projects dealing with diverse topics such as the behavioral effect of the environment on people with dementia, children's museums, and homeless shelters. His design research findings have been presented at more than 200 professional and scientific conferences, as well as more than 60 university lectures and symposia. He has served on the editorial or advisory board of 9 journals or professional magazines.

As a teacher, Professor Regnier is the only architecture faculty member at the University of Southern California to have won university-wide teaching recognition—being named a University of Southern California Mortar Board Professor in 1995. He is well known as a mentor, as well as a stimulating and knowledgeable teacher. He also heads the school's summer Executive Education program.

As a designer and practicing architect, he has provided consultation advice over the past 30 years on more than 400 building projects in 38 states in the United States, as well as in Canada, Germany, and England. Projects on which he has consulted have won more than 50 state and national design awards in the last decade. Professor Regnier is considered one of the world's leading authorities on housing for the elderly.

Rick J. Scheidt: Your work in environmental gerontology has focused consistently on ways that physical design can improve the quality of life of older residents here in the United States and abroad. Your research practice and teaching have earned many awards from diverse and distinguished professional associations, so I'm going to take advantage of your experience and long-sightedness here.

Can you describe three or four ideas or people that have influenced your own work the most, what made them so special, and perhaps illustrate their impact with some examples?

Victor Regnier: My professional life has been highly influenced by Northern European long-term care examples. In fact, I really can't imagine my professional life without that exposure. It clearly changed the way I think about what is possible. It changed the way I assess liability and the appropriateness of codes and regulations, and it introduced me to a lot of differing cultural attitudes that were represented by a range of professions, including clinicians, architects, managers, and home care providers. All of them had assumptions and attitudes that were fundamentally different from what we hold sacred in the United States. I believe the northern Europeans (specifically Denmark, Sweden, Norway, Finland, and the Netherlands) have a more enlightened approach toward the individual. Also, you find people in positions of power and influence who run facilities and feel they've got the ability and permission to do creative things that take advantage of opportunities that lead to much more satisfying environments for older people. It's just kind of amazing. That influence is multi-layered. They recognize they have the creativity, ambition, and permission to do things that we in the United States think about—but frequently dismiss.

Probably the most important building/care hybrid that I've watched evolving for the past 15 years is the Apartments for Life movement in Rotterdam. I visited the first building that used this philosophy—The Humanitas Bergweg building—shortly after it was completed in 1999, and I have been monitoring that building, going back every few years to see what it's like and how it has changed over time. Since then, 20 or 30 of these building types have been constructed, primarily in the southern part of the Netherlands, although there are a few in Amsterdam, Germany, and Australia, as well as other places. The building, to describe it simply, is an urban building, relatively large in size and scale. Generally, there are 150 to 200 units, like a large apartment building. It's generally mid-rise, so it can take advantage of vertical transportation and short corridor lengths from the elevator core to the entrance of a resident's unit. The big idea is to keep people in a conventional apartment until they die—period. Residents fit into one of three competency categories. They have a process for establishing or indicating people for a certain level of care. In Bergweg, about one-third are independent older people (55 years and older). Another one-third are assisted-living residents, and the final one-third are people who are medically dependent (those who would likely be in a nursing home in the United States). That would be typical—one-third, one-third, one-third, with all of them living in a 700-square foot unit designed from a universal design perspective to accommodate their needs as they change physiologically over time. More importantly, the services they require to stay happy and function well are plugged in and can be increased over time. Independent residents often move in with an ailing spouse. Services can be provided to the spouse in the beginning. If the spouse dies, the remaining individual will grow older in the unit and may take services when needed later. That individual may become less capable and may require more help and support until, perhaps, they're in a hospice-like situation and die in their unit. Recently, they have created a small group cluster environment for people with dementia. Although, most of the people who live here have come from the outside community rather than from inside.

It is such an amazingly simple idea—but here in the United States it is very difficult to implement because our codes are tied to specific occupancy categories. When we think of the most advanced building types around, we think of the continuing care retirement community, and say, "Oh, that's the way to do it!" It's always made me a little uncomfortable that in CCRCs we move people when they have the least amount of power and ability to make decisions about their future. We push them into assisted living or dementia or the nursing unit without really having them participate in that decision. It's done as a clinical decision—sometimes involving the family.

RJS: Residents are also making physical transitions between residential care levels, often hanging on by their fingernails, hoping to remain in their present environment.

VR: That's right. So, the Northern European option affords continuity of care and environment. At 700-square feet, the dwelling unit is big enough for a family member to stay overnight. Units have enclosed balconies, which is common in the Netherlands, so they can use it as a wintergarden space for plants when it is cold or they can open it up in the summer for outdoor use. The dwelling unit has an independent kitchen, a good-sized living room, and a small second bedroom that could be used as a study or for overnight visitors. This is compared with the typical U.S. nursing home where two people share 400 square feet. This larger unit allows you to hold onto furniture, artwork, and possessions—those items that are really important to you. Possessions that allow you to reflect on your past and on the people who are important to you are there. Continuity is important, as are community and surrounding context. In many buildings, services are provided on the first floor for residents, as well as people living in the surrounding neighborhood. These spaces might include a bar, a restaurant, a computer center and other spaces for special activities. Many buildings have large atrium spaces where all types of fun things can happen. These buildings invite other people to participate in the life of the place. Outside participation makes the setting varied and interesting to watch. It's a setting open to people living in the surrounding community and neighborhood, so everybody feels comfortable. It almost always has a daycare component. Daycare is typically targeted toward people living in the surrounding neighborhood that need a lot of attention or have memory loss. However, they also have a lot of other people who come there to volunteer their time and participate in the spirit of the place. This makes it more eclectic—much more of a community setting. It doesn't look or feel like an institution. It's a place that is lively with people participating from all over—young people and old people and volunteers and people who are repairing the local telephone lines or just having lunch. It is a place that is far more interesting to live. It's also been accepted by the Dutch people as a great way to age in place. The building is purpose built, so everything is thought out from an aging-in-place perspective, but at the same time residents view it as a real home where you can put down roots, get to know people, and participate in community life.

Another thing I love is the level of volunteerism that occurs. People feel committed to helping one another, and they exercise a sense of interdependence. The Dutch culture in general focuses on this idea of doing as much as you can for yourself with a presumption that if you can't do what you need to do for yourself, there will be somebody to help you. But as Powell Lawton would say, they're always working on the idea of challenging individuals to do as much as they can for themselves. As a result, they not only encourage residents to be more independent, but also help them exercise their remaining ability so they can fight the inevitable decline in competency that aging normally brings. If we could build the perfect building, it would operate in some of these ways.

RJS: A predominant shift to this model in the United States would push beyond our culture change perspective.

VR: Yes, I think so, and it is a differing culture, and interestingly enough, you don't find the Apartment for Life idea replicated in quite the same way in Sweden or Denmark. They'll say something like "Well, this building is like a Dutch Apartment for Life format," but in each country it is operationalized a little differently. However, most northern European countries are far more committed than we are to keeping people in their own homes. The village strategy (like that in Beacon Hill Village in Boston, Massachusetts) has been active here for 50 years. Therefore, their interests are fundamentally different, and they aren't as involved in the production of purpose-built housing for people who are active adults. You see some of it, but much of the housing stock is not as fully outfitted with services and is designed in a way to produce the kind of continuity and longevity you get in an Apartment for Life building.

RJS: Did the Dutch housing ethic evolve historically out of their own tortuous experience with a medical model of residential care?

VR: Well, the story is actually pretty interesting. Hans Becker, the CEO of Humanitas, the largest non-profit provider of housing in Rotterdam, decided that he wanted to build this Apartment for Life concept but there were no precedents in the Netherlands, and it didn't neatly fit into a conventional housing/service category. Hans is an interesting and controversial spokesperson—he is always being quoted in the press. He reminds me of an elderly male version of Oprah Winfrey. His philosophy is quite unique. He was able to create this unusual building type despite the regulatory agencies. Toward the end, when regulatory officials started to ask questions about how they were going to manage care, he explained to them the concept that he had in mind and they said, "You know what, I don't think we can let you do that" because it is unprecedented. The story he tells is that he not only had people ready to move into the building, he had 3,000 people on a waiting list that wanted to get in, and he said, "If you'd like, I will write them all and tell them that you don't want them to move into this building." Thinking about the potential for a major flap, they folded and said, "Hmmm, you know, let's just try it and see what it's like," thinking all along that it probably wouldn't work out. Because Humanitas had 50 facilities and had been operating for 200 years, it was not an organization that the central government in the Netherlands was willing to take on. Once it was implemented, everybody embraced it, thinking, "Wow! This is it! This is what it should be." So it took a bold person taking risks, but also someone who knew this was the right thing to do. The other thing that's amazing about this building is that it costs less to operate than a conventional Assisted Living Facility (ALF) or Skilled Nursing Facility (SNF). Because Humanitas owns a lot of psychiatric facilities and a lot of conventional nursing homes, they have the ability to make side-by-side comparisons. They claim it costs 15% to 20% less for somebody of a comparable dependency level to live in an Apartment for Life than in a more conventional institution. It is cheaper, and residents are happier and have much more freedom. They also feel more connected to the surrounding community. Generally, when you create something that's cheaper and better, it's pretty hard to keep it a secret. So Hans had good intuition, he had the right kind of political influence, and he was good with follow through. His vision was one which the Humantitas organization was also committed to implement. It's one of those great stories and makes you think, "How could we do that here?" I think it is possible to find a progressive state in the United States that would allow something like this to be sanctioned and set up as a demonstration. At least, I hope that is possible because we have to start thinking about how to deinstitutionalize long-term care. We simply can't afford it in the future.

RJS: So you think it would have to win approval with stakeholders at the state level?

VR: I think so. In northern Europe, most of these settings are non-profit, which makes it a little easier to test by avoiding the inevitable assumption that it's just not another way to make money. We have strong proprietary providers who are inventive but also are jerked around by Wall Street and the demand for profitable returns.

RJS: Yes, what Carroll Estes once described as "the aging enterprise."

VR: You're right. So that is my favorite housing/service type, but if you look at what else they do in northern Europe, there are many approaches and lots of concepts that are worth testing in this country. For example, the idea that privacy and communality are stressed as necessary components of lifestyle. They've embraced both. People live in dwelling units that are single-occupied, yet they believe there should be natural and easy ways for people to come together and create new friendships and celebrate a social life with one another. The idea of being able to keep people at home as long as they possibly can is reflected in the home care systems that they have designed as well.

The emphasis on small group clusters is amazing and has been around for decades in northern Europe. I gave a presentation at American Association of Homes and Services for the Aging (AASHA) last year and showed examples of small group clusters from Danish long-term care examples that were 35 years old. They organized small groups of between 10 and 12 people in larger buildings that were decentralized in these clusters. Small group clusters of units are always linked to a community care system, which connects residents with the surrounding neighborhood. In the United States, we see institutions—people and organizations—that have separated themselves from the surrounding context and operate like little mini-hospitals. It's refreshing when you see an approach to housing that involves helping people in the community age in housing they find satisfying and familiar.

RJS: Well, I know that you've been championing this idea for some time in your work and in your own training program, and I suppose we could do a whole separate interview on the implementation of this idea within a country like the United States and what it would take at various levels to do that.

VR: So maybe we'll do that in the future [laughing].

RJS: Are there other major influences you would like to share?

VR: You asked about people too. There are two people who really influenced me. One was a student and one was a mentor, and, of course, my mentor who is probably your favorite mentor and everybody's favorite mentor is Powell Lawton. Powell was powerful because he cared about me as an individual and gave me really good fatherly advice about my career and about what he considered to be the most important attributes associated with quality housing for older frail people. I loved the way that Powell operated on two different planes. Here was a clinician working for the Philadelphia Geriatric Center with responsibilities as a psychologist to think and operate every day about how to make life more satisfying for the older people who were living there. While at the same time he had an intellectual life dedicated to unraveling the mysteries of measurement and understanding how environments could be better understood and dimensionalized so they could be better understood and made more satisfying for a broad range of frail older people. His ability to think about interrelationships between theory and practice affected me a great deal. I just thought, "What a great way to do it!" . . . where you have a commitment to people, and you have a commitment to ideas and to a bigger and broader agenda. It's just a great way to structure your academic/professional life.

RJS: He had a unique combination of qualities. He was a compassionate person, a kind and caring individual on the one hand, yet was very tough-minded when it came to doing good science.

VR: Yes, he was really a great scientist, I think, in terms of the kind of self-discipline that he had and his training and his insistence that research be performed at the highest quality level as well. He was always thinking creatively about how to measure and control for influences that would distort our understanding of a phenomena.

The other person I have long-term affection for is David Hogland, who was a student of mine at Illinois and who is now President of Perkins Eastman Architects, which is the one of the largest design firms in the country with dedicated studios throughout the world dealing with senior housing. The great thing about David is that he is never satisfied. He is always trying to figure out how to do the job better, and improve his understanding of the work from what he's done with the last project. There are always greater challenges, and he also operates at that same level. He's now created a nonprofit research group for Perkins Eastman because they feel strongly about gathering information from projects they've created and to learn more formally about their own work and try to figure out how to capture insights from that work going forward. He is a great pleasure to be with and to talk to and is like Powell except, kind of the opposite. Where Powell was interested in the larger issues of research and understanding phenomena at a higher level that could be applied to test ideas, David is much more interested in testing the ideas and then stepping back and saying, "What did we learn from that?" and how can we use that as a point of departure for our work in the future? Both of them are wonderful people and great colleagues.

RJS: You've partly answered the question I was going to ask you next. Whose work excites you the most right now?

VR: Well, you know, I continue to go back to northern Europe. I just returned from 6 weeks in Denmark, Sweden, and the Netherlands where I visited 45 buildings. Typically, in each building I spend 3 hours interviewing a slate of people, touring the place, and talking about what they are trying to achieve. Often, I get a chance to do some observations or have some conversations with older residents or with their families. For me, it's a great way to understand more about how settings differ one from another. I'm always interested in how unique these places can be, and also the emphasis on both volunteerism and community care. The issue I always think about is how can frail people be supported in settings that make them as independent as they can possibly be for as long as possible. I guess the other aspect I look for is how they influence affect and pleasure seeking. I think that's something we give up on with older people. Having visited a lot of buildings in my life, I find many of them unfriendly and unhappy places. When you see a setting where there is genuine affect and where the families are happy to be there and where the older people seem as if they're well cared for on one level, but also feel good about getting up in the morning and living life to its fullest—you recognize how powerful that can be.

RJS: That's a very interesting metric or barometer to use—the bottom line feeling about the level of morale and affect one can pick up from observing and interacting with the staff and residents when you enter a residential care setting. I always ask myself "Could I live here? Would I have a loved one live here?"

VR: It's one of the qualities—just as you described—that makes a big difference. When you go into a setting, you can feel and sense it. It has a lot to do with the art of management and how residents are engaged and how well trained the staff is, in terms of making it a friendly place. The intrinsic commitment is not just a job but a way of performing a mission that is helpful to people and dedicated to making them feel better about themselves and life in general. I do find it kind of interesting. A lot of consulting work I did with Sunrise Senior Living was centered on a building plan that was similar. The replication of that prototype over again was something I found interesting. Even though the plan had some fairly predictable rooms, connections, and relationships that were well recognized and identified in terms of how they were supposed to work, each place had its own life. It was always interesting to me how an individual manager and the care providers who were working within that building could make it better or [laughing] could take something that was really nice and screw it up. So it's interesting to me. I find it fascinating that there is a certain beginning stage where everything is in flux but the history of how you intervene, how you use the environment, and how you create community can have lasting effects. How people come together and feel they're part of a larger whole is powerful and sometimes can last for a long time. It's almost like your own life, where the history of what you have experienced in the last year or two or three influences the way you go forward and the choices that you make. The influence of your past history is always fascinating.

RJS: I think we're both aware of self-proclaimed "culture change" settings where the style and tone of the policy environment by itself can completely override good physical design.

VR: Yeah, that's exactly right. What's interesting about some of the Dutch and Danish examples is that they have these decentralized settings but then they challenge the leader who has responsibility for that cluster to custom fit that social setting around the people who happen to live there. Group leaders go out of their way to find out what type of food residents want or what types of activities or games they want to be involved with or how they want to live their lives. You know, this cut-to-fit attitude is pervasive throughout northern Europe; they feel committed to making the place familiar and comfortable to every resident. Some may want to skip their breakfast and have tea and toast at 10:00 a.m. For those residents, you don't wake them up at 7:00 a.m. and say, "It's time for you to eat your scrambled eggs." They cherish the attitude that every person can be accommodated and their differences can be celebrated, yet their common needs for interaction and community are respected and supported. It's a hard thing to do, I think, but because everybody has the challenge of doing that in the most artful way, they don't have rigid policies. It's really important to try and understand how to implement a collective lifestyle in a way that's consistent with what people would like to do on their own.

RJS: Trying to balance the autonomy/security continuum that Powell Lawton focused on so much?

VR: Right, that's right.

RJS: ... and moving that needle back and forth to accommodate individual differences within and across specific places. There's room for some flexibility there, I suppose.

VR: One of the things I find disturbing when I go into an old style nursing home—although it's a little less common now—is the presumption that everybody wants to play Bingo or that everybody wants to do this or that. In these places, there is less sensitivity and interest in trying to understand the individual, who they are, what they're about, how they've lived their lives, and what has brought pleasure to them over time. Also, how they have maintained a semblance of continuity in this last part of life, right? That aspect of culture change I really like. I like the idea that we are treating people like they are individuals and not assuming for the moment that they all have the same types of interests or they have the same point of view. That, I think, is very hard to do.

I noticed when I was in Sweden this spring that there was a lot of emphasis on gathering information about the person from the family, especially for people with dementia, to try and understand how to unlock what those preferences and desires were in ways that increase the individual's level of engagement with the surrounding environment and other people. There was a serious approach to gathering that information and using it in an almost semi-clinical way to figure out how to make the place more satisfying for the individual. Sometimes it involves leaving the place. Sometimes it's saying, "Okay, let's all go down to the local bar and billiards tavern and have a good time and enjoy it like we used to." There's this attitude that everybody is a little bit different from one another and most people have led a full life. Continuity is considered beneficial, especially when many are trapped in a setting where they're doing things that have little meaning—things they would not select on their own to do.

The green house or a smaller cluster is now becoming popular. This idea that you can accommodate individuals and their interests in a small group setting of 10 people is, I think, powerful. One of the places I visited in the Netherlands is the Hogeway in Weesp—it always had this attitude. They administer a questionnaire that you or a family member answers. They have 20 to 25 questions about the individual's past, their preferences, and their interests. The result of the answers to that questionnaire allows them to recommend one or two clusters (out of 20) that you may find a little bit more comfortable because there are people like yourself or individuals who share the same habits, tastes, or ideas.

It's a good way to create continuity at a time when it's sometimes tough to do that. More people are thinking creatively about how to do that type of matching. I think for me the small-scale cluster can also be a little bit deadly as well. I think it's a good idea to live with 10 people. It's a decent scale setting when you're with nine others who are similar to you, and conversations with them and with their family members come easy. You can feel a level of comfort. But then you know, it's also not so great to have only nine people you can interact with [laughing] and have your social world narrowed in that way. I think that is one of the great dilemmas. How do we benefit from the intimacy and the customizing that can occur in a small group setting while at the same time allowing us to have the type of choices that would occur if you had 60 people and the types of events or activities that could be staged for groups of that size? Or just the idea of having a more eclectic group of individuals who you can interact with on a daily basis. Continuity is wonderful, but it's also good to have it mixed up a little bit on occasion. When you see both of those things happening in a positive and constructive way, it does make you feel like they're addressing the downside of being in a setting with your ten closest friends ... forever.

RJS: Well, I suppose it's a continuation of the life you've known. The group setting affords the same types of life experiences—forming attachments and intimacies, making and losing friends, and transitioning to different phases in life.

VR: Right. You had mentioned earlier about the overall look or feel of the environment as well, and I really feel strongly about that. Partly, I guess because it's been so uniformly rejected by my Northern European colleagues for so many years. They have been dogged about "let's make sure it's personal and appears residential and comfortable. Let's make certain family members feel a level of comfort when they visit, make it feel like visiting grandma in her house." That is such a powerful concept, and sometimes it doesn't take much to make it work. However, it takes what it takes to make you feel that way, and if the environment has the wrong set of surfaces, textures, materials, or furniture or if the layout of the kitchen is one that looks more commercial than it does familiar, it can really mess it up. It can make the whole experience seem foreign and kind of strange to the family, the staff, and the older person. Therefore, it is important to use those components in a creative way, to give people comfort, make them feel relaxed, and give them a reason to behave in a way that's more like how you would act at home than in a hospital or an institution. It's just really important. You can see the difference sometimes in how the staff treats residents if they have a uniform or if they don't have a uniform. It's just odd, but that one thing can make a big difference. I don't think the individuals are necessarily that different, but they perform differently. They see themselves and their role in a different way, and that makes a difference.

RJS: It seems that you're describing a holistic culture change philosophy implemented within a micro-level scale compared with the larger scale settings we're so familiar with here in the United States.

VR: The thing to keep in mind in Northern Europe is that most of the people who live in planned small group settings have memory loss. If you walk into any setting, typically at least 75% of the residents are there because they have dementia or some type of memory loss that makes it impossible for them to live independently.

Most of the physically frail but cognitively intact people who would be in a setting like that in the United States are being supported in the community through home healthcare. It's cheaper, better, and maybe smarter for us to help people live in their own environment, in their own apartment, in their own house, for as long as they possibly can. They move when it's uncomfortable for them because of a lack of security or because they have such a strong collection of needs or they want the security of caregivers nearby who can attend to them. In fact, in those environments, partly because of the high quality of the environment, securing a place in a nursing home or assisted-living building is hard to do. There are lots of people who want to move into nursing homes, or their version of a nursing home, and move from the farm where they're living or the apartment on the third floor that they're struggling to try and gain access to in a walkup. So it's interesting when they say, "We have this long waiting list, but we really want to help these people." Some people who are insecure psychologically could really benefit from a more contained and secure environment, yet they are low on the totem pole because they don't have high needs. They don't have as many places as they should for this burgeoning population. It's different in the United States. Most people are reticent to move into any kind of a long-term care setting. It's scary and alienating to most.

RJS: In terms of developing an agenda—formal or informal—that might guide future research training or practice in this area, from your experiences and vantage point, where do you see things going in the future in this arena?

VR: That's an excellent question, and I think about it a lot. I ask myself, "Am I just fascinated with these purpose-built northern European settings because they are more attractive and comfortable because I think qualitatively, they're better, or is there something about the systematic approach they have taken that makes sense?" Actually, I believe that both are true. The idea of being able to keep people in their own environment in a comfortable context where family members, neighbors, and community institutions are available to help them, look after them, and support them is very powerful. I think it happens in the United States as well when the next door neighbor gets paid a few dollars to help out. When we start to cut all of those ties and we move somebody into an independent environment where we have to reproduce everything and provide everything for that individual, it's pretty expensive, and pretty disruptive—which is what the northern Europeans discovered more than 40 years ago.

We've seen a lot of community-based health care solutions develop in the past 20 years. We don't have hospitals where people go in and spend 3 days after a hernia operation or after having a child. We get them in and out quickly because it costs several thousand dollars a day to support somebody in a hospital. I believe that is what will happen with long-term care. To do this more effectively, we will need a stronger system for homecare support. I think it is probably the most important single, long-term care initiative we could implement, and it's something a lot of older people would like to see in place. Speaking as an architect, I may be talking out of turn by saying it's not all about building something new—that's perfect, but having a balanced approach that supports community care as well. That can also involve a better transportation system or a sidewalk repair program that makes it a little bit safer for people to walk or even focusing on the civic entitlement side. This would encourage older people to volunteer and make a contribution to the local community in a positive way. They may even feel some obligation to do that, but we need to help them exercise it appropriately. I do think we are stuck with care settings for people with dementia (at least in the foreseeable future).

Back to my Apartments for Life strategy. I find that approach appealing because these purpose-built environments have ad hoc service and care systems. In that type of apartment environment, a care professional visits you based on the needs you have. Unlike an institution, you're not being checked on every 20 minutes by a nurse who has to do it because that's what the regulations require. It's a much more natural way of allowing the older person to have security when they need it, but autonomy when they don't. Choice is respected, and you live in a more normal environment with friends you have a reciprocal obligation to help and feel appreciated and valued. When you see that happening, you think, "This is the way to do it. This is the right way to do it." You don't over support. If you do anything, you slightly under support people. You stimulate them to be as independent as they possibly can be. You stamp out every bit of learned helplessness that you can and make people feel as if they have control over living a satisfying lifestyle, that is not that different than what they've had during the first 75 years of life.

RJS: Do you believe that the field of gerontology and environmental gerontology in particular are paying enough attention to physical design and spatial issues as opposed to a historical focus on the "P" component of the person–environment equation?

VR: If you don't have a well-designed environment, you can't do a lot of things. So you may have all the best ideas, but if the kitchen counter is one where you can't go behind to get a glass of water or if it is inaccessible, it is a problem. The truth is that it is about both environment and management. These two are interrelated in long-term care settings. Earlier, we were talking about how habits develop and how those habits become a sort of ad hoc culture. That is, sometimes very good and sometimes not. However, it is really important for us to be more mindful about what we're doing and think about what the possibilities are for individuals. I think one solution has to do with people being trained to use the environment in creative ways. I sometimes will visit a building and see the staff doing something just kind of zany, you know, maybe some ad-hoc dancing in the middle of the room, or residents watching the staff do something. I visited a building in the United Kingdom 6 months ago where all of the staff members were wearing a costume. The residents formed a committee and a process for assessing their costumes as well as their deportment—how they handled the costume, whether they were really playing the part that they were dressed up to be, and it was fun and interesting.

RJS: Well, this brings up kind of an interesting issue because I know that in Kansas and other places, there are many "mom and pop" facilities, and they're looking at what's going on and they're hearing about culture change and they're in facilities designed as and serving the goals of the old medical model. So I'm wondering, without significant redesign of the physical environment, can you grow a successful culture change program?

VR: Yeah, that's a good question. I'm a really strong believer in decoration, you know. When I go into settings and they are decorated for a special event—Cinco de Mayo or 4th of July or maybe a special event they have invented on their own, like a family day or birthday—I'm always surprised at how they can transform the setting with $20 worth of items they pick up at the local Hallmark or Walmart that can make the place seem very different than it is.

RJS: I see.

VR: Almost any major change can make a difference—moving the furniture in a slightly different way, tinkering with the light fixtures, or hanging something in a prominent location, creating a stronger focus to the room because they've rearranged it in a certain way. I do think there are a lot of things you can do that aren't dependent on moving the four walls that enclose the space. This type of change is dependent on creating interesting things to look at or to pay some attention to. In fact, I will often assess buildings before all of the furniture and accessories are installed because once all the furniture and accessories are in, it's hard to see flaws. You can't see construction flaws because all of this other stuff is competing for your attention. It's a type of camouflage that robs your of ability to see whether the trim is done exactly right or the detailing of the carpet pattern is managed properly. I think it works that way with everybody. I think you can make a place much more playful, interesting, and fun through careful placements of items. I designed a three-sided triangular kiosk once, which I think is a really great idea. It was designed to be placed in a corridor where people would bump into it without anticipation. One side had documentary photos of events (e.g., the hayride, the kids who came over in Halloween costumes, or the dogs and cats that visited a month and a half ago). All of the positive memories that make up the past life of the place life which everyone enjoyed. Maybe a staff or family member dressed up or wearing a wig and acting silly. It was a side that documented and represented fun times in the immediate past. The second side was reserved for notices, maps, and descriptions of events planned for the immediate future (within the next month or so)—the opportunities for activity and engagement. Announcements that they were going to go on this kind of trip, that these people are coming in to visit/perform, or that they will have the chance to cook cookies for the 3rd graders in the local primary school two weeks from now. All of those things that are anticipatory in nature that I think people really look forward to and if it's there and you can refer to it, you know, "Oh yeah, that's next Tuesday, isn't it? Boy! That will be fun." On the third side, we would always put jokes and cartoons and funny stuff—anything that was amusing that just made you laugh when you looked at it, whatever that might be. It just seemed to me that kind of prop had great promise. It is pretty simple—all it requires are three pieces of plywood and a lot of imagination. But that is the kind of object that can make a big difference because there are aspects of the lifestyle that are just intrinsically interesting. They stimulate your memory and make you feel good about the future and make you just chuckle when you need to do that.

RJS: Those are nice examples. We really appreciate you giving us your views and your time today.

VR: I enjoyed talking to you Rick. I know we are both passionate about these issues, and we all feel committed to improving the status quo. Thank you for asking me to do this interview. I found it interesting as well as fun—which it the whole point of life—right?

Design for Dementia Care: A Retrospective Look at the Woodside Place Model

STEFANI DANES

Perkins Eastman Research Collaborative, Pittsburgh, Pennsylvania, USA

This retrospective study looks at the evolution of the Woodside Place model as it was applied to three later facilities, Copper Ridge and the memory-support units at the Gardens at William Hill Manor and NewBridge on the Charles. All four facilities were designed by Perkins Eastman. Woodside Place and Copper Ridge are both early projects, opening within 3 years of each other. The Gardens at William Hill Manor and NewBridge on the Charles both opened approximately 20 years later and embody lessons learned from the Woodside Place model over the intervening years. The investigation for this study was done through a series of post-occupancy evaluations by the Research Collaborative at Perkins Eastman. Each of the facilities was visited. Interviews with the administration, care and facilities staff, and families were conducted. Facility tours were taken with administrators and care and facilities staff, with follow-up questionnaires. In addition, archived information from earlier post-occupancy evaluations at Woodside Place and Copper Ridge were used. The study found that the Woodside Place model had been successfully adapted to a variety of contexts, populations, and programs. Several improvements have been made since the original building was opened. Based on these findings, the article provides design recommendations for current residential dementia facilities.

INTRODUCTION

In the past two decades, we have seen a revolution in dementia care. The culture change movement has brought with it an increasingly important role for the design of the physical environment (Cohen & Day, 1993; Brawley, 2006). This article looks back to design ideas that were introduced at the outset of the culture change movement with the creation of Woodside Place in Oakmont, Pennsylvania. To understand how the design concepts in the original model have evolved and how well they have stood the test of time, we conducted post-occupancy evaluations of four dementia care facilities based on the Woodside Place model that were built between 1990 and 2010. The article discusses the findings from those studies and looks at concepts for care facilities that are currently being developed on the basis of this experience.

THE WOODSIDE PLACE MODEL: DESIGN INTENTIONS

In the late 1980s, the best hope for families looking for a place to care for their relatives with Alzheimer's disease was to find a nursing home where restraints were not used frequently and where a sympathetic roommate might be found. Compared with the wards in mental hospitals 50 years before that, this represented a real advancement in humane care (Lacey, 1999). In the mid-1980's, Charles Pruitt of the Presbyterian Association on Aging (now Presbyterian SeniorCare) in western Pennsylvania assembled a multidisciplinary team, including specialists in dementia, geriatrics, and architecture from West Penn Hospital, Perkins Eastman Architects, the University of Pittsburgh, and Carnegie Mellon University. They saw the need for a better kind of therapeutic environment for the increasing number of people with dementia, who were placed in nursing homes despite their otherwise good health because no other care was available for them.[1] In nursing homes at the time, it was a commonly accepted practice to deal with dementia-related behavioral issues with physical or psychotropic restraints.[2] To find a better solution, Pruitt's team initiated research into alternatives that eventually led to the creation of Woodside Place. With lessons learned from visiting the few state-of-the-art facilities at the time, such as Corinne Dolan in Ohio, Gardiner House in Maine, the Lefroy Hospital in Australia, and Woodside in Birmingham, England, the team conceived a non-institutional, resident-focused model (Figure 1).

The design goals for the facility were integrally related to the philosophy of care and plans for programming and staffing. The central insight was that a social model of care rather than a medical model would sustain residents by affirming their personal dignity and supporting their capabilities instead of focusing on their deficiencies. The principles the team developed were an early articulation of the values that would be widely adopted in the Culture Change movement:

- Enable residents to maintain their independence for as long as possible without jeopardizing their safety.

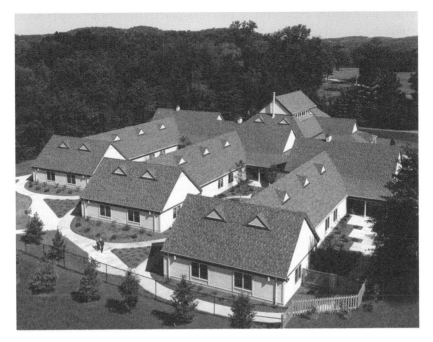

FIGURE 1 Woodside Place (courtesy of Perkins Eastman, 2011).

- Respect the dignity of every person.
- Acknowledge everyone's needs for both privacy and community.
- Provide individualized care, permitting flexible daily rhythms and patterns.
- Offer focused and appropriate stimulation and avoid both sterile monotony and excessive distraction.
- Instead of trying to discourage wandering, find opportunities to engage residents along their path.
- Create small-group environments that support building relationships.
- Introduce alternative way-finding systems into the environment.
- Design a residential (non-institutional) environment in layout, scale, and architectural language.
- Encourage family and caregiver participation.

Today, 20 years after the opening of Woodside Place, many examples exist of resident-centered, residential-style care for people with dementia. What distinguishes the Woodside Place model among residential facilities derives from its fundamental spatial organization rather than its finishes or style:

- The facility is divided into households of 8 to 12 residents. Small dining rooms, sitting spaces, and residential kitchens are part of the households.
- The environment conveys the message that it "belongs to" the residents. For example, the entrance leads right into the residents' living space, not to

administrative space. Households provide places for residents to participate in activities of everyday life.

- Recognizing that the primary responsibility of the direct care staff is to build close, caring relationships with residents, the environment facilitates their engagement with residents by distributing rather than centralizing work space and supplies.
- The environment recognizes the difference between the public and private spaces in a home. Common spaces are more public than residents' rooms, which are in more private hallways and are not between public destinations. Private rooms open onto private hallways, not onto common spaces.
- To respect the hierarchy of privacy, specialized common spaces that are used by everyone, such as a larger assembly room, a spa/bathing/beauty center, or activity rooms, are provided outside the households.
- Activity spaces are kept open to circulation paths so that residents can see what's going on and more easily get involved. In the common area, circulation paths are integrated into the habitable space, rather than separate, institutional-like corridors.
- Residents have the option of going outside into a secure yard or courtyard from several places in the facility. Paths form continuous "loops" with interior circulation and offer options for longer or shorter travels.
- Large windows and sheltered porch spaces connect residents and staff with the outside.

The four dementia care facilities that are considered in this article are Woodside Place, Copper Ridge, and the memory-support units at William Hill Manor and NewBridge on the Charles. They were designed by Perkins Eastman based on the Woodside Place model. Woodside Place and Copper Ridge are both early projects, opening within 3 years of each other. William Hill Manor and NewBridge on the Charles opened in 2009 and 2010, and embody lessons learned from the Woodside Model over the intervening years.

The investigation for this study was done through a series of post-occupancy evaluations by the Research Collaborative at Perkins Eastman. During 2011, each of the facilities was visited by a researcher (S.D.) accompanied (except at Woodside Place) by a project architect who had taken part in the project. The 2-day trips were planned approximately 6 weeks in advance with the help of a liaison from the administrative staff, who set up meetings with administrators, care staff, facilities and support staff, and families. The goal was to obtain information and insights from a variety of perspectives. In some instances, we met with a single individual and at other times, with a group of as many as six participants. These interviews took between 45 to 90 minutes. They began with a set of questions that were asked at all facilities and subsequently broadened to an open-ended discussion of issues important to the participants. The research team toured the facility with administrators and care and facilities staff, making first-hand observations that were documented by taking notes and photographs. The tours were also particularly useful for raising questions and pointing out issues that had not been identified in interviews. At the end of the visit, time was set aside to have meetings with key staff members to reflect on the observations and insights from the visit. The documentation from each visit was organized into an in-house report. Follow-up questionnaires were sent back to the liaison in each facility to obtain clarifications and other specific information. Additionally, archived information from earlier post-occupancy evaluations at Woodside Place and Copper Ridge were used to prepare the final report.

THE FOUR FACILITIES

• Woodside Place is a freestanding, specialized assisted.living (personal care) facility run by the Presbyterian Association on Aging (Presbyterian Senior-Care) in Oakmont, Pennsylvania, on their Hulton Road campus (assisted living and skilled care). It was opened in 1991 and was designed to serve individuals in mid-stage dementia who are mobile, are at least partially continent, and require no more than one person for assistance. Thirty-six residents were located in three households of 12 residents in 8 single rooms and 2 double rooms. The building area is 23,000 gross square feet (gsf) which includes 600 square feet (sf) of interior space per resident (not including service, support, or inaccessible space). It also has a secure outdoor area that is approximately 8,000 sf in size (Figure 2).

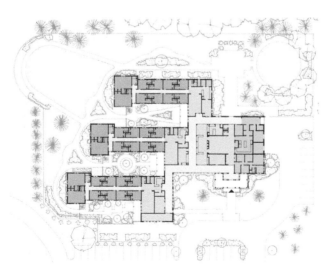

FIGURE 2 Woodside Place floor plan (courtesy of Perkins Eastman, 2011).

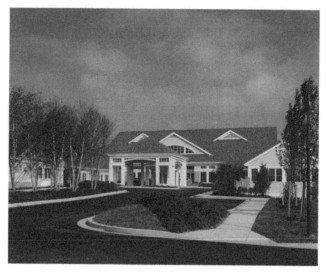

FIGURE 3 Copper Ridge exterior view (courtesy of Perkins Eastman, 2011).

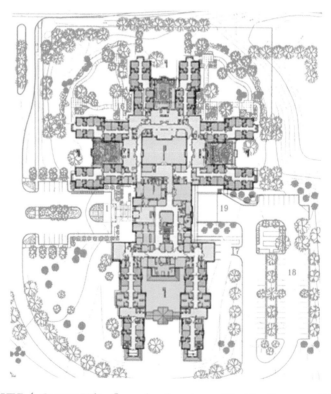

FIGURE 4 Copper Ridge floor plan (courtesy of Perkins Eastman, 2011).

Innovative features include residential households, private rooms, private half-baths, dutch doors, plate shelf, open activity spaces along walking paths, access to outdoor space, elimination of nurses' stations, and cuing with themed finishes and artwork.

- Copper Ridge is a freestanding, specialized assisted-living (domiciliary care) and skilled care facility run by the Episcopal Ministries to the Aging in Sykesville, Maryland, that is adjacent to EMA's Fairhaven Retirement Community. The facility was opened in 1994 and was designed to serve individuals with early to mid-stage dementia. Sixty residents were located in assisted-living units in 6 households and 60 residents in skilled care. The building area is 33,855 gsf, which includes 537 sf of interior space per resident (in domiciliary care wing), and a secure outdoor area of 27,000 sf in size (Figures 3 and 4).

Innovative features include shared spaces that link households, window seats in rooms, cuing with furniture as well as finishes and artwork, common areas linked around a courtyard, and the Copper Ridge Institute (on-site research partnership with Johns Hopkins University).

- *NewBridge on the Charles* is a specialized care unit in the assisted-living building that is run by Hebrew SeniorLife in Dedham, Massachusetts, in a continuing care retirement community. It was opened in 2009 and was designed to serve individuals with early to mid-stage dementia. Forty residents lived in four households (two households on two floors). The area of the unit is 27,800 gsf, which includes 663 sf of interior space per resident and a secure outdoor area 2,400 sf in size (Figures 5 and 6).

Innovative features include integration of the residential model into a larger building, multi-floor facility, open central kitchen, paired households connected at ends of bedroom hallways, a screened-in balcony, as well as a secure yard and showers in the bathrooms.

- The Gardens at William Hill Manor is a specialized care unit in an assisted-living building run by the Episcopal Ministries to the Aging in Easton, Maryland, on the campus of William Hill Manor. It was opened in 2010 and was designed to serve individuals with early to mid-stage dementia. Twenty-four residents live in one household, which, along with three other households, were created as an addition and renovation of an existing building. The area of the household is 12,500 gsf, which includes 479 sf of interior space per resident and a secure outdoor area 3,400 sf in size (Figures 7 and 8).

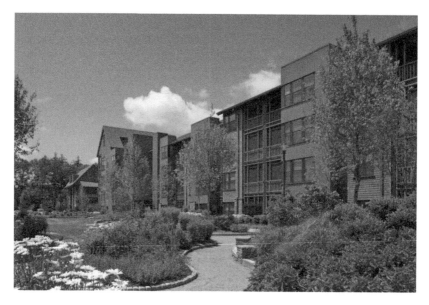

FIGURE 5 NewBridge exterior view (courtesy of Perkins Eastman, 2011).

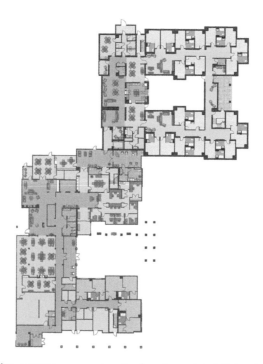

FIGURE 6 NewBridge memory support unit plan, in assisted living building (courtesy of Perkins Eastman, 2011).

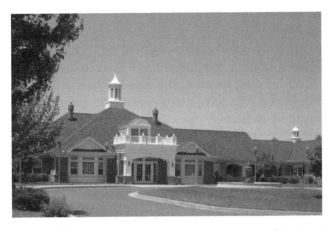

FIGURE 7 Gardens at William Hill Manor exterior view (courtesy of Perkins Eastman, 2011).

Innovative features include the adaptation of an existing building, two households merged into a single household (single dining area, sitting area, continuous bedroom hallway), internal courtyard, room refrigerator, and controlled access into kitchen, as well as an on-site geriatric psychiatrist, Copper Ridge Institute memory clinic, short-stay evaluations, grand rounds, and respite care.

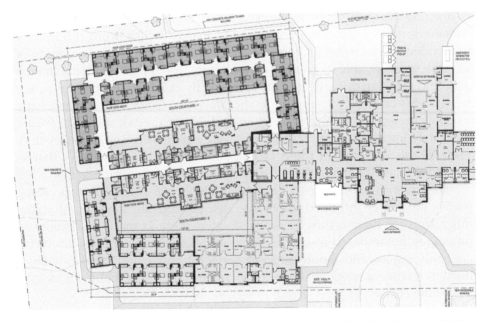

FIGURE 8 Gardens at William Hill Manor floor plan (courtesy of Perkins Eastman, 2011).

THE CHANGING CONTEXT OF DEMENTIA CARE

In the 20 years since Woodside Place opened, the culture change movement has taken root, expectations for dementia care have increased, and medical research has discovered more about the disease itself and its effects on both cognition and behavior. We have also seen major changes in the social and economic context of dementia care. For example, the average household income in the United States has decreased, and families are less secure in their prospects for a secure retirement. Public support for the care of the elderly remains a relatively high priority, but government spending on social programs of all kinds continues to be cut back. This evolving contextual backdrop is critical to understanding the effectiveness of the design concept over the years. The need for appropriate and affordable care that was addressed by Woodside Place is as great today as it was then, but many of the challenges are even greater. Among them are five that have a significant effect on the design of dementia care today.

Extent of Impairment

Residents today are not entering dementia care facilities at the "early-mid-stage" of dementia, which was characteristic of residents 20 years ago. In all four facilities, residents are entering with extensive cognitive impairment, along with more incontinence, behavior problems, and mobility impairment. For example, at Copper Ridge, staff recalled that the residents' acuity level on opening was markedly higher than that of the population today. All residents in the domiciliary care (assisted living) facility were moderately independent; all were ambulatory; one-third were continent; and a portion of the residents were able to do their own laundry, use the kitchen on a limited basis, and enjoy many activities off campus. By contrast, the current acuity level in assisted living, according to the Maryland Guidelines for Assessing Residents in Assisted Living, only 1% are mildly impaired (level 1), 28.5% are moderately impaired (level 2), and 66.7% are extensively impaired (level 3). Residents are accepted in these facilities today with characteristics that in 1991 would have qualified them for discharge to a skilled care facility.

The reasons are likely to be a combination of several factors: some families are better informed about the disease and are more comfortable with caring for their relative at home longer; there is more availability of community home-based resources, including home care services, adult day care, and respite and family support services; and many families cannot afford to pay for a residential care program and must forestall it for as long as possible (Figure 9).

The effect on designing and running the facility is readily observable. In general, residents cannot participate in as many daily activities and need

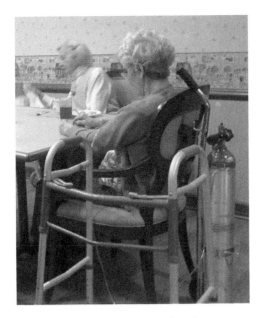

FIGURE 9 Residents today (courtesy of Perkins Eastman, 2011).

more supervision and attention. More residents are passive observers rather than active participants. Staff finds that prompting is rarely effective and that consequently they are initiating more of the activities for residents. Less able to navigate their surroundings, residents tend to cluster around staff members, and some of the care staff tends to keep them closer to them, whether to provide assistance or to minimize the likelihood of out-of-sight falls or other mishaps. At Copper Ridge, where their reputation for expert care now attracts residents deemed too difficult by other care facilities and younger people with other kinds of dementia, the staff is dealing with new kinds of psychiatric and physically aggressive behaviors, as well as with the different interests and capabilities of the younger residents.

Staff also responds differently to the greater frequency of inappropriate behaviors. At Copper Ridge, as residents more often handled food and dishes improperly, the household kitchens were modified to enable staff to limit residents' access. At Woodside Place, faced with the same problem, the staff chose to keep an eye on residents in the kitchen and, whenever needed, follow up by running dishes through the dishwasher a second time or removing food from the refrigerator. All of the facilities reported that they have adapted their programming substantially to find ways to support and engage the more impaired residents.

Understanding of Alzheimer's Disease and Other Dementias

Research into the physiology and chemistry of the diseases of the brain has yet to uncover their causes, although we understand more about the process that we did 20 years ago. By the mid-1990s, four of the genes associated with Alzheimer's disease had been discovered. Research in the past decade has increasingly focused on the role of beta-amyloid and tau proteins in the production of the characteristic plaques and tangles that progressively disrupt normal brain functions and kill brain cells. Current research is aimed at earlier detection of Alzheimer's disease, as well as developing interventions to halt the chemical changes in the brain, with the expectation that earlier interventions are more likely to be successful.[3]

Other research in the late 1990s addressed the psychological, cognitive, and behavioral aspects of dementia. For example, studies showed that people with Alzheimer's disease retain the ability to read far longer than assumed (Hopper, Bayles, & Kim, 2001). Still more interestingly, the research of Dr. Cameron Camp and others (2006) at the Myers Research Institute in conjunction with developing Montessori Based Dementia Programming has demonstrated that people even in mid-stage Alzheimer's disease have the ability to learn and adapt their behaviors. These insights have far-reaching implications for the design of both programming and the physical environment, including the possibility of better approaches to wayfinding.

Financial Stresses

When Woodside Place was conceived, one of the goals was to demonstrate a more cost-effective alternative to nursing home care. The situation is only more critical today. Private providers and state and local governments are concerned about the impact of inadequate Medicaid reimbursement, unfunded mandates and regulations, inconsistent interpretation of regulations, and a lagging payment cycle (Ullman, 1984).

Most people live for 4 to 8 years after a diagnosis of Alzheimer's disease, but some people survive for 20 years or more (Alzheimer's Association, 2011). Given the high cost of long-term care, this brings financial challenges to both families and society that are mitigated by delaying entry into a specialized or long-term care facility. According to the Alzheimer's Association (2011), Medicaid payments for seniors with dementia are nine times higher than for seniors without the disease. The Alzheimer's Association (2011) estimates that Medicaid spending in 2011 on individuals with Alzheimer's and other dementias will total $37 billion, and that it will increase by almost 400%, before inflation, by 2050. But the alternative of caring for a relative at home has its own costs, ranging from the expenses of making home improvements to the added medical costs related to the caregiver's heightened stress level.

These conditions have intensified the pressure on dementia care facilities to contain costs, as well as maintain a high level of occupancy. The issue of affordability directly affects staffing and programming, and indirectly affects the use of the facility. To the extent that the building layout contributes to staffing efficiencies, high-quality care is kept more affordable.[4] Economies of scale tend to drive meal and laundry services. Aligning the benefits of a small-scale environment with the advantages of larger-scale systems affects site planning, building programming, and the size and organization of households. These factors tend to shift over time, so designing to optimize the balance before the building is constructed may preclude the flexibility needed for later adaptations as the economics change.

One response by providers and the public sector to the high cost of care is to substitute electronic technologies for personal engagement. However, social engagement is a particularly important factor in the well-being of older people. According to a long-term study of adults from 55 to 85 years, social support is strongly correlated with a lower mortality risk (Penninx et al., 1997). Although it is not as apparent as the cost savings, the long-term effects of linking people through a computer screen on their health and well-being need to be considered.

Health Insurance Portability and Accountability Act and Reporting Regulations

The Health Insurance Portability and Accountability Act (HIPAA)[5] was passed 5 years after Woodside Place opened. Because of HIPAA's requirements for maintaining stricter confidentiality, care staff has to keep records and other information where it is not available to be seen or heard by others. At some facilities, this has tended to push staff, who had been encouraged to take care of this work at the kitchen counter or at a table in the living room where they could be with residents, back into an office and away from both residents and families (Figure 10). With limited staffing resources, this has been particularly stressful, both individually and organizationally. Although confidentiality is in the resident's interest, this pressure is counter to the goals

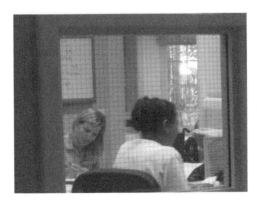

FIGURE 10 Staff working in office (courtesy of Perkins Eastman, 2011).

of resident-centered care, a philosophy that discourages staff from retreating to a centralized nursing station. Some providers are trying to overcome it by introducing electronic record-keeping and hand-held data entry devices that enable staff to do their reporting without leaving the residents' space. In the years since the Woodside Place model was developed, HIPAA has added not only a challenge to meeting the goal of resident-centered care, but also a greater complexity to programming the design of resident-centered dementia care facilities.

Dementia Care in Non-Western Cultures

In 1995 and in 1998, the Woodside Place model was replicated in Edmonton, Canada. As demonstrated in a follow-up study, the model adapted success-fully to the modest change in cultural context (Milke, Beck, & Ledewitz, 1999). Today, as developing countries around the world address the care of elderly in their societies, facilities for dementia care are being introduced in much different cultural contexts. This is raising new issues, requiring cultur-ally specific reinterpretations of design for resident-centered care. In some places, local codes have a great effect on the facilities. For example, in China, whether by code in the south or by market expectations in the north, resident rooms are required to face the south. This dramatically constrains the possible options for the layout of a household, as well as challenging western ideas of home and privacy. In both China and India, it is considered impolite to view the toilet from the bedroom. Mementos and belongings can have different meanings, social roles may take on a new significance, and activities of everyday living need to be understood within their local context.

LESSONS LEARNED

In 20 years of dementia care, the population served has changed, economic and regulatory constraints are more challenging, new diagnostic and thera-peutic methods are evolving, and new technologies are being tested. At the same time, the concept of a residential model for dementia care has become well-accepted and widespread. It is used in renovating older institutional environments, as well as in building new freestanding buildings or additions for dementia care. Wherever the principles of culture change have been adopted, the residential facility model is also accepted. But how appropriate is this model to today's context? Our study suggests that the fundamental features of the model are still valid today, but some limitations and poten-tial conflicts need to be addressed. The answer is often finding a balance between different goals.

Organize the Facility into Households that are as Small as Staffing and Servicing Efficiencies Will Permit

Inherent in the residential model is the idea of small groups of residents living in households with their own space for dining and common activities. Households in the four facilities we studied serve either 10 or 12 residents. We found that this grouping supports personal relationships among the residents, their families, and the direct care staff and facilitates resident-centered care. However, as residents age and decline in cognitive abilities, the burden on direct care staff increases, yet the cost of adding staff has been prohibitive. To the extent that the physical environment supports the staff, increasing the effective staff-to-resident ratio, its function has become even more important over time. Bringing supplies and services closer to where residents spend time, for instance, enables staff to spend less of their time on logistical errands.

At Woodside Place, where the focus was on breaking down the large-scale spaces of institutional facilities, the 12-resident houses are each entirely independent, but this makes it difficult for staff to assist each other across households. The later facilities connect pairs of households with a common kitchen and at a second point (Figure 11). Both William Hill and NewBridge connect two households at the far end of the bedroom corridor and at the kitchen. Copper Ridge connects households diagonally through the den. These facilities, although designed on the small-scale household model, are also attached to larger buildings. All four facilities are part of larger senior living organizations, which provide operational (e.g., meals and laundry) and administrative (e.g., human resources and accounting) services. The

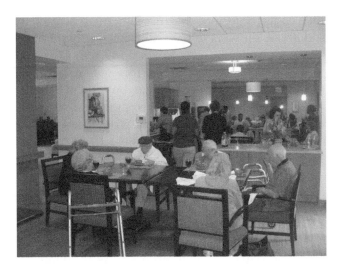

FIGURE 11 Connection between households (courtesy of Perkins Eastman, 2011).

functional, administrative, and physical linkages have been advantageous to maintaining the small-scale households.

Provide Private Rooms with Full Bathrooms

There was universal agreement that private rooms are beneficial, even essential. In the few instances of double rooms, finding pairs of residents to live together was more difficult than expected, and some of those rooms have been converted into either two small singles with a shared bath or a deluxe single room. Experience has shown that a private room does not have to be large because residents spend little waking time there. It was observed in the early study of Woodside Place that residents spent 90% of their waking hours in the common areas. Similarly, it was observed in the recent post-occupancy evaluations at all the facilities that residents' rooms are rarely used during the day except for naps, which limits the need for space. On the other hand, the increasing prevalence of mobility devices does require more space. The net area of a typical private bedroom ranges from 120 to 170 sf, and those sizes have tended to increase over time.[6] A popular space-saving feature is the window seat, which was introduced at Copper Ridge. It provides an efficient alternative to chairs and a storage cupboard, as well as adding character to the room. The built-in drawers are used primarily by staff. Other appreciated features of the rooms are the view of the toilet from the bed, the high shelf that is visible from the hallway for displaying residents' personal items, the dutch door, the large photo/name plate at the door, and the ways they can be personalized. Whether the dutch door is used seems to depend on the staff in charge.

An attached private bathroom should provide a shower and should be large enough for at least one assisting staff member (50 to 60 sf). Because of the greater incidence of incontinence, an additional storage cabinet or closet is needed, which is factored into the recommended size of the bathroom. One issue raised about showers in the bathrooms is the importance of good drainage for European style showers to keep the water from spreading and making the floor slippery (Figure 12). Mirrors got mixed reviews because some residents are frightened by their image, but others like it for grooming. It was suggested that a solid door hinged to the mirror could be opened or closed as needed. The warm radiant floors in Woodside Place are particularly appreciated in the bedrooms and bathrooms.

Separate Bedrooms from Common Spaces with Hallways but Keep them Short and Visible

The bedroom hallways are important in separating the residents' bedrooms from the more public parts of the household. As residents age or decline in mobility, distances between bedrooms and common areas become more

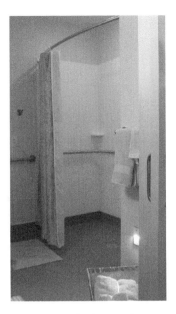

FIGURE 12 Shower in resident's private bathroom (courtesy of Perkins Eastman, 2011).

critical. For obvious reasons, residents are not relocated to different rooms but instead age in place. At Copper Ridge and William Hill Manor, the visibility of bedroom corridors from the common areas was a significant staff concern because they felt they had to be more vigilant about the residents' whereabouts. In one facility, where part of the corridor is out of eyesight from the common area, the care staff took the extreme measure of locking residents out of their rooms during the day. They no longer do so, but they and the families are concerned about the potential for unseen falls or other mishaps if no one is in that area. The bedroom hallways at Woodside Place are about 75 feet long; at NewBridge, no room is more than 60 feet from the common area, although the privacy of two of the rooms is compromised by opening onto the common area. It is important to keep hallways as short as possible without losing the privacy the hallway affords.

Open the Household Kitchen to Dining and Gathering Spaces but Allow for Controlled Access into It

The homelike kitchens at Woodside Place were integral to transforming a facility from institutional to residential. Balancing concerns for safety with opportunities they provide for engagement, the kitchen was intended to serve several functions: to make it easy for staff to offer breakfast and snacks to residents when they want to eat, to provide a familiar setting for everyday activities in which the residents can participate or just watch, and to give

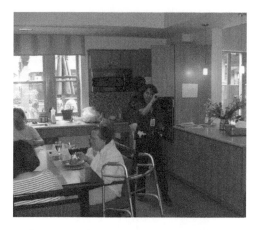

FIGURE 13 Residents at kitchen table (courtesy of Perkins Eastman, 2011).

staff a place to do their work without losing touch with the residents. The kitchens are still used as a place for the household staff to keep records, though they are particularly attentive to maintaining confidentiality.

The household kitchens at Woodside Place continue to be a focal point of resident–staff interaction, where residents help fold laundry and load the dishwasher. At Copper Ridge and William Hill Manor, the care staff has felt it necessary to regulate residents' access to the kitchens. They have eliminated one of the entrances into the kitchen and added a gate at the other. They also increased visibility between the kitchen and dining areas by widening the openings in the walls. At William Hill Manor, sliding doors were installed to close off the kitchen. At NewBridge, the kitchen is central and more open to the dining areas, yet seems to be maintained as the staff's territory. A table in the kitchen, although generally used just by staff, is sometimes occupied by residents or family members who are invited to sit down there (Figure 13). Staff said they remind everyone entering the kitchen to wash their hands but feel that the arrangement is working well. Whether kitchens offer table space, it's a good idea to provide open counters that are low enough for residents to sit at and participate in kitchen activities from the adjacent space.

The design of the household kitchen presents in microcosm many of the overall issues and tensions: supporting residents' independence and dignity while ensuring safe and sanitary conditions, providing for daily activities while recognizing residents' limited functional abilities, creating opportunities for relationship building while facilitating staff's administrative responsibilities, and complying with building and licensing regulations while providing a familiar residential setting for residents and their families. The four facilities offer several examples of household kitchens that are generally successful in addressing these issues, and the variations point out the differences in staffing culture and philosophy.

Provide Several Activity Spaces Open to a Common Circulation Path

An open circulation path is important to linking common spaces, activities, and people together. Each facility offers several loops that residents can walk without getting lost or reaching a frustrating dead end. In the early study of Woodside Place, residents were sometimes observed walking with a staff person, a family member, or other residents, and it was described as "social walking." It was also observed that other residents would regularly sit in the chairs that they had pulled into a row along the path, as if they were "porch sitting" and residents walking by would sometimes greet them. These casual but routine activities were the source of more social interaction than programmed activities. Today, because the residents are older, more impaired, and more frail, there are more residents in chairs, and those who walk are moving more slowly. However, the pattern of circulating through the facility was still observed in all the facilities, although the porch sitting behavior was unique to Woodside Place, where the generous circulation space was designed with room for seating. Family members and staff have observed that the routes residents are walking are generally shorter now.

Openings among the common spaces along the path are integral to the vitality there. At Woodside Place today, we saw the same pattern as we did 20 years ago: residents are most often seated along the circulation path that wraps around three open activity areas: the library and two areas with tables on either side of it (Figure 14). The armchairs have been replaced by larger electrified loungers, which residents occupy for longer times. At NewBridge, residents spend much of the day in the cluster of common spaces near the kitchen. Anyone in the kitchen can look across the counter to the dining and sitting spaces and to the views through the windows beyond. Walking from their bedroom to the dining room, residents at William Hill Manor can look not only into the courtyard, but also into small activity rooms on their way. Staff report that they like the ability to see where residents are and family

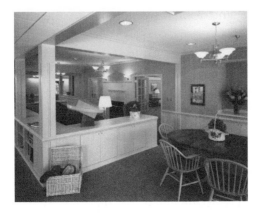

FIGURE 14 Open common spaces (courtesy of Perkins Eastman, 2011).

members like the openness without feeling that everyone has to be in the same place.

One of the important findings is that few common spaces in the facilities are used exclusively for what they were intended. In some instances, rooms are used for compatible multiple purposes, such as a small dining room that is used for staff conferences or a family's jigsaw puzzle. Other spaces have been transformed for new uses, some of which were not considered in the original design: a family dining room turned into a fitness gym or a "quiet" room used for daycare. The use of the building may change if the therapeutic approach (such as engaging residents in small groups) on which it was based is replaced by another approach (large group activities). Ongoing research will continue to introduce new ideas and approaches to dementia care that cannot be anticipated in advance.

Create a Hierarchical Wayfinding System, Including Personalized Cues

In the four facilities we studied, getting lost is more often due to mistaking which household to go to rather than which room to go to. Today, just as 20 years ago, residents are sometimes found in the "right" room in the wrong household. It was noted in the Woodside Place study that residents respond more to personalized than to generic landmarks. That is, a picture or familiar possession is more likely to be useful in orienting a resident than a color or an unfamiliar object, and the more concrete (less abstract) it is, the better. Rooms tend to be personalized and, not surprisingly, are more personalized than common spaces. Perhaps a display cabinet at the entrance to the household could be as useful as the nameplate or memory box at the residents' rooms. Because we now understand that recognition of words and numbers is retained longer than many other kinds of memory (Paque & Warrington, 1995), it would be appropriate to add identification of houses by name and rooms by number to the kinds of cues already offered.

Accommodate Televisions, Computers, and Mobility Devices

Today, it is more likely that families will furnish a resident's room with a television. Some families have indicated that they like having television in a resident's room, and Woodside Place rewired the building to permit television and computer connections in all rooms. Residents' televisions tend to be used when families visit more than at other times. The television in the common den is used occasionally, but particularly by individual residents or families (Figure 15). At Copper Ridge, William Hill Manor, and NewBridge,

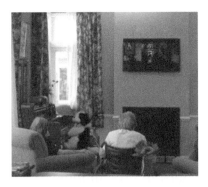

FIGURE 15 Residents watching television (courtesy of Perkins Eastman, 2011).

televisions have been installed in the household living rooms. Televisions need to be located where daylight and glare do not compromise viewing, but also where the sound will not intrude on other people or activities. Although we do not have evidence about their prior lifestyles, it may be that residents today were more accustomed to watching television than those 20 years ago, or it may be that their families simply want them to have amenities.

Newer residents are starting to bring computer skills, and some activity programs use interactive computer games. NewBridge provides a computer station for families. The more prevalent use of computers is by staff, and computer workstations have to be integrated into the facility. In earlier facilities where computers were not planned for, mobile stations for computers and other technologies can become obtrusive features that are out of place in a residential environment and present a "parking" problem. These carts get moved around a lot, and they are often parked in residents' sitting areas or in hallways. They are used too frequently to be put away in closets, but small conveniently located alcoves with outlets and data ports (if not wireless) would perhaps keep the carts out of the way.

More generally, residential facilities have to deal with the kinds of equipment once found only in more institutional settings. The increasing use of walkers and wheelchairs is creating a storage problem. This may involve simple actions like removing chairs from tables, but it also entails factoring in space for parking walkers where they can be conveniently retrieved without the danger of being left in someone's path. Low shelving units can also be storage units for mobility devices.

Provide Spaces for Walking and Exercise

At all the facilities, walking is no longer treated as a pathological behavior but rather as a healthy exercise. Residents are encouraged to walk to help maintain cardiovascular and muscular strength. At Copper Ridge, an activity room facing the courtyard is now a small fitness facility. It is intended to serve all of the residents but was introduced to provide an outlet for the physical energy of the younger residents they have started accepting. NewBridge on the Charles offers an individualized fitness program for residents, including those in the skilled nursing center. With the increasing understanding of the interaction between cognitive and physical health, fitness facilities are more likely to be built into dementia facilities in the future.

Provide Safe Opportunities to go Outdoors

Access to protected outdoor space has become a widespread practice, providing benefit for health, mood, and social engagement. Most facilities combine different types of spaces, including courtyards, terraces, yards, and balconies. The total areas vary from 2,400 to 27,000 ft^2, which is equivalent to 60 to 450 sf per resident. Even at the smaller end of that range, residents were able to go outdoors and participate in outdoor activities. Although there is sometimes concern over appropriate dress in inclement weather, it is generally understood that residents benefit from the freedom to choose to go outdoors. All of the facilities arrange picnics, gardening, and other events outdoors. Sheltered space makes such activities more pleasant and more likely to occur. With the help of generous donations, Woodside Place has added a large gazebo, a canopy, and a lot of outdoor furniture. Copper Ridge holds many events in the courtyard at umbrella tables and recently installed soft paving. NewBridge, which occupies two floors, offers residents both an enclosed yard and a screened-in balcony (Figure 16).

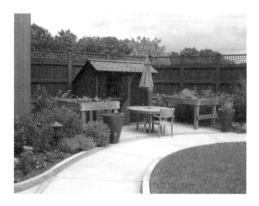

FIGURE 16 Residents' outdoor space (courtesy of Perkins Eastman, 2011).

Create Quiet and Cheerful Interiors

All of the four facilities offer carpeted living areas and hallways, wood trim, upholstered furniture, lamps, and artwork. Many of the spaces are also naturally lit through the large windows. The ambience is residential. NewBridge is furnished in a contemporary style, whereas the other three are traditional. People respond positively to both; it seems they are less concerned with style than with warm colors and soft materials. Strong contrasts are avoided. Several family members and staff remarked that they enjoyed the sense of calm that they usually feel in their facility. Residents are generally sitting quietly, walking, or participating in an activity.

Materials for interior flooring and exterior paving have improved during the past 20 years. Woodside Place was unusual in providing wood-look vinyl flooring in residents' rooms and in common dining rooms. At the time, carpeting was considered disadvantageous because of the difficulty in keeping it clean. Solution-dying and improved filaments have made carpeting more resistant to odor and stains. Because it is softer and quieter, carpeting has been used more extensively at William Hill Manor and NewBridge.

The soft residential lighting and domestic color palette at Woodside Place distinguished it from institutional settings and were noticed favorably by families and visitors. However, 20 years later, the blue and mauve color theme in the common area is seen as somewhat dated and too restrictive for redecorating. It is also felt that the colors made the interiors dimmer and less cheerful than they should be. Recently, the walls have been lightened to ivory with new wallcoverings and paint. Residents' rooms, which were also blue, are being re-painted off-white as they are vacated to give families an opportunity to personalize the rooms with residents' preferred colors.

In contrast to the strong ceiling lights of nursing homes, Woodside Place has soft lighting, often indirect. Lamps provide residential lighting. Care was taken not to over-light the spaces, and, particularly at that time, the substitution of fluorescent for incandescent lamps often led to less light. According to the administrator there, many people find the lighting, particularly in the non-daylit spaces, a little dim, so they are in the process of increasing light levels in some areas, such as the bedroom hallways. At William Hill Manor, the windows, especially those looking into the courtyard, bring abundant daylight into the interiors. There is a variety of soft colors, but they are generally light in value. The lighting is considered sufficient. Similarly at NewBridge, where the color palette is somewhat richer and the colors a little deeper in tone, the daylight and the artificial lighting provide enough light to be satisfactory. Options in lighting levels should be provided with a variety of sources and, if possible, dimmable fixtures.

The furniture today is in some ways better designed for seniors in the durability and cleanability of fabrics and configuration of armrests and legs. What has added a challenge to the design of the interiors is the introduction of large lounge chairs or recliners that occupy more space than the furniture 20 years ago. They can dramatically change the scale of a room, as well as limit its use, because they are not only big but heavy. At NewBridge, staff felt that the large dining tables inhibited flexibility and their ability to adapt to residents' different meal schedules and preferences. They would like small tables that could be either placed together as a single large table or kept separate. In general, furniture should be selected not only for its durability, but also for its flexibility.

Allow for the Integration of Outreach Services

The role of the dementia care facility is evolving to encompass services such as daycare, respite, assessment, and education. Two years after opening, Woodside Place introduced a daycare program, a major change that was made possible by using space that was not needed for the residential program. To meet licensing requirements, the daycare program was required to have a separate area that could be closed off from the rest of the building. Doors were added to the corridor just past the entry to Star House, and what had originally been the Oasis Room and the Music Room were opened to each other and became the daycare space. The daycare program, which continues today, serves up to 13 individuals per day. In practice, the daycare participants mingle with the residents and participate in activities together. It has been beneficial for the daycare participants in providing high-quality care and programming. Conversely, the higher-functioning daycare participants bring greater engagement and help the permanent residents take part in more of Woodside Place's life. It also has turned into a good "feeder" for the residential program: about three people a year have been admitted as residents. This development, which had not been anticipated in designing the building, was made possible by the size of the building and the multiple activity spaces that had been built in.

The Copper Ridge Institute, which arose out of EMA's partnership with Johns Hopkins, provides assessment, as well as research and education, at both Copper Ridge and William Hill Manor. The assessment clinic serves the larger community. Recently, at William Hill Manor the program was expanded to provide a 2-week extended stay, during which time an individual is not only evaluated with standard assessment tools, but also observed in a setting of everyday activities with other people. The extended assessments are limited to openings in the facility between full-time residents, so occur on an irregular basis.

Design for Resilience

We have noted some of the ways in which these facilities have changed and the many reasons for those changes. If only because approaches to dementia care are evolving, it is important for a dementia care facility to be adaptable. If the design is a highly specific response to a program or an extensive and detailed collaborative process, the facility may be so tightly fit to one particular approach that it is not resilient enough to adapt to changes over time. This retrospective suggests several general strategies. Private bedrooms with bathrooms are a good "chassis" for the building. Structural blocking for grab bars and lifts, as well as conduits for future wiring, can save money later. In terms of priorities, several smaller activity rooms are likely to provide more versatility than one large one, and "habitable" circulation spaces can provide even more advantageous social settings than an activity room. In general, a facility that is a little more generous spatially will probably offer more resilience over time. Woodside Place, which has been successfully adapted to new uses, new programs, and a changing population, was built for 36 residents at a net area of 600 ft^2 per resident.[7]

THE WOODSIDE PLACE MODEL TODAY AND IN THE FUTURE

Many of the ideas pioneered in Woodside Place have become familiar features not only in dementia care facilities, but also in a broad range of senior living environments, particularly in the many assisted-living buildings that were developed in the 1990s (Regnier, Hamilton, & Yatabe, 1995). Mild cognitive impairment is common in such facilities, and features that provide memory support through enriching the environment, rather than sterilizing or institutionalizing it, are attractive to residents, families, and providers, especially if such supports can help delay the need for higher-acuity care. Private rooms or suites, good toileting and grooming cues, personalized entrances, common spaces that are intimate in scale yet open and visible, and even details like plate shelves have become standard. Designing for people with dementia or with other disabilities has often led to innovations that eventually improve the quality of life for people in general (Schwarz & Brent, 1999).

Today, thousands of older people with dementia are experiencing a better quality of life in dementia care facilities or memory support units that provide resident-centered care (Milke, Beck, & Danes, 2006). Through the Pioneer Network, the Eden Alternative, and the small house movement, an increasing—although still relatively small—number of nursing homes has adopted the same principles and in some cases have adapted their philosophy of care, as well as their physical facilities, to reflect the principles of models such as Woodside Place.

At the time the Woodside Place model was being developed, we were also seeing the beginnings of a trend away from institutional care. Americans, who continue to envision growing old at home as their best future, tend to see nursing home care as a last resort. The cost of long-term care is, on average, more than $70,000 per year (Genworth Financial, 2011). Although residential dementia care programs have been shown to be more cost-effective than comparable care in a nursing home, monthly fees of $4,000 to $7,000 are unaffordable for most families. On the other hand, the limited number of specialized facilities that provide high-quality dementia care at lower costs is also a factor. Similarly, shifts in healthcare policy from insti-tutional to community-based care have contributed to the trend (O'Brian & Elias, 2004). With diminishing reimbursements from public sources, the cost of such care is out of reach for most people. The effect of these trends is multiplied by the projected growth of the elderly population over the next 30 years. For all of these reasons, even the small-scale alternatives to institutional care such as Woodside Place will not answer the need for dementia care.

A large and increasing percentage of older individuals with dementia are living at home and receiving community-based care services. Today, infor-mal caregivers—spouses and other family members, which number approxi-mately 15 million in the United States—provide an estimated 17 billion hours of care annually for individuals with Alzheimer's disease. The Alzheimer's Association (2011) estimated the value of that care in 2010 totaled more than $202 billion. Between 2006 and 2016, the increase in home care is expected to create a demand for 1 million new direct care workers.[8] Although limiting out-of-pocket expense, the costs of informal care are paid in other ways. The stresses on dementia caregivers will result in $7.9 billion higher annual health care costs for caregivers during the current year, according to 2011 Alzheimer's Disease Facts and Figures (Alzheimer's Association, 2011).

The principles of Woodside Place are now guiding the design of facilities that take the original intentions further in a new generation of community-based dementia care. The House for Betty and Marian's House both address the shift toward in-home and community-based care for dementia.

The House for Betty is a prototype created by Perkins Eastman that rein-tegrates the design concepts of the household model back into the design of the single-family house to support aging-in-place. It would let a person with dementia continue to live at home with a spouse or caregiver instead of moving into a care facility. The freestanding two-bedroom house, which is designed to fit into a cluster of cottages on the campus of a retirement community or on a suburban neighborhood street, provides a secure and supportive environment for a person from early- through middle-stage cog-nitive decline. The caregiver or spouse is also relieved of the anxieties of trying to protect that person from the hazards that eventually make it impos-sible to keep him or her at home. The house is intended to be altered over time to meet increased care needs. A vestibule with a double set of locking doors, built-in display shelves for landmarks, a dutch door to a protected garden, strategically varied lighting, convenient bathrooms, and appropriate interior materials all contribute to a familiar and comfortable home while quietly serving important prosthetic functions (Figure 17).

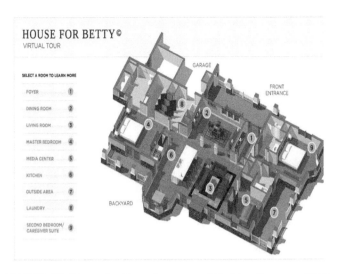

FIGURE 17 House for Betty (courtesy of Perkins Eastman, 2011).

Some of the features familiar from the Woodside Place model are its small-scale rooms, the visible activity areas, the abundance of controlled daylight, the looped walking paths, soft materials to reduce distracting sounds, open wardrobe and glass-faced cabinets, connections to a secure outdoor space, unobtrusive doors, alarm, lockable doors and drains, and its adaptability to mobility devices. The first built example of the House for Betty is in planning in partnership with Asbury Communities, Inc., the Alzheimer's Association, and Leading Age (Figure 18).

Marian's House is a project of Jewish Senior Life of Rochester, New York. It is a small free-standing residential building that combines a daycare facility with an apartment for a resident caretaker (Figure 19). It is envisioned as a facility that will provide a day program for a population of up to 20 adults with early- to mid-stage dementia, as well as occasional respite care and community education. The 5,400 ft^2 building has a residential common area, including kitchen, dining, and sitting spaces for the daycare program. In addition, in a part of the building that can be closed off are two respite bedrooms and the one-bedroom caretaker's apartment. The common space has the key features of the Woodside Place model: an open arrangement of small-group settings that support active engagement in a variety of everyday activities, continuous circulation paths, access to a porch and secure outdoor yard, visibility throughout, display shelves, and exits that are tucked out of sight. This is similar to the area in Woodside Place where residents spend most of their waking time. With a commitment to individualized attention and respect, Marian's House offers the potential for residents and their families to enjoy most of the benefits of a residential care facility at far less cost.

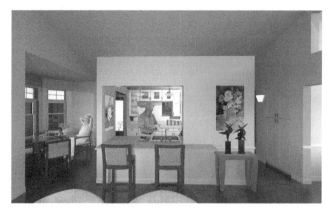

FIGURE 18 House for Betty interior (courtesy of Perkins Eastman, 2011).

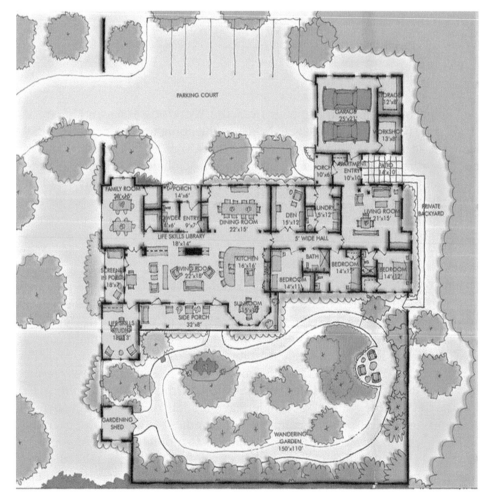

FIGURE 19 Marian's House plan (courtesy of Perkins Eastman, 2011).

Because both of these projects are in the planning stage, they can only suggest prospectively what the next generation of dementia care facilities may offer. It will be important to see how they work once they are built and to share the lessons learned. Customized houses and local day care facilities may provide affordable options that extend people's connectedness to their families, enable them to continue living in familiar environments, and have the care they need without exhausting their families or their means. As next steps toward fulfilling these goals, these prototypes would be new ways of accomplishing what Woodside Place set out to do 20 years ago. Woodside Place and its successors provide their most important lessons not as facilities to be replicated but as innovative ideas that give rise to new interpretations and adaptations as new challenges arise.

NOTES

1. For more information, see Silverman et al. (1995)

2. See Lacey (1999). The average use of restraints in nursing homes was 40%; in individual instances the use was as high as 80%. OBRA was established in 1987 to address, among other issues, the overuse of restraints and inconsistent quality of care in nursing facilities.

3. http://www.alz.org/research/science/alzheimers_disease_causes.asp

4. Similarly, although not the focus of this article, a well-designed building should also limit facility operating costs through resource and energy conserving strategies.

5. The Health Insurance Portability and Accountability Act of 1996 provides federal protection for personal health information, including limits on access to workstations, files, and electronic media. See http://www.hhs.gov/ocr/privacy/hipaa/understanding.

6. Area does not include closet or bathroom, but does include window seat.

7. The net area excludes administrative, service, and any other non-resident space. The gross area of the building is 640 ft^2 per resident.

8. www.phinational.org PHI Facts Number 1.

REFERENCES

Alzheimer's Association. (2011). 2011 Alzheimer's disease facts and figures. *Alzheimer's & Dementia, 7*(2), 208–244.

Brawley, E. C. (2006). *Design innovations for aging and alzheimer's*. New York, NY: John Wiley & Sons.

Camp, C. (2006, November 30). Paper presented at the Neuroscience of Facilities for the Aging and People with Alzheimer's. Academy of Neuroscience for Architecture and the American Institute of Architects, Washington, DC.

Cohen, U., & Day, K. (1993). *Contemporary environments for people with dementia*. Baltimore, MD: Johns Hopkins Press.

Genworth Financial. (2011). 2011 cost of care survey. Retrieved from http://www.genworth.com

Hopper, T., Bayles, K. A., & Kim, E. (2001). Retained neuropsychological abilities of individuals with alzheimer's disease. *Seminars in Speech and Language, 22*, 261–273.

Lacey, D. (1999). The evolution of care: A 100-year history of institutionalization of people with alzheimer's disease. *Journal of Gerontological Social Work, 31*, 101–131.

Milke, D. L., Beck, C. H. M., & Danes, S. (2006). Meeting the needs in continuing care of facility-based residents diagnosed with dementia: Comparison of ratings by families, direct care staff, and other staff. *The Journal of Applied Gerontology, 25*, 103–119.

Milke, D. L., Beck, C. H. M., & Ledewitz, S. (1999). A five-site comparison of care settings built on the 'Woodside Place model': An evaluation of resident needs and outcomes and their relationship to physical features, staffing, and programming. *Capital Care Group Technical Report.*

O'Brian, E., & Elias, R. (2004). *Medicaid and long-term care.* Retrieved from http://www.kff.org/medicaid/loader.cfm?url=/commonspot/security/getfile.cfm&PageID=36296

Paque, L., & Warrington, E. (1995). A longitudinal study of reading ability in patients suffering from dementia. *Journal of the International Neuropsychological Society, 1*, 517–524.

Penninx, B. W., van Tilburg, T., Kriegsman, D., Deeg, D., Boeke, J. P., & van Eljk, J. (1997) Effects of social support and personal coping resources on mortality in older age: The longitudinal aging study Amsterdam. *American Journal of Epidemiology, 146*, 510–519.

Regnier, V., Hamilton, J., & Yatabe, S. (1995). *Assisted living for the aged and frail.* New York, NY: Columbia University Press.

Schwarz, B., & Brent, R. (1999). *Aging, autonomy, and architecture: Advances in assisted living.* Baltimore, MD: Johns Hopkins University Press.

Silverman, M., Ricci, E., Saxton, J., Ledewitz, S. D., McAllister, C., & Keane, C. (1995). *Woodside Place: The first three years of a residential Alzheimer's facility.* Oakmont, PA: Presbyterian Association on Aging.

Ullman, S. G. (1984). Cost analysis and facility reimbursement in the long-term health care industry. *Health Services Research, 19*, 83–102.

PART V: INTO THE LIGHT: POPULATIONS AND TOPICS DESERVING MORE ATTENTION

Understudied Older Populations and Settings in Environmental Gerontology: Candidates for Future Research

RICK J. SCHEIDT

School of Family Studies and Human Services, Kansas State University, Manhattan, Kansas, USA

CAROLYN NORRIS-BAKER

Center on Aging, Kansas State University, Manhattan, Kansas, USA

Environmental gerontologists from several disciplines focus on an overarching primary goal: to discover and apply information about person–environment transactions to produce more sanguine relationships between older adults and the environments they inhabit. As we move into the second decade of the 21st century, it is appropriate to conduct a roll-call of populations of older individuals who deserve but have not yet received adequate empirical attention. The purpose of this paper is two-fold. First, we contrast benefits derived from an environmental gerontology of the usual with those associated from conducting research on understudied populations and their environmental contexts. We also offer reasons that may explain why environmental gerontology has not placed the study of these older individuals and settings more prominently on the empirical radar screen. Second, we present two understudied subpopulations of elders living in voluntarily and involuntarily selected environments—older male and female prisoners and older residents of declining and dying small rural towns. We provide some examples of issues and research questions of potential relevance to environmental gerontologists who may be interested in entering each of these venues.

269

USUAL PROBLEMS, POPULATIONS, AND SETTINGS

Across the past half century, environmental gerontologists from several disciplines have focused on an overarching primary goal—to discover and apply information about person–environment transactions to produce more sanguine relations between older adults and the environments they inhabit (Scheidt & Windley, 2006).

As this Special Issue of JHE illustrates, there is new and exciting work occurring on several fronts in the ecology of aging. This progress has been based on data drawn from older populations with environmentally related problems associated with primary and secondary aging. Much of our data collection has been guided by nomothetic values or what might be called central tendency criteria; that is, we have targeted our research efforts at the adaptive challenges posed by more typical problems experienced by more usual populations of older adults who reside in more representative environmental conditions. Thus, because many elders express a strong desire to age-in-place and spend the majority of their time in their residences, a focus on housing or the near-environment is vital and has prompted considerable research and policy attention on housing for the elderly, home modification programs, place meaning, and place attachment (Scheidt & Schwarz, 2010).

We have developed problem-oriented criteria defining elders who exhibit health-related functional declines that lower the quality of life. We have developed comparable criteria that define supportive and more potentially harmful environmental features associated with these conditions. Here, problem-guided person–environment concerns have naturally led many disciplines to focus on more highly visible special populations of vulnerable elders, such as those who reside in long-term care settings.

BENEFITS OF STUDYING THE UNDERSTUDIED

It is fitting that an environmental gerontology of "the usual" should capture the lion's share of attention and resources. However, we believe there are definite benefits that may result from research with populations of elders who do not live beneath the taller peaks of the frequency distribution of environmentally associated need but rather at the margins. First and most obvious, a direct focus on these rarely studied populations may generate findings useful for improving the quality of their lives. Many would agree with the moral position that attainment and maintenance of health is a basic human right and that social conditions that produce inequities among groups of people violate this premise and deserve to be redressed (De Negri Filho, 2008). Second, we may find that this research on understudied populations may broaden and solidify the base of science on environmental gerontology. Purposive focus on less studied populations of elders may allow us to test the range of applicability of our theories and models. Critical case studies drawn from understudied populations may tell us much about the range of generalizability of our long-held theoretical assumptions (Flyvbjerg, 2001). Using only one arena of research (e.g., that of subjective well-being), what might research on these populations tell us about the functionality of disjunctures among conditions that produce "the good life" (i.e., psychological well-being, perceived quality of life, behavioral competence, and the objective environment) (Lawton, 1983) or about how and why social and cultural environmental conditions affect appraisals and set points of facets of subjective well-being (Diener, 2009). Also, as Iwarsson and her colleagues have demonstrated, emergent methods for data collection can be derived from in situ research on critical populations (Iwarsson, 2004).

Similarly, exploring person-environment transactions in understudied settings that seldom are a target for aging-environment research can refine and expand our understanding of the nuances of the transactional frameworks used by much of existing theory in the field (Lawton & Nahemow, 1973; Norris-Baker & Scheidt, 1994; Rowles & Watkins, 2003; Scheidt & Norris-Baker, 1990). Arenas of research include small rural communities at risk, adapting new technologies for experiencing environments for the oldest-old whose sensory abilities are limited, and identifying and meeting diverse cultural needs and expectations of elder in-migrants from different nations.

REASONS WHY SOME OLDER POPULATIONS REMAIN UNDERSTUDIED

Many reasons exist for why understudied older populations retain an excepted status among researchers. Research and policy actions in gerontology are incentivized by resources and values that lead us to select high profile topics and populations that may lead to research over years of study and, not unusual, for entire careers. Research agendas are often set at national levels, where funding opportunities serve as a magnet for both new and established professionals and may push research activity into relevant and long-lasting directions. Some populations of older adults may be viewed as interesting but as presenting fewer critical needs, especially in an era where triage-guided thinking directs limited resources to more deserving targets; conversely, under a triage-type logic, the level of need may be viewed as serious but the absolute numbers of affected individuals may be seen as too low to warrant sustained and wide-spread scrutiny. Older residents in small, rural towns in the heartland of the nation illustrate such a population (Scheidt & Schwarz, 2010). Some populations may be excluded from attention because of the difficulty in clearly defining a parent population; this poses challenges for targeting, accessing, and recruiting sufficiently numerous and representative participants, such as elders who are undocumented aliens who have relocated to the United States to be near family. Other enclaves are ignored due to stigmatization that creates and reinforces a devalued status reflected in both research and popular culture. We believe that older male and female prisoners, despite increases in their numbers, remain understudied among environmental gerontologists largely for this reason. Other groups of elders in need may receive less attention because rapidly changing environmental conditions and complex population composition pose unique challenges for the study of person–environment dynamics. For example, we know little about the meaning of environmental transitions, behavioral adaptation, and sense of place for older in-migrants transitioning into new cultural settings. Conversely, we might find that the emergent populations are tied to the evolution of novel environments populated by "new settlers" who have not yet captured the full imagination of behavioral ecologists. This is illustrated by those older residents of "instant towns" or simulacra (Scheidt, 2007), as well as "avatar elders" who regularly visit and develop a sense of place in virtual environments (Rowles, 2009).

In the article, we offer illustrative candidates of populations and settings that we believe deserve more serious attention within environmental gerontology. We place a brief but suggestive focus on little-studied populations and settings that might benefit directly from research-informed interventions and, at the same time, benefit the field through the research and practice challenges they pose. We can conceptualize these populations and settings in terms of a matrix that considers relocation versus aging in place as one dimension and the involuntary or voluntary aspects of relocation versus aging in place decisions as a continuum along the second dimension, all within the framework of space and time continua. Thus, the older prisoner might be characterized as involuntarily aging in place in a highly restrictive institutional setting, whereas some classic nursing home relocation studies (e.g., Heller, 1982) represent voluntary moves to institutional settings. Understudied groups such as ex-patriots retiring internationally could be classified as voluntarily relocating community dwellers, whereas elder refugees arriving in the United States could represent the involuntary end of this continuum. The extensively studied community dwellers preferring to age in place can be contrasted with the less studied population of small town elders whose inability to sell their home, caregiving obligations, or similar circumstances make their aging in place involuntary. Time, as characterized by cohort membership, is a critical dimension of this framework because the rapidly changing ways of representing and interacting with environments, both actual and virtual, can be expected to effect the young-old and the oldest-old differently.

UNDERSTUDIED POPULATIONS: TWO PRIME CANDIDATES STILL IN THE SHADOWS

Older Prisoners: Persistent and Growing Challenges

Although incarcerated populations present challenges to almost every nation, the United States incarcerates more people than any other country in the world (The Pew Center, 2008). At the end of 2009, more than 1,613,656 prisoners were being held in state and federal prisons and correctional facilities in the United States (Bureau of Justice Statistics, 2010). Approximately 1,500,000 were men and 113,500 were women. Although this represented a slowing rate of growth over 2008, the federal prison population actually showed an increase of 3.4%, whereas the state prison population continued a 3-year trend of declining annual growth rates. As of January 19, 2012, a total of 216,899 inmates were housed in federal facilities. Almost 28,000 of these inmates are housed in 16 privately managed secure facilities, located primarily in Texas, California, and Georgia (Federal Bureau of Prisons, 2012).

In 2009, the male imprisonment rate was 14 times higher than that of females. As of June 2009, Black, non-Hispanic males had incarceration rates 6 times higher than White, non-Hispanic males and almost 3 times higher than Hispanic males. The incarceration rate of Black, non-Hispanic females was 1 in 703 compared with 1 in 1,987 White females and 1 in 1,356 Hispanic females (Bureau of Justice Statistics, 2010).

The Bureau of Justice Statistics (2010) reports that the number of people 55 years or older in state and federal prisons increased 76.9% between 1999 and 2007, whereas the cohort of those 45 to 54 years increased almost 68% (Vera Institute on Justice, 2010). Dramatic increases in the number of older prisons reflects the general aging of society, mandatory minimum sentences, three strike rules, and the fact that prisoners are living longer (Abner, 2006). It is difficult to find specific rationale for chronological or cohort definers of "elderly" used by federal agencies and information gathering organizations. There are a variety of age definers of "old" or "older" for inmates used by different states. The National Commission on Correctional Health Care uses age 55 years as the chronological threshold. The Vera Institute on Justice (2010) maintains that this lower threshold, compared to the U.S. Census Bureau of age 65 years, reflects the accelerated effect of secondary aging processes on physical and mental health of these inmates. These include the hits imposed by pre-prison factors (e.g., substance abuse, lack of access to adequate health care, poverty, and lack of education) as well as confinement-associated factors such as separation from family and friends, the anticipation of living a large part of one's life in prison, the threat of victimization (Vera Institute on Justice, 2010), and adjustment to the culture of the prison environment, or "prisonization" (Aday & Krabill,

2011). Also in 2009, 198,000 (approximately 13% of inmates) were 50 years or older; about 7,000 of these inmates were women 50 years or older (approximately 5% of the older inmate prison population) (Aday & Krabill, 2011). It is estimated that by 2030, inmates 55 years and older will comprise about one third of the U.S. prison population (Enders, Paterniti, & Myers, 2005).

Who is the more usual older prisoner? According to Aday (2003):

> An aging long-termer imprisoned today typically is someone who entered prison as a poor young male, is usually black, and committed a violent crime such as murder or rape. Legally ignorant and undereducated, the defendant is often poorly served by an appointed counsel. At trial, the defendant generally pleaded guilty, was convicted, and was given a life sentence. For years the inmate may have made only a minimal effort to be released. The inmate did his time, worked, and settled into the prison routine. His family now has forgotten him or is unable to help. The only ones who remember are his victims and legal system officials. (p. 119)

Environmental Gerontology and Older Prisoners

Several recent international sources document higher rates of physical disease (particularly infectious diseases) and mental disorders (e.g., depression, post-traumatic stress, and cognitive impairment) among older prisoners compared with their non-institutionalized peers (Baillargeon, 2011; Kingston, Le Mesurier, Yorston, Wardle, & Heath, 2011). Data drawn from many countries show higher rates of suicide within prison, as well as increased mortality from all causes on release (Baillargeon, 2011). These morbidity and mortality outcomes are due to preexisting risk factors and ailments of inmates, as well as impacts due to the direct effects of incarceration.

Environmental gerontologists have a well-established track record attempting to reverse the harmful effects of institutionalization. Although other professional fields have targeted older prisoners, few environment-aging specialists have directly engaged the health-related needs of prisoners, regardless of age. Why? It is possible that, for some professionals, the threshold for involvement may be connected to the social devaluation and stigmatization of this population, reflected and reinforced by attitudes shared in wider popular culture (Tornstam, 2005). Incarceration is designed to remove and restrict opportunities to exercise one's legal and constitutional rights. The total prison milieu—physical, social, psychological, and cultural—is often viewed as deservedly punitive, despite the fact the "right to safety inside prison is constitutionally guaranteed and protected" (Wolff & Shi, 2009, p. 405). Health-related declines may be viewed as justified, judged against a value of "the punishment must be proportional to the crime." The politicization of health derives from disagreements surrounding the core value of health as a basic human right, which often presupposes an ethic that embraces the absolute value of life (De Negri Filho, 2008). If health is a basic human right, it must be accorded unconditionally to prisoners. More active discussion of these issues and how they affect more vigorous study of this and other understudied population is needed.

Environmental gerontologists have played an important role in demonstrating how specific person-environment transactions can aid or inhibit successful or optimal aging among community-based populations. Importantly, in recent years, we have extended these efforts to elderly residents of nursing homes in an attempt to "deinstitutionalize" settings bound by a strict medical model of long-term care (Rahman & Schnelle, 2008). Institutional environments pose obvious challenges if the goal is to extend an absolute model of successful aging (Rowe & Kahn, 1998) into institutional settings. What best outcomes model should guide the work of environmental gerontologists within prison settings? What components of optimal aging are possible to install in environments with higher levels of institutional constraints? What institution-specific metrics should be applied to evaluate the success of such efforts?

At the broadest level, almost all research conducted within prison environments is ecological in nature given the unique context and population. At a more specific level, research conducted in prisons within the environment-behavior perspective has occurred for approximately 50 years but has focused almost exclusively on non-elderly prison populations. For example, Glaser (1972) noted the challenge confronting prison architects in their attempts to achieve an appropriate balance between the goals of rehabilitation and punishment. The development and application of measures of the psychosocial climate of prisons (Ajdukovic, 1990; Moos, 1968; Ross, Diamond, Liebling, & Saylor, 2008) have been actively pursued for more than four decades. At the conceptual level, the General Ecological Model (Lawton & Nahemow, 1973) has been used to describe differences among prison environments, particularly with respect to environmental press. Aday (2003) observed that chronic environmental demands force adaptive responses from prisoners that may grow less effective as losses occur in general health, sensory-motor functions, and cognitive capacities. Physical design issues, crowding, and noise in high-demand environments such as maximum-security prisons designed for younger offenders may exceed the ability of older prisoners to adapt emotionally and physically. Conversely, highly regimented prisons may be under-challenging, producing boredom, sensory deprivation, withdrawal, depression (Aday, 2003), and excess disability (Kahn, 1965), where functional capacity is greater than that warranted by the actual impairment. Aday (2003) noted the major person–environment dialectic that occurs between autonomy and security, where attempts to insure the safety and security of inmates may dangerously affect their sense of autonomy and choice.

Designing an effective balance between autonomy and security in special environments for the elderly is a familiar challenge to behaviorally oriented designers and housing specialists targeting older populations (Golant, 2011; Parmalee & Lawton, 1990). Both environmentally and individually targeted interventions have risen in recent years to meet the needs of the increasing numbers of older prisoners in the United States and abroad. Indeed, although not discussed in these terms, naturally evolving "categorical care" has emerged in recognition of differences in special needs among older prisoners. A recent survey (Sterns, Lax, Sed, Keohane, & Sterns, 2008) of 41 responding states found that most have not created any dedicated facilities for older offenders, which ranged from simply having beds for the old and infirm among general inmate populations to stand-alone, secure medical facilities and hospices. Aday (2003) claimed that many states currently house older prisoners in age-segregated environments (e.g., geriatric facilities and secure nursing homes) based on their distinct needs. This extends to preventative care, chronic care clinics, assisted living units, and hospice programs, as well as to recreational, faith-based, and work opportunity programs. The costs and benefits of these largely age-specific programs continue to be actively debated. Aday and Krabill (2011) reported that removal of older women prisoners from the general prison population increases feelings of safety; it reduces higher demands for activity and exercise and increases more sedentary pursuits. The Federal Bureau of Prisons (2009) reports that "several facilities offer intensive treatment programs" designed to aid female inmates with histories of chronic sexual, emotional, or physical abuse by teaching them strategies to handle victimization, facilitate grieving over lost relationships, and develop positive relationships. A special population module was created to aid training of both civilian and custody staff in the management of geriatric offenders from custody to the end of life (Federal Bureau of Prisons, 2009). From a purely educational standpoint, environmental gerontology would have much to contribute to this type of training mission. Prisons were not designed with older people in mind, evidenced by "the stairs and steps and walkways, the distances, the gates, the football pitches and gymnasia; the serveries and queues; the communal showers, the incessant background noise" (Crawley & Sparks, 2005, p. 350).

Aside from these more familiar applications and discoveries that parallel those within mainstream environment-aging research, prison settings invite applications of environment-behavior models less frequently observed in environmental gerontology. Both chronic and temporary mismatches between individual needs and capacities and environmental demands and resources may require thinking in terms beyond or outside of usual "goodness of fit" models. Kahana (1982) delineated several underutilized congruence models designed to predict health-related outcomes associated with varying degrees of goodness of it between environmental demands and competence attributes of older individuals. In addition to their own classic congruence model, she also posed several other models "for considering the relation-ship of congruence to outcome" (Kahana, 1982, p. 109), where positive and negative personal outcomes might vary with the size and direction of mismatch between personal needs and environmental resources. These include cumulative difference, critical difference, and optimal discrepancy models. Prison environments may be described and predicted best by mod-els that assume person–environment mismatch or incongruence. The efficacy of these models for increasing our ability to understand and modify these environment-behavior outcomes for older prisoners cannot be determined without our empirical involvement. Although congruity models have been used to more effectively guide educational and treatment interventions for juvenile offenders (Brill, 1978), we are currently unaware of efforts to apply person–environment matching models to older prisoner populations.

Despite a paucity of research on older male and female prisoners, there are many research-rich issues that await further study by the many disciplines within environmental gerontology. These include transition into and release from prison life (Crawley & Sparks, 2006), end-of-life medical decisions (Phillips, Allen, Harris, Presnell, DeCoster, & Cavanaugh, 2011), predictors of post-traumatic stress and depression (Maschi, Morgen, Zgoba, Courtney, & Ristow, 2011), predictors of prisoner suicide (Marzano, Hawton, Rivlin, & Fazel, 2011), caregiving behind bars (Williams et al., 2009), age segregation (Kerbs & Jolley, 2009), feelings of safety (Wolff & Shi, 2009), victimization and distress (Hochstetler, Murphy, & Simmons, 2004), environ-mental "niches" that ameliorate stress (Seymour, 1980), ethnic, gender, and cohort differences (Shah, Plugge, & Douglas, 2011), environmental design and environmental modification (Moore, 1989), and health-related attitudes and self-care management (Loeb & Steffensmeier, 2011). Systematic study of the effect of the physical, policy, social milieu, and culture on the mental and physical health of older prisoners deserves high priority. Environmental gerontologists entering the research milieu will find multiple models target-ing factors responsible for "prisonization," the "consequences of exposure to inmate society prisoner" (Aday, 2003, pp. 119–120). Research on prisoner assimilation has modeled the attributes they carry into the environment, the social construction of a meaningful life in prison, and more macro-level background variables such as age, race, socioeconomic status, and criminal history (Aday, 2003). Worth noting, much research on prison populations uses chronological age as an index or proxy variable for processes and conditions that are not directly assessed. Thus, the age variable may carry different meanings across different studies. Environmental gerontologists are perhaps more prepared to unpack these underlying meanings given their age-specific interests in distinguishing between more modifiable secondary aging and less modifiable primary aging influences.

In addition to the opportunities that prison environments offer for more objective measurement-bound environmental assessment and evaluation, there is research-based and anecdotal evidence to indicate that prison environments have much to offer professionals interested in place experience or sense of place (i.e., subjective environmental perceptions and processes). This includes adjustments of self-to-place, as well as re-configuring the meanings of self within prison environments. For example, Rowles and Watkins (2003) suggested that history, habit, heart, and hearth are psychological and behavioral components sequentially applied by community-based elders when converting spaces to places. Are these components necessary or sufficient ingredients in the conversion of spaces to places when entered involuntarily by prisoners? Indeed, longitudinal study of the psychological construction of place would address such a question. Incarceration imposes both sequential (chronos) and within-time (kairos) opportunities to form personal history, as well as habitual regimens. The construction and meaning of place-in-time is an important and appropriate target for future study. Although routine, ritual, and habit may be an anodyne against the fear of the unpredictable or unexpected events within prison, there is evidence that "institutional thoughtlessness" created by over-regimentation of routines, rules, and time-tables (or traditional regimes) can harm prisoners by failing to recognize their health and social care needs (Crawley & Sparks, 2005). Oddly enough, anecdotal evidence indicates that even aversive places may have psychological valences that are positive (Pierson, 2006), as in "the place I love to hate." Leon "Whitey" Thompson, an Alcatraz convict, spent 4 years on Alcatraz Island as a prisoner and, following his release, became a celebrity by voluntarily returning to the former prison to share his views and memories of his prison experience to tourists. The signifiers of home and hearth in this scenario are interesting to consider in terms of place attachment and place dependency.

Behavioral programming and modifications of prison environments must accommodate the specific differences among prisons, their behavioral purposes, level of security (custody requirements), planned programs and services, the profile of the target population, and facility relationships with other parts of the corrections system (e.g., reception and release). The Bureau of Prisons within the U.S. Department of Justice uses five different security levels to confine offenders. Four of these can be located on a security con-tinuum from low to high. Minimum security institutions (or Federal Prison Camps) are work- or program-oriented with dormitory housing and limited to no perimeter fencing. They are often located near larger institutions or close to sites where the inmates can meet their labor demands. Low security Federal Correctional Institutions have double-fenced perimeters, dormitory or cubicle housing, and heavy emphasis on work and program compo-nents. The staff-to-inmate ratio is higher than in minimum security facilities. Medium-security Federal Correctional Institutions have higher security in place, usually use double fences with electronic detection systems, often have cell-type housing, offer both work and program components, and use greater internal controls with a higher staff-to-inmate ratio than the previous facilities. Penitentiaries in the United States are high security institutions, featuring perimeters secured with walls or reinforced fences, multiple- and single-occupant cell housing, the highest staff-to-inmate ratio, and close control and monitoring of inmate movement. Distinguished by their multiple functions, Federal Correctional Complexes locate institutions with different missions and security levels near one another, allowing for the sharing of services, staff training at diverse facilities, and enhanced emergency preparedness. Finally, currently, there is one Secure Female Facility located in West Virginia specifically designed to house female inmates. Programming is designed to promote personal growth and address the unique needs of this population (Federal Bureau of Prisons, 2012). Currently, female offenders are located primarily in Satellite Prison Camps and Administrative facilities, including metropolitan correctional and detention centers. The missions associated with these multiple functions—indeed, the array of environmental variations they encompass—are well-suited to the wide scope of environmental influences and interventions pursued by the multidisciplinary fields in the ecology of aging. For example, community-based studies on elders have shown that older people spend about three-fourths of their daytime in the home and immediate home environment (Oswald & Wahl, 2005). A considerable amount of research documents activity patterns in both accommodating and constant environments across a wide range of housing types and levels of functional ability. How does involuntary confinement in these settings affect adaptive functioning of inmates across these prison types? What contrasts exist between the involuntariness imposed on housebound community elders confined by disability and older prisoners involuntarily confined by incarceration? What might we discover about the strategies that older prisoners use to enhance sense of control in micro-residential spaces? Sixty years of research on the ecology of aging among more "usual" elderly residents provides a deep background of theory, method, and person–environment outcomes that will enrich the way we conduct research on older prisoners.

Finally, we raise one last issue here. Negative connotative and denotative meanings of prison may discourage some professionals from trying to enter this realm of research. Many researchers report little difficulty gaining access to this research venue, although prisoners are a protected population under federal regulations. This means that researchers must have their protocols reviewed and approved initially by an Institutional Review Board, as well as by personnel within federal or state correctional facilities. Prisoners have a protected status within the Code of Federal Regulations 45CFR46 (2005) under the National Institutes of Health because they may be "under constraints because of their incarceration which could affect their ability to make a truly voluntary and uncoerced decision whether or not to participate as subjects in research" (Code of Federal Regulations 45CFR46, Subpart C46.302). At least one member of the Institutional Review Board must be a prisoner or a prisoner representative with appropriate experience and background. In addition, an Institutional Review Board may approve a research protocol with prisoners provided that: (1) the advantages of participation are not of such a magnitude that his or her ability to weigh the risks of the research against the value of such advantages in the limited choice environment is impaired; (2) the risks are commensurate with risks that would be accepted by non-prisoner volunteers; (3) information is presented in understandable language; (4) prisoners are informed in advance that participation will have no effect on her or her parole and that adequate assurance exists that parole boards will not take into account a prisoner's participation in the research in making decisions regarding parole; and (5) adequate provision is made for follow-up care, if found necessary, that takes into account the varying lengths of individual prisoners' sentences and for informing the participants of this fact (Code of Federal Regulations 45CFR46, Subpart C46.305).

Research conducted or supported by the Department of Health and Human Services is permitted pursuant to restrictions on the study goals (e.g., causes, effects, and processes of incarceration; prisons as institutional structures; conditions affecting prisoners as a class; and practices and programs intended to improve the health or well-being of the prisoner) that pose no greater than minimal risk to the prisoner participant. Those intending to conduct research with prisoners should become familiar with the conditions for the protection and participation of this population (Code of Federal Regulations 45CFR46, Subpart C46.305).

Older Residents of Small Dying Towns

It is more difficult to provide a demographic profile for the second area on which we will focus—elders who currently reside or have resided in a diverse range of high risk small town settings. These communities include not only those with a chronic shortage of resources (such as the declining Kansas communities in our previous research; Norris-Baker & Scheidt, 2005), but also those experiencing physical threats—the tornadoes, fires, and floods that have struck many rural communities in the recent past, and the changes resulting from some aspects of economic development. In these cases, national statistics are less helpful than the careful selection of specific communities and settings that provide the best crucible for studying a particular research question. Given the relatively uncharted populations and settings discussed here, the research questions outlined below are exemplified with anecdotal illustrations.

Revisiting the small towns described in our earlier research (Norris-Baker & Scheidt, 1994; Scheidt & Norris-Baker, 1990) indicates that they continue to face economic stress and declining and aging populations, having lost from 10% to over 20% of their already few residents in the past decade. Place remaking and compensation for lost residents and settings create ongoing challenges (Scheidt, 2010). A variety of research questions could benefit from studying these settings and their elders at the scale of transitions for the community and for individual elders. In earlier research (Norris-Baker & Scheidt, 2005), we concluded that in terms of community, these elders increasingly "may cling to the meanings of a personal and shared past, remaining attached to and continuing reminiscent relations with places and people that survive only in memory" (p. 292). The long-term costs and consequences of such efforts, combined with those of helping sustain the functioning of what community settings remain, are relatively undocumented. Studying such settings longitudinally provides a basis for further understanding the processes and social capital involved in neighborhood and community place making and remaking, reculturation, and the evolution of community covenants over time. It also allows for the discovery of ways that these settings may shape or fail to shape the behavior and place attachment of in-migrants who may bring social values that differ markedly from those of long-time residents. Such initiatives contrast residents who may be aging-in-place involuntarily with both in-migrants and life-long residents who perceive their place of residence is primarily by choice. For example, life-long residents may support community institutions, such as public schools, even if they experience no direct benefits, whereas many immigrant elders may not be supportive of settings from which they derive no obvious direct benefit (Berkman & Plutzer, 2004).

Scheidt's (2010) documentation of the efforts of the two elderly sisters in Ramona, Kansas, to bring together both kinds of residents through cooperation on agreed on values (welfare of local children and "Redneck Day," a culture-making event) exemplifies the need to better understand these processes and how they may further our understanding of the roles of different types of residents in place-making as culture-making and social integration at the community scale. Another focus for coming together is the immediate threat to many small rural communities of 3,700 Post Office locations in the United States closing by 2015, including those in Ramona and Neosho Falls, Kansas. As discussed in our previous research (Norris-Baker & Scheidt, 2005), the loss of a post office represents not only a loss of the community's place identity, reducing it to a rural neighborhood, but loss of a key setting for social interaction and critical community functions. Older residents have rallied to prevent such a loss in the past, and Ramona is currently meeting to plan their response to the threat. We could expect that this kind of threat would again bring together both older life-long residents and newer in-migrants in ways that could prove instructive for environmental gerontology.

The creation or failure to create material and symbolic legacies for rural elders merits attention at several different scales. Legacy creation is a multifaceted, complex phenomenon, embedded in an individual's culture, which can enable personal contributions to the future (Hunter & Rowles, 2005). However, at times there is no family to accept the material legacy, and elders attempt to find community-based recipients, such as county museums, willing to accept artifacts such as photo albums (Ekerdt & Sergeant, 2006). Hunter and Rowles' (2005) research suggested that although passing on a legacy of personal values might be the most important form of legacy transmission for the majority of their participants, elders without children focused legacy transmission at the community rather than the individual level. This finding appears to fit with the efforts of the Ramona sisters and suggests that further research with samples of elders who have no close ties to younger family members may provide additional insight into the functions of creating cultural place-related legacies.

At a different scale, the natural scenic environments represent a major economic asset for many small rural towns. Those located in areas with scenic beauty and recreational amenities often attract not only tourists, but also in-migrants, especially the third age young-old, seeking retirement in amenity Naturally Occurring Retirement Communities (NORCs). Successfully maintaining and preserving the natural environment may be seen by some rural elders as a form of creating a symbolic legacy of cultural value and material substance. At the same time, these communities are typically experiencing net out-migration and loss of economic viability through resource-related manufacturing and agriculture, leading to efforts to attract economic development, even at the cost of natural amenities. Empirical research has confirmed the relevance of place attachment and meaning for understanding responses to environmental changes such as development proposals, including housing and energy projects (Devine-Wright, 2009, 2011; Stedman, 2002). The effect of the tensions between these conflicting goals, and the roles older residents may play in mitigating or exacerbating such conflicts with small rural communities, could provide greater insights into the community and individual level processes and outcomes related to place making and environmental legacy.

Among the settings ideal for the study of such phenomena are small northern New England towns, where energy-related development issues threaten these scenic resources by the construction of mountain-top wind farms or swaths of high-voltage power lines to transmit energy to distant urban centers. Personal and community efforts to protect the scenic milieu take forms ranging from yard signs to fundraising to media initiatives, testimony before government bodies, and web and Facebook presences. One example can be found in the North Country of New Hampshire. The Northern Pass proposal to construct 180 miles of high-voltage transmission line from Canada through northern New Hampshire has been met with substantial resistance by local residents and environmental groups over the 40 miles of new right-of-ways needed for the project. The northernmost portion of this right-of-way lies in a sparsely populated county with 10 of the 12 communities with 100 to 1,000 residents, declining populations, residents whose median age is higher than the state average, and where incomes and home values are substantially lower than the state median. Although the age and location of residents devoting personal resources to this resistance is not documented, it can be assumed that a meaningful number of them are older residents of the small communities at risk. Their efforts highlight the need to consider the ways in which residents use emerging technologies and more traditional strategies in efforts to sustain place, and the role cohort factors may play in the participation of elders in such initiatives.

A related issue is the effect of efforts to sustain community viability on the daily activities and social networks of elders in such small communities. Does the time invested in activism, whether to preserve a post office or prevent environmental degradation, mean they are learning new technologies that enable them to increase interactions not only with neighbors but with distant family or that they have less time for social interactions in general or less time to contribute to volunteering for other projects in their community or for creative pursuits? With initiatives such as Northern Pass, whose timeline extends for many years, the cumulative effects of such efforts could have important consequences for health and well-being, as well as social networks.

At the same time, other residents view the Northern Pass initiative as helpful economic development for the region, which also can lead to the sale of property for substantial profits. For some residents, being able to sell a homestead or small business and relocate from the community where they might otherwise be forced to live out their lives as involuntary aging-in-place residents could be a positive outcome of such development. For example, Northern Pass officials recently purchased a 118-acre family campground near the Canadian border. According to the former owner's attorney, the $2,300,000 purchase price for the land with an assessed value of $653,300 allowed the owner, whose father started the campground in the 1960s, to retire (Timmons, 2011). At the same time, the sale was "celebrated by Franklin officials for its tax benefits, which Northern Pass officials have projected at $4.2 million annually. The campground paid the city about $14,000 a year in taxes" (Timmons, 2011).

The construction of the Kingdom Community Wind Project in the Lowell Mountains of northern Vermont has created a similar year-long controversy involving needed permits, viewshed, wildlife habitat, and stream erosion (Gardner, 2011). Although several residents of Lowell, a town of about 700 residents, apparently approve of the project and even have rallied about 100 people to show their support, some residents in adjacent towns have protested the construction through civil disobedience at the construction site. A 59-year-old member of the Lowell Select Board, who has lived his entire life in this community, said he felt many of the protesters were being selfish because the project will bring tax revenue and potentially additional jobs. The only real downside of the 21 turbines on the ridge line, he said, "is the appearance" and noted that "when his 91-year-old mother was younger, people were opposed to the utility poles and wires that are now everywhere.

'We've accepted it. We don't even notice them anymore,' he said. 'That's what will happen with these wind turbines, eventually'" (Ring, 2011).

Studying the effects of such opposing dynamics within a community or cluster of adjacent communities may provide valuable insights into place identity, possible cohort differences in response to such initiatives, and potentially ways of coming to terms with a changing landscape through culture-making and place therapy (Scheidt & Norris-Baker, 1999).

At a more personal and community scale, the natural disasters of 2011 offer arenas for small town place-related research. As Rowles (2009, p. 8) points out, "If a sense of being in place and well-being is threatened by in situ environmental change, it can be completely disrupted by relocation (Sims, 1994)." Although in most cases relocation involves a combination of involuntary and voluntary factors (Oswald & Rowles, 2007), moving temporarily or permanently following a natural disaster falls at the involuntary anchor of the continuum. Older adults generally have been found to experience more negative effects and have higher mortality and morbidity rates than younger cohorts, but there is limited research on the mental health effects and psychosocial needs for these elders (Tuohy & Stephens, 2012). There is increasing recognition of the need to regard relocation from experiential and life-course perspectives and to understand the processes involved in successfully reestablishing a sense of place after losing a home through relocation (Rowles & Watkins, 2003).

One target region might be small towns in Vermont, which recently suffered the worst floods in 84 years and where approximately 40% of its communities have populations of less than 1,000 residents. Unlike the endemic threat of a tornado for the small communities in Kansas, most small town residents in Vermont had not experienced such a threat of natural disaster in their lifetimes. Older residents who unexpectedly lost their possessions, and in some cases their homes and land as rivers changed course, represent a group worthy of study in terms of not only of the effects on their psychological and physical health, but also the roles of place identity and attachment (Carroll, Morbey, Balogh, & Araoz, 2009; Fullilove, 1996), coping with loss of heirlooms valued for reminiscence, possible archiving and legacy (Hunter & Rowles, 2005; Ekerdt & Sergeant, 2006), and place remaking skills and adaptation (Rowles & Watkins, 2003) in outcomes. In general, these residents were forced to move unexpectedly and involuntarily, whether within their community or to an entirely different location closer to family or with greater resources for aging-in-place. They were abruptly deprived of any sense of security provided by their neighborhood and dwelling, as well as the desired perception that one has choice and control over relocation decisions and the transferring treasured possessions (Oswald & Rowles, 2007). The potential population for study should probably include not only full-time elders who lost homes and possessions, but also the cohort near retirement, whose retirement plans and timing may have been radically effected (Norris, Kaniasty, Conrad, Inman, & Murphy, 2002).[1] If possible, research might also extend to residents of the same age cohort who owned second homes and intended to become in-migrants at retirement.

There is a substantial area of existing research related to the loss of home and possessions and relocation that may inform research questions here (Campbell, 2007/2008, Rowles, Oswald, & Hunter, 2003; Rubinstein, 1987; Rubinstein & Parmalee, 1992; Tapsell & Tunstall, 2008). Carroll et al. (2009) concluded from previous research and their study of displaced flood victims ages 30–70 years that psychological health effects may be more long-lasting and severe than those on physical health, and the loss of personal possessions may be more devastating than the damage to the dwelling it-self. Those in their study who experienced temporary relocation while their homes were repaired experienced psychological distress not only from the direct damage of the floods to home and possessions, but from disputes with insurance companies and contractors and from a loss of a perceived sense of security, comfort and privacy of home, and concern about being stuck in a repaired home in the future because it could not be sold. By contrast, Tuohy and Stephens' (2012) research on a small group of elders who had experienced devastating floods in New Zealand suggested that they were not necessarily vulnerable victims, but could contribute their life experiences as community social resources to aid recovery and help people come to terms with the flood. For example, one of the community-dwelling elders narrated themes of personal responsibility and self-efficacy, her actions having been facilitated by previously experiencing a flood.

Older residents who experienced sudden disasters like the floods in the Northeast would seem ideal candidates to study some of the questions growing out of the issues raised by Rowles and Watkins (2003), and Rowles (2009):

- Why do some elders develop strong resilience for place-making as part of the relocation process, whereas for others relocation is linked to crisis and negative outcomes, and what happens if place making fails?
- What skills do experienced place-makers use in recreating abandoned spaces, especially when many if not all familiar possessions are missing?
- How are social strategies used by experienced place-makers employed when an entire community may be disrupted? Are new technologies used for communication?
- What role does time play in these processes, and what time frame should be used to evaluate outcomes?
- Are there significant cohort differences in the processes and degrees of success with which they transform new spaces into places?

Another area of logical investigation is the role of locus of control in such outcomes because the flash flooding would typically be perceived as an event beyond one's control but the ways in which one handled the outcomes could influence both physical and mental health outcomes. Using the life-course model of environmental experience (Rowles & Watkins, 2003) could provide valuable insights into the role of previous events and adjustments in coping with the loss of home and possessions through unexpected natural disasters. It is critical that such research extend longitudinally to document longer term outcomes and to explore ways in which the experiences of such place loss shape future place-making and place attachment. Tuohy and Stephens (2012) noted that the narratives they obtained may not only be an effective way of studying the outcomes of such losses, but also could potentially provide a therapeutic tool, creating meaning, facilitating the interpretation of the self in terms of past experiences, and sharing what one has learned with others.

A final area of exploration within the context of small rural communities is that of seasonal migrants, who live in a circle of migration and, for the most part, do not migrate permanently (McHugh & Mings, 1996). Most of these elders probably fall on the voluntary end of the continuum, striking a balance between aging-in-place and relocation. However, for some young-old elders in declining communities, seasonal migration may represent the pragmatic alternative because they are unable to sell a life-long home and move permanently to a more amenity rich locale. Although extensive research has been done on migration decisions and processes (Bradley & Longino, 2009; Cuba, 1991; Cuba & Hummon, 1993; Haas & Serow, 1993; Litwak & Longino, 1987; Longino, 1990, 2006; Watkins, 1999) and more recently on downsizing and household disbandenment processes over time (Ekerdt & Sergeant, 2006; Luborsky, Lysack, & Van Nuil, 2011), rural small town seasonal migrants should be studied longitudinally to explore changes in their place-related experiences as they age. They represent a group of experienced place-makers who have honed their skills over time and should provide valuable insights into the role of the life-course perspective in adaptive place-making. In addition, the ability to contrast the permanent relocation experiences of seasonal migrants with residents of the same communities who age-in-place could help identify critical influences in successful adaptation post relocation to more supportive settings.

CONCLUSION

We have shared our views about two older populations within settings deserving more attention from environmental gerontologists. There are other equally deserving candidates. These include new domains such as virtual reality, including the creation of virtual environments, cultures, and identities by older individuals (Boellstorff, 2008; Rowles, 2009). Improvements in medical technology and the management of associated health problems has produced the first generation of aging individuals with intellectual disabilities and developmental delays (Merrick, Kandel, Lotan, Aspler, Fuchs, & Morad, 2010). There is little research on environmentally oriented interventions targeting these adults and their caregivers. As noted above, we believe that migrating and migrant elderly deserve more study, including those who migrate voluntarily and involuntarily. This extends to the effect of chronic migration and its effects on health of temporary residents in transitional environments (de Orca, Garcia, Saenz, & Guillen, 2011). Although more difficult to access, there is little systematic evidence on environmental transactions of elderly illegal immigrants. Although there is an increasing number of studies on homeless elderly (Shibusawa & Padgett, 2009) and aging Native Americans (Jervis, 2010), few deal directly with person–environment interactions. We urge environmental gerontologists to place greater focus on these and other subpopulations deserving of empirical attention. These efforts may enrich the theoretical, methodological, and applied knowledge base of each population and, it is hoped, offer transferable suggestions for intervention models designed to improve the quality of life of elders who live in environments that pose more challenging and unusual demands.

NOTE

1. Identified the 55–65 age cohort to be more vulnerable to disasters than some other age cohorts.

REFERENCES

Abner, C. (2006). *Graying prisons: States face challenges of an aging inmate population.* Retrieved from http://www.csg.org/knowledgecenter/docs/sn0611GrayingPrisons.pdf

Aday, R. (2003). *Aging prisoners: Crisis in American corrections.* Westport, CT: Praeger.

Aday, R., & Krabill, J. (2011). *Women aging in prison: A neglected population in the correctional system.* Boulder, CO: Lynne Rienner Publishers.

Ajdukovic, D. (1990). Psychosocial climate in correctional institutions: Which attributes describe it? *Environment and Behavior, 22,* 420–432.

Baillargeon, F. (2011). The health of prisoners. *Lancet, 377,* 956–965.

Boellstorff, T. (2008). *Coming of age in Second Life: An anthropologist explores the virtually human.* Princeton, NJ: Princeton University Press.

Bradley, D., & Longino, C. (2009). Geographic mobility and aging in place. In P. Uhlenberg (Ed.), *International handbook of population aging* (pp. 319–339). Dordrecht, The Netherlands: Springer Netherlands.

Berkman, M., & Plutzer, E. (2004). Gray peril or loyal support? The effects of the elderly on educational expenditures. *Social Science Quarterly, 85,* 1178–1192.

Bureau of Justice Statistics. (2010). *Prisoners at yearend 2009: Advance counts.* Retrieved from http://www.pewcenteronthestates.org/report_detail.aspx?id= 35904

Campbell, C. (2007/2008). On belonging and belongings: Older adults, Katrina, and lessons learned. *Generations, 31*(4), 75–79.

Carroll, B., Morbey, H., Balogh, R., & Araoz, G. (2009). Flooded homes, broken bonds, the meaning of home, psychological processes and their impact on psychological health in a disaster. *Health and Place, 15,* 540–547.

Code of Federal Regulations 45CFR46. (2005). *National Institutes of Health, Office of Human Subjects Research.* Retrieved from http://ohsr.od.nih.gov/ guidelines/45cfr46.html

Crawley, E., & Sparks, R. (2005). Hidden injuries? Researching the experiences of older men in English prisons. *The Howard Journal, 44,* 345–356.

Crawley, E., & Sparks, R. (2006). Is there life after imprisonment? How elderly men talk about imprisonment and release. *Criminology and Criminal Justice, 6*(1), 63–80.

Cuba, L. (1991). Models of migration decision making reexamined: The destination search of older migrants to Cape Cod. *The Gerontologist, 13,* 63–67.

Cuba, L., & Hummon, D. (1993). A place to call home: Identification with dwelling, community and region. *Sociology Quarterly, 34,* 111–131.

de Orca, V., Garcia, T., Saenz, R., & Guillen, J. (2011). The linkage of life course, migration, health, and aging: Health in adults and elderly Mexican migrants. *Journal of Aging and Health, 23,* 1116–1140.

De Negri Filho. (2008). A human rights approach to quality of life and health: Applications to public health programming. *Health and Human Rights, 10*(1). Retrieved from http://www.hhrjournal.org/index.php/hhr/article/view/29/95

Devine-Wright, P. (2009). Rethinking NIMBYism: The role of place attachment and place identity in explaining place-protective action. *Journal of Community and Applied Social Psychology, 19,* 426–441.

Devine-Wright, P. (2011). Place attachment and public acceptance of renewable energy: A tidal energy case study. *Journal of Environmental Psychology, 31,* 336–343.

Diener, E. (2009). Assessing subjective well-being: Progress and opportunities. New York, NY: Springer.

Ekerdt, D., & Sergeant, J. (2006). Family things: Attending the household disbandment of older adults. *Journal of Aging Studies, 20,* 193–205.

Enders, R., Paterniti, D., & Myers, F. (2005). An approach to develop effective health care decision making for women in prison. *Journal of Palliative Medicine, 8,* 432–439.

Federal Bureau of Prisons. (2009). *State of the bureau 2009: The bureau's core values.* Retrieved from http://www.bop.gov/news/PDFs/sob09.pdf

Federal Bureau of Prisons. (2012). *Prison types and general information.* Retrieved from http://www.bop.gov/locations/institutions/index.jsp

Flyvbjerg, B. (2001). *Making social science matter: Why social inquiry fails and how it can succeed again.* New York, NY: Cambridge University Press.

Fullilove, M. (1996). Psychiatric implications of displacement. Contributions from the psychology of place. *American Journal of Psychiatry, 153,* 1516.

Gardner, T. (2011, December 28). Year in review: Embezzlement story headlines year's news. *The Hardwick Gazette, 122*, 1, 5, 7–9, 12–14.

Golant, S. M. (2011). The changing residential environments of older people. In R. H. Binstock & L. K. George (Eds.), *Handbook of aging and the social sciences (7th ed.,* pp. 207–220). New York, NY: Academic Press.

Glaser, D. (1972). Architectural factors in isolation promotion in prisons. In J. Wohlwill & D. Carson (Eds.), *Environment and the social sciences: Perspectives and applications* (pp. 105–113). Washington, DC: American Psychological Association.

Haas, W., & Scrow, W. (1993). Amenity retirement migration process: A model and preliminary evidence. *The Gerontologist, 33*, 212–220.

Heller, T. (1982). The effects of involuntary residential relocation: A review. *American Journal of Community Psychology, 10*, 471–492.

Hochstetler, A., Murphy, D., & Simons, R. (2004). Damaged goods: Exploring predictors of distress in prison inmates. *Crime & Delinquency, 50*(3), 436–457.

Hunter, E., & Rowles, R. (2005). Leaving a legacy: Toward a typology. *Journal of Aging Studies, 19*, 327–348.

Iwarsson, S. (2004). Assessing the fit between older people and their physical home environments: An occupational therapy research perspective. In H. W. Wahl, R. Scheidt, & P. Windley (Eds.), *Annual review of gerontology and geriatrics (Vol. 23, 2003): Focus on aging in contexts: Socio-physical environments* (pp. 85–109). New York, NY: Springer.

Jervis, L. (2010). Aging, health, and the indigenous people of North America. *Journal of Cross-Cultural Gerontology, 25*, 299–301.

Kahana, E. (1982). A congruence model of person-environment interaction. In M. Powell Lawton, P. G. Windley, & T. O. Byerts (Eds.), *Aging and the environment: Theoretical approaches* (pp. 97–121). New York, NY: Springer.

Kahn, R. S. (1965). *Comments. Proceedings of the York House Institute on the mentally impaired aged.* Philadelphia, PA: Philadelphia Geriatric Center.

Kerbs, J., & Jolley, J. (2009). A commentary on age segregation for older prisoners: Philosophical and pragmatic considerations for correctional systems. *Criminal Justice Review, 34*, 119–139.

Kingston, P., Le Mesurier, N., Yorston, G., Wardle, S., & Heath, L. (2011). Psychiatric morbidity in older prisoners: Unrecognized and undertreated. *International Psychogeriatrics, 23*, 1354–1360.

Lawton, M. P. (1983). Environment and other determinants of well-being in older people. *The Gerontologist, 23*, 349–357.

Lawton, M. P., & Nahemow, L. (1973). Ecology and the aging process. In C. Eisdorfer & M. P. Lawton (Eds.), *Psychology of adult development and aging* (pp. 619–674). Washington, DC: American Psychological Association.

Litwak, E., & Longino, C. (1987). Migration patterns among the elderly: A developmental perspective. *The Gerontologist, 27*, 266–272.

Loeb, S., & Steffensmeier, D. (2011). Older inmates' pursuit of good health. *Research in Gerontological Nursing, 4*, 185–194.

Longino, C. (1990). Retirement migration streams: Trends and implications for North Carolina communities. *Journal of Applied Gerontology, 9*, 393–404.

Longino, C. (2006). *Retirement migration in America* (2nd ed.). Houston, TX: Vacation Publications.

Luborsky, M., Lysack, C., & Van Nuil, J. (2011). Refashioning one's place in time: Stories of household downsizing. *Journal of Aging Studies, 25*, 243–252.

Marzano, L., Hawton, K., Rivlin, A., & Fazel, S. (2011). Psychosocial influences on prisoner suicide: A case-control study of near-lethal self-harm in women prisoners. *Social Science & Medicine, 72*, 874–883.

Maschi, T., Morgen, K., Zgoba, K., Courtney, D., & Ristow, J. (2011). Age, cumulative trauma and stressful life events, and post-traumatic stress symptoms among older adults in prison: Do subjective impressions matter? *The Gerontologist, 51*, 675–686.

McHugh, K., & Mings, R. (1996). The circle of migration: Attachment to place in aging. *Annals of the Association of American Geographers, 83*, 530–550.

Merrick, J., Kandel, I., Lotan, M., Aspler, S., Fuchs, B., & Morad, M. (2010). Aging with intellectual disability. Current health issues. *International Journal on Disability and Human Development, 9*, 245–251.

Moore, E. O. (1989). Prison environments and their impact on older citizens. *Journal of Offender Counseling, Services and Rehabilitation, 13*, 175–191.

Moos, R. (1968). The assessment of the social climates of correctional institutions. *Journal of Research in Crime and Delinquency, 5*, 173–188.

Norris, F., Kaniasty, K., Conrad, M., Inman, G., & Murphy, A. (2002). Placing age differences in cultural context: A comparison of the effects of PTSD after disasters in the United States, Mexico, and Poland. *Journal of Clinical Geropsychology, 8*, 153–173.

Norris-Baker, C., & Scheidt, R.J. (1994). From "Our Town" to "Ghost Town?" The changing context of home for rural elderly. *International Journal of Aging and Human Development, 38*, 99–120.

Norris-Baker, C., & Scheidt, R.J. (2005). On community as home: Places that endure in rural Kansas. In G. Rowles & H. Chaudhury (Eds.), *Home and identity in later life: International perspectives* (pp. 279–296). New York, NY: Springer.

Oswald, F., & Wahl, H.-W. (2005). Dimensions of the meaning of home in later life. In G. D. Rowles & H. Chaudhury (Eds.), *Home and identity in later life: International perspectives* (pp. 21–46). New York, NY: Springer.

Oswald, F., & Rowles, G. (2007). Beyond the relocation trauma in old age: New trends in elders residential decisions. In H. Wahl, C. Tesch-Romer, & A. Hoff (Eds.), *New dynamics in old age: Individual, environmental, and societal perspectives* (pp. 127–152). Amityville, NY: Baywood.

Parmalee, P. A., & Lawton, M.P. (1990). The design of special environments for the aged. In J. Birren & K. W. Schaie (Eds.), *Handbook of the psychology of aging* (3rd ed., pp. 464–488). New York, NY: Academic Press.

Phillips, L., Allen, R., Harris, G., Presnell, A., DeCoster, J., & Cavanaugh, R. (2011). Aging prisoners' treatment selection: Does prospect theory enhance understanding of end-of-life medical decisions. *The Gerontologist, 51*(5), 663–674.

Rahman, A., & Schnelle, J. (2008). The nursing home culture-change movement: Recent past, present, and future directions for research. *The Gerontologist, 48*, 142–148.

Ring, W. (2011, November 4). Lowell, Vt., leaders, residents support wind farm. *Bloomberg Business Week*. Retrieved from http://www.businessweek.com/ap/financialnews/D9QPUQ880.htm.

Ross, M., Diamond, P., Liebling, A., & Saylor, W. (2008). Measurement of prison social climate: A comparison of an inmate measure in England and the USA. *Punishment & Society, 10*, 447–474.

Rowles, G. (2009). Making and remaking place in old age. Unpublished manuscript, Sanders-Brown Center on Aging, University of Kentucky, Lexington, KY.

Rowles, G., & Watkins, J. (2003). History, habit, heart, and hearth: On making spaces into places. In K. Schaie, F. Wahl, H. Mollenkopf, & F. Oswald (Eds.), *Aging independently: Living arrangements and mobility* (pp. 77–96). New York, NY: Springer.

Rowles, G., Oswald, F., & Hunter, E. (2004). Interior living environments in old age. *Annual Review of Gerontology and Geriatrics, 23*, 167–194.

Rowe, J., & Kahn, R. (1998). *Successful aging*. New York, NY: Random House.

Rubinstein, R. (1987). The significance of personal objects to older people. *Journal of Aging Studies, 1*, 225–238.

Rubinstein, R., & Parmalee, P. (1992). Attachment to place and the representation of the life course by the elderly. In A. Altman & S. Low (Eds.), *Place attachment* (pp. 139–163). New York, NY: Plenum Press.

Scheidt, R. (2007). Review of Melissa Holbrook Pierson, "The Place You Love is Gone: Progress Hits Home." *Canadian Journal of Urban Research, 16*(1), 135–136.

Scheidt, R. (2010). *Place-making interventions and aging-in-place in small dying towns: A report from the Great Plains*. Poster session presented at the meeting of the Gerontological Society of America, New Orleans, LA.

Scheidt, R., & Norris-Baker, C. (1990). A transactional approach to environmental stress among older residents of rural communities: Introduction to a special issue. *Journal of Rural Community Psychology, 11*(1), 5–30.

Scheidt, R., & Norris-Baker, C. (1999). Place therapies for older adults: Conceptual and interventive approaches. *International Journal of Aging and Human Development, 48*, 1–15.

Scheidt, R., & Windley, P. G. (2006). Environmental gerontology: Progress in the post-Lawton era. In J. Birren & K. Warner Schaie (Eds.), *Handbook of the psychology of aging* (6th ed., pp. 105–125). New York, NY: Academic Press.

Scheidt, R., & Schwarz, B. (2010). Environmental gerontology: A sampler of issues and applications. In J. Cavanaugh & C. Cavanaugh (Eds.), *Aging in America (Volume 1): Psychological Aspects* (pp. 156–176). Santa Barbara, CA: Praeger.

Seymour, J. F. (1980). *Niches in prison: Adaptation and environment in correctional institutions* (Doctoral dissertation). Available from ProQuest Dissertations and Theses database. (Document ID 749722741).

Shah, S., Plugge, E., & Douglas, N. (2011). Ethnic differences in the health of women prisoners. *Public Health, 125*, 349–356.

Sims, G. (1994). *Leaving Alaska*. New York, NY: Atlantic Monthly Press.

Stedman, R. (2002). Toward a social psychology of place: Predicting behavior from place-based cognition, attitude and identity. *Environment and Behavior, 34*, 561–581.

Sterns, A., Lax, G., Sed, C., Keohane, P., & Sterns, R. (2008). *The growing wave of older prisoners: A national survey of older prisoner health, mental health, and programming*. Retrieved from http://nicic.gov/Library/024470

Tapsell, S., & Tunstall, S. (2008). I wish I'd never heard of Banbury: The relationship between 'place' and health impacts of flooding. *Health and Place, 14,* 133–154.

The Pew Center. (2008, February). *One in 100: Behind bars in America 2008.* Retrieved from http://www.pewcenteronthestates.org/report_detail.aspx?id=35904

Timmons, A. (2011, December 12). *Northern Pass buys 118-acre plot.* Retrieved from http://www.concordmonitor.com/article/297826/northern-pass-buys-118-acreplot?CSAuthResp=1326126281%3Am47qn3gg129lvenh9ian78sku4%3ACSUserId%7CCSGroupId%3Aapproved%3A443474CED252E3C60A4A12DDDE59A7E6&CSUserId=94&CSGroupId=1

Tornstam, L. (2005). *Gerotranscendence: A developmental theory of positive aging.* New York, NY: Springer.

Tuohy, R., & Stephens, C. (2012). Older adults' narratives about a flood disaster: Resilience, coherence, and personal identity. *Journal of Aging Studies, 26,* 26–34.

Vera Institute of Justice. (2010, April). *It's about time: Aging prisoners, increasing costs, and geriatric release.* Retrieved from http://www.vera.org/content/its-about-time-aging-prisoners-increasing-costs-and-geriatric-release

Watkins, J. (1999). Life course and spatial experience: A personal narrative approach to migration studies. In K. Pandit & S. Withers (Eds.), *Migration and restructuring in the United States* (pp. 294–312). Boulder, CO: Rowman & Littlefield.

Williams, B., Lindquist, K., Hill, T., Baillargeon, J., Mellow, J., Greifinger, R., & Walter, L.C. (2009). Caregiving behind bars: Correctional officer reports of disability in geriatric prisoners. *Journal of the American Geriatric Society, 57,* 1286–1292.

Wolff, N., & Shi, J. (2009). Feelings of safety among male inmates: The safety paradox. *Criminal Justice Review, 34,* 404–427.

The Dark Side: Stigma in Purpose-Built Senior Environments

REGINA HRYBYK, ROBERT L. RUBINSTEIN, J. KEVIN ECKERT,
ANN CHRISTINE FRANKOWSKI, LYNN KEIMIG, MARY NEMEC,
AMANDA D. PEEPLES, ERIN ROTH, and PATRICK J. DOYLE
*Department of Sociology and Anthropology, Center for Aging Studies, University of Maryland,
Baltimore County, Baltimore, Maryland, USA*

*This paper focuses on stigma in collective living environments for
older adults. We contrast two design profiles, a purpose-built campus which opened in 1997, and an older setting that grew by accretion over decades. The separation by care levels in both sites
is reflected in their cultures as residents and staff relate to levels
of care through a vocabulary of fear. Residents of the independent living building on the purpose-built campus refer to the assisted living building as "the dark side." In this setting we observe
stigma assigned to a place in the built environment. By contrast,
the older setting features a less-structured clustering of independent living and assisted living. We have observed less stigma associated with levels of care in this older building. Grounding our
analysis in data drawn from ongoing ethnographic research, we
focus on the built environment as it relates to stigma in the social
environment.*

This article derives from a 5-year study *Stigma and the Cultural Context of Residential
Settings* supported by NIA R01 AG028469, conducted in the Mid-Atlantic region (J. Kevin
Eckert, PI). Five of the co-authors on this article contributed to the fieldwork: Ann Christine
Frankowski, Lynn Keimig, Mary Nemec, Amanda D. Peeples, and Erin Roth. Their insights, and
those of the other team members, shaped the discussion of stigma in the built environment
and broader issues relating to senior housing. All sites and data discussed in this article have
been de-identified to protect anonymity.

INTRODUCTION

Over the past two decades, the United States has seen growth in the number and complexity of housing settings for the elderly. These are mostly purpose-built; that is, settings designed and built to address the social and health needs in housing for older adults. Although some buildings are constructed to provide housing for residents needing one particular level of care, many are built as multi-level campuses, such as continuing care retirement communities that offer a continuum of care with independent living, assisted living, and skilled nursing care. Purpose-built long-term care settings are generally designed and used as intended with few additions or substantial changes to the built environment. These more recent housing options stand in direct contrast to older long-term care settings that different proprietors have made changes to over time. Often constructed for purposes other than elder care, these traditional settings have been modified, with sections added, renovated, or demolished. Thus, housing built by accretion has been transformed, sometimes several times, to accommodate changing needs and meet current trends. This article will compare two settings—one purpose-built (The Riverside) and one built by accretion (Stonemont)—and examine the presence and evolution of social stigma in these environments.

We provide a brief introduction to the built environment and stigma in senior housing, present an overview of our field research and methodology, compare and contrast stigma in two multi-level long-term care campuses, and discuss the significance of this topic and its implications for the quality of life for residents in senior housing. This article seeks to address the question of how emotions, social categorizations, and other personal and social meanings get attached to physical space within long-term care settings. We believe the question must be more thoroughly investigated in studies of housing for the elderly.

THE BUILT ENVIRONMENT IN AGE-BASED HOUSING

Housing for older adults has experienced rapid changes over the past 20 years as the assisted-living culture morphed into various interpretations of aging-in-place. The social model of assisted living, a change from the medical model of nursing homes, was reinforced by the types of structures and the arrangement of the buildings designed and built as collective living settings (Carder, 2002). Facilities that had been nursing homes were retrofitted to accommodate apartment-style living, with added amenities such as assistance with meals and laundry. The market demand for smaller living spaces combined with opportunities to mingle with age peers drove the development of purpose-built senior housing in the suburban landscape. In continuing care retirement communities, the benefit of aging in place added to the lifestyle allure. Older adults and their families expected that a move to one of these settings would be the last move because the setting would provide for their changing needs (Eckert, Carder, Morgan, Frankowski, & Roth, 2009).

Moving into age-based housing is often precipitated by the fear of changes in physical or mental health conditions, be they actual or anticipated. In addition, changes in health status that require higher levels of care may lead to moves within a multi-level facility, which can be seen as representing a degree of loss of control. Because one needs more assistance to meet daily needs, one becomes more dependent on others. Family members may be conflicted about moves that are evidence of age-related changes. Both fear and the desire to avoid a higher care level complicate the social dynamics in multi-level settings (Nakashima, Chapin, MacMillan, & Zimmerman, 2004).

STIGMA AND THE BUILT ENVIRONMENT

Stigma may be defined as the assignment of negative worth and social distancing on the basis of group or individual characteristics. Groups of people or individuals may distance themselves from other groups or individuals based on some negative attribute or social worth, real or perceived (Crocker, Major, & Steele, 1998; Goffman, 1963). Major and O'Brien (2005) noted that "Stigma is relationship- and context-specific; it does not reside in the person but in a social context" (p. 395). In theory, stigma may be mitigated in senior living settings because other residents are experiencing similar age-related changes. However, in some settings, especially those with a mix of both higher and lower functioning individuals, stigmatizing behavior may be exacerbated as residents and staff monitor physical or mental declines that mark a person as "going downhill" and may prompt a move to a higher level of care. The genesis of such stigma is found in both the fears stemming from a dreaded and assumed inevitability of decline and in the ease with which we characterize other people as different.

The key to stigma is seeing others as different from oneself; that is, the key is found in the social process of othering. We other people out of fear—be it fear of those people or fear of what we ourselves might become (a form of self-othering). Labeling others or characterizing them in some way is part of general social life, and as such it is brought into the senior environment by residents, family, and staff. Labeling others as different from oneself is a critical component of stigmatizing behavior. Becker (1963) suggested that we have little control over how we are labeled, but that the power and status of the labeler and the one who is labeled define social grouping.

Rubinstein (1998) described how objects and places in the physical environment derive "meaning by the culture into which they are meaningfully embedded" (p. 91). We propose that within the two senior housing settings presented here, stigma can be assigned to a specific place. This stigma is reflected in the social context of relationships between and among residents and staff. As a consequence, the place itself, along with the people living there, is devalued and to be avoided. Our analytical focus here is how the purpose-built environment of The Riverside and the environment of a century-old structure, Stonemont, influence social grouping and the process of othering. We discuss the stigmatizing behavior that exists in two multi-level settings for insight into our over-arching question: How does social meaning such as stigma become attached to a particular space?

BACKGROUND

This article derives from ethnographic data collected over the course of a 5-year study—*Stigma and the Cultural Context of Residential Settings*. Names and identifying details of places and people throughout the article have been changed to preserve anonymity. The central focus of this ethnographic project is to examine the existence and nature of stigma in the larger context of social relations in seven diverse senior housing settings representing a range of living options (e.g., multi-level continuing care retirement communities, age-restricted housing developments, and various combinations of independent living, assisted living, and licensed nursing). Although we have chosen to focus our discussion of stigma and the built environment on two of the seven sites, we draw on insights developed in the other settings in which we have worked.

The research team for this project included several principle investigators, analytic staff, and the five field ethnographers who are coauthors of this article. In-depth participant observation and ethnographic interviews with residents, staff, and family members presented a grounded view of the social environment. Teams of two or three ethnographers spent an average of 6 months at each site and shared detailed observations with the entire team through extensive field notes and exact transcripts of research interviews. Field updates and in-depth case presentation in biweekly meetings occurred throughout the duration of the study. The team discussions led to a continuous and reflexive examination of the material. Documents were analyzed thematically using codes that emerged from team discussions of transcripts and field notes. To date, we have completed fieldwork in five of the seven sites. Our data include 273 interviews and 376 field notes. For the purposes of this article, 87 transcribed interviews and 141 field notes from the two sites were analyzed. Using the qualitative program Atlas.ti (Atlas.ti, Berlin, Germany), sections of text labeled with codes *physical setting, belonging or not belonging,* and *exclusion/inclusion* were pulled from the 228 documents. Discussions relating stigma to the built environment at team meetings directed the development of this analysis.

Although the general findings of the larger study are complex and beyond the scope of the current article, germane here is that we discovered stigma and related identity issues, such as self-isolation, in all of the settings in which we have worked. The nature, type, and extent of the stigma varied widely between and within sites. Many issues related to stigma were contextual and local, and thus not generalizable to other settings. We found stigma attached to particular units, especially units for individuals who are cognitively impaired, at several of our research sites. However, even though this finding was consistent across the settings, local variations of this unit-specific stigma existed.

This article details the local articulations of environmental stigma in two settings. In The Riverside (a modern, purpose-built, multi-level campus), stigma was attached to the assisted-living building that included a locked unit designed to house individuals who were cognitively impaired. At Stonemont (built by accretion over time), stigma toward residents in assisted living and individuals who were cognitively impaired, although present, was not as strongly attached to a particular unit in the same manner as it was in The Riverside.

Again, the study aims were to examine and explore the social dynamics of stigma as it operates in multi-level senior living environments. Our ethnographic research methods presented an insider's view of the people who live in and work at The Riverside and Stonemont. Through excerpts from field notes and in-depth interviews, we will hear from residents, family members, and staff in both the assisted living and the independent living buildings at The Riverside. Following this, we will similarly examine Stonemont, an affinity-based long-term care community. We refer to affinity-based housing as collective-living environments where residence is based on a cultural kinship of religious or fraternal spirit. We will explain the culture of the affinity group and explore how shared experiences over the life course may mitigate some of the troubling effects of a move to a collective living setting. We will describe the built environment as we experienced it during our fieldwork, and hear Stonemont residents, staff, and family members describe the social environment in this rambling and often confusing maze of additions and wings.

The cultures of these particular settings appear to be influenced by the physical environment. By contrasting these two sites, we hope to show how higher functioning residents, staff, and family members in the purpose-built setting ascribe stigma to the place, as well as to the residents, in assisted living. In addition, we note how the shared spaces and activities at the setting built by accretion encourage interactions between residents of varying care levels. We assert that any discussion that juxtaposes the built environment with the social environment must be reflexive in nature in that the culture and social dynamics of a place reflect its physical structure and vice versa. Stigma can be subtle and require one to look and listen deeply, or stigma can be overt and so embedded in the place as to evoke a distancing of independent residents from what is jokingly referred to as "the dark side" of assisted living. Using what we have learned at The Riverside and Stonemont, we examine the effect of the built environment on social grouping.

STIGMA AT THE RIVERSIDE

"She'll say to me if she loses something or she can't remember something that she knows she should, she'll say, 'Joan, my memory is getting so bad I don't know what they're going to do with me, but please don't put me away. Please don't put me on that other side.' ... And I mean my mother was adamant that she was not going; 'I'm not even walking through there. Those people are crazy.' And I'm like, how do you know? ... That's where the hair salon is and I wanted her to get a perm and I finally did. But she kept telling me, no, she wasn't going over; she absolutely would not go over there."
—Daughter of an independent resident in The Riverside

The Riverside's web site describes how the founders looked to nostalgic inns and picturesque homes for inspiration to express their senior housing vision. They successfully created a large-scale residential community that incorporates visual cues to an era when the residents were younger. The cultural meaning of Victorian porches and themed gathering places may speak of home (or at least a posh hotel) but seem to confer a somewhat contrived effect to the setting. The tree-shaded walks and quaint common areas appear to mitigate the reality for residents wherein the social and physical manifestations of levels of care reflect their fears of increased dependence.

The campus consists of two buildings connected by a second floor link. Seldom will independent living residents venture to visit former friends who have made the transition across the link to assisted living, and few assisted living residents visit former neighbors on the independent living side. One ethnographer described the stigma she observed:

"We have learned that despite the attractive link, independent living residents remain in their building and noticeably stigmatize assisted living. Many residents refer to assisted living as 'over there' and 'the dark side.'

Independent living residents form cliques who sit in common areas and evaluate residents on their side, often speaking loudly, as to who should be 'over there.' Residents are labeled for negative traits, such as memory loss, personality disorders, obesity, body odor, and repeating stories. Residents then tell staff who should move to assisted living. In fact, to these independent living residents, all of assisted living is somewhat suspect. The only practical use for the link for independent residents is to provide an inside passage to the hair salon in assisted living and then back home."

This facility purports a social model of assisted living care. Services are provided to help older adults adjust to age-related losses, both physical and cognitive. The Riverside assisted living includes a locked dementia care unit (DCU), and we have observed stigmatizing behavior, including labeling and avoidance, aimed at the DCU by the assisted- and independent-living residents. However, the most salient stigmatizing discourse that was documented at this site was directed by the residents of the independent-living building and its residents toward the assisted-living building and its residents. An excerpt from an interview with an independent living resident demonstrated the stigma attached to the loss of cognitive ability and aimed at assisted living:

> Respondent: Well, we have an older resident that's really now, is really getting more forgetful. She's been here a while, so they seem to think she'll be going on the other side, but I hope she doesn't because she likes it on this side.
> Ethnographer: Now "the other side," I keep hearing that a lot. That's the Assisted Living?
> Respondent: Right.

Another independent living resident feels that the assisted-living residents are different from "them" (those in independent living) because "they" (those in assisted living) are "managed by health care workers." In an interview with an upper-level administrator, the ethnographer probed about residents who make recommendations as to who should be moved to assisted living. The administrator confirmed that the independent living residents will advise the staff: "'They have to go over to the other side.' [or] 'You really might want to look at THAT one.' You know, and you're thinking, 'Um-hmm, and you're not long behind them.'" Later she continues, "It's fear. It's loss of control ... sometimes you have to look at that fear." A former independent living resident now in assisted living characterized independent living as the place "where everybody has their sense." At another point in the conversation, she called independent living "the better part." Still she says "I'm very contented here [in assisted living] and very lucky."

The staff at The Riverside was aware of the tendency toward stigmatization and has made attempts to mitigate it. There is no lock on the link between independent living and assisted living, and the doors at both ends are kept open. A few independent living residents come over to assisted living for the morning exercise program, and assisted living residents will occasionally attend the Bingo games in independent living because, as an independent living resident explained, "They prefer our method better. We play for money. They play for a bag of popcorn or some such thing." Although some shared activities exist, each care level at The Riverside has a separate activities calendar.

Another independent-living resident recognized the cultural disconnect, "In a community like this, where you've got the three divisions—residential, assisted, and [DCU] communities; that puts up some barriers right away. We don't see that much of people from the other two communities." An administrator described the culture of stigma, "Over the years, it has not changed as far as the stigma of assisted living. The independent living residents do not want to go to assisted living as a general rule. One of the hardest things in our community, really, is to get people to transition from one area to the next. It's very challenging."

The Riverside's locked DCU is located in one part of the assisted-living building. Residents who live in other parts of the assisted-living building stigmatize the DCU. Again, the phenomenon of othering and the desire to distance oneself from devalued housemates were documented by the ethnographers:

> "Staff was in the process of wheeling in residents. One woman placed near the opening of the circle periodically screamed a piercing 'Help me!' Ms. Harmon, in a stage whisper, commented that she does that a lot and felt that this woman should be placed in the area [the DCU] for people like that. . . . She felt this resident had no business living in assisted living with them."

The examples above are selected from many interviews and field notes that reiterate the same theme, attributing a spoiled identity to both the building that houses assisted living and the DCU and to those who live on "the dark side." With these examples, we see how, in collective living segregated by care levels, social meaning may become attached to a particular space.

STONEMONT AND THE EFFECT OF AFFINITY-BASED HOUSING ON STIGMA

Stonemont, built by accretion over time, has a dated institutional appearance with various additions, some in matching granite and some in mismatched yellow brick. Originally a private estate, Stonemont was purchased in the

1920s by an affinity group who renovated and added to the existing mansion to create a home for elderly, indigent members of the group and their widows. Currently, safe and affordable living in this community is offered to eligible members and their families. Eligibility is determined by membership in the regional affinity group or kinship to a member, with 20 eligible kinship relationships identified. There are three wings, built or renovated at various times, connected by glassed-in breezeways and a maze of interior hallways. Although there are no locked areas, certain units have security alarms that are activated when people exit without entering a pass code.

Currently, Stonemont houses people at three levels of care: independent living, assisted living, and higher needs assisted living. Residents of different levels mix in several common areas, both informally and for shared planned activities. Such places can be thought of as social ecotones defined by Doyle, de Medeiros, and Saunders (2011) as "a tension and transition area between two or more adjacent social environments." They suggested that these ecotones could "create a bridge" between social groups and "expand social connectedness" (p. 9).

During one of the renovations at Stonemont, independent apartments with full kitchens and private assisted-living rooms were retrofitted into two wings that had existed as dormitory-style units with rows of beds. The large dining hall on the second floor serves as a link between the two wings and is shared by assisted living and independent living, although independent living residents tend to come for the evening meal only. A sitting area where residents wait to enter the dining room prior to meals is located on the assisted living side of the dining hall. Adjacent to the dining room is a grand hall used for meetings and family gatherings. Another shared space is a large lounge on the first floor where regular, facility-wide Bingo games are held. All of these places serve as social ecotones, where it is possible for residents from independent living and assisted living to interact.

The most recent addition to Stonemont is a three-floor wing that includes a terrace-level assisted-living unit and two upper floors for residents who need more extensive care than can be provided in the assisted-living wing. The upper floors also provide temporary rooms for independent and assisted living residents recuperating from hospitalization. This most recent wing appears more like a medical unit than the rest of the campus, as an ethnographer describes:

> "The design of the health care unit appears to be from the 1980s with central nurses' stations, wide corridors, and glass walkways connecting back to the historic building. On both floors one and two, I detected strong odors where residents were gathered at the nurses' station. These residents appeared to be among the most impaired, cognitively and physically, at [Stonemont]. Few people seemed to be in their rooms, and nearly all of the doors were open."

An excerpt from a field note shows how another ethnographer explained the lack of clear boundaries between the care levels at Stonemont:

> I'm beginning to understand the fuzziness between the terrace level of assisted living and health care [on the two upper floors of the most recent wing]. It appears as though those in the terrace level of assisted living want to participate and align more with the assisted living/independent living folks. It makes sense since many of them ... were residents there before they moved to the terrace. ... When I asked [the activity director] if the terrace was included in the assisted living-independent living calendar, she indicated by her protracted answer that it was an association that she didn't think worked but said, "They like to be included."

In an interview with an independent living resident, the fluidity of movement at Stonemont is discussed, as follows:

> Ethnographer: Is there much visiting back and forth do you notice ... between the different levels? Like if your neighbor, if someone you know moves, do people go back and forth to visit?
> Respondent: Yeah, because there's no problem to go downstairs. Like a real good friend of ours in assisted living had to go down on the terrace, which is like the lowest level of assisted living ... and we've been down to visit her. Of course, she can't wait to get back to her own room.
> Ethnographer: So there's a chance that ... people move back?
> Respondent: Back and forth. Well, if they have a real bad spell or a fall or something that sets them back then ... they used to put them right in health care, but now they try to put them on the terrace, which is the in-between.

Although care levels are housed in different areas of the building, there is no locked DCU, but memory of what was once a locked DCU persists. Several years ago, one of the floors of the most recent wing was a locked dementia floor, and this floor continues to be negatively regarded. One administrator referred to it as "the ghetto," noting how "nobody wants to go there." Residents who were aware of its history did not want to be placed there, and staff continued to make generalizations about residents who lived on that floor. The floor appears to retain this negative cachet from the time it was a locked DCU, despite the fact that residents of varying cognitive abilities are mixed together on both upper floors of the wing. There seems to be residual stigma ascribed to this floor because of its past as a locked DCU.

Stigma was attached to other areas in the medical care unit. Many residents preferred to sit near the central nurses' stations. These areas were referred to by some higher functioning residents as the "sleeping zone." A resident who had come from the independent apartments but was now living in this unit because of mobility issues said, "I call this thing out here 'Death Valley.' The [staff] don't like to hear me call it that but that's what it is." Roth and Eckert (2011) explored the unintended use and experience of spaces in assisted living, referring to such places as vernacular landscapes. Similar to The Riverside's "dark side," Stonemont's "Death Valley" demonstrates the stigma people can and do attach to a place. However, we note that the built environment at Stonemont appears to lessen the power of stigma as it is attached to place. Although the nature of stigma in this site built by accretion appears to be less focused on a particular place than in The Riverside (a purpose-built environment), sociocultural factors may work to mitigate othering and must be considered in any discussion of stigma.

Stonemont is embedded within an affinity community where the fraternal culture encourages relationships among the generations. Clearly, for purposes of anonymity, we cannot disclose the specific affinity group here. Residents who share affiliation with the affinity group share values and experiences passed along within families. These values may also be shared with people who have been indirectly associated with the group through kinship with a member. Membership confers a strong sense of belonging, as the director of Stonemont tells us, "You needed to have that early on to make you who you are today and [if you didn't belong] you don't have an understanding of that because you weren't involved."

Stonemont is adjacent to the headquarters of the affinity organization that, for nearly a century, has hosted events for affinity clubs from around the region. Local clubs associated with the group regularly visit the home. Families attend these traditional events and volunteer their time with Bingo and other activities, even though they may not be related to residents. Many of the residents we met had visited Stonemont throughout their lives. This association over the life course influences many of the people who choose to live in the home and may serve to mute any tendency to other co-residents.

During interviews, several residents mentioned that they came to the home as children or young adults to visit the elders living there. A daughter of a resident told us how her father "had been going there for years because they had events up there. ... So we went there." An ethnographer noted that "Mrs. James jumped right in to tell me how she and her husband had selected [Stonemont]. Her father was a [member of the group] and her sister had moved in about three years before they did. She knew the place well before she and her husband decided to move there."

Residents who share a common culture and intergenerational contact with the home may have formed a bond that lessens or diffuses the stigma we have seen at more recently built sites that lack the longevity and cultural connectivity of Stonemont. However, not all residents have a strong association with the affinity group. Because various kin of members are eligible, some residents are not members of the affinity group and may be excluded and shunned. One of the administrators explained the social dynamic:

"For those individuals that ... the brother's wife's niece is the tie to this person coming in, being admitted, there is a barrier there with some residents, especially with the men ... where they are reluctant to [include outsiders]—not that they wouldn't talk to them, but they aren't going to include them [because they] don't know what it's all about."

Although it appears that stigma exists at Stonemont, we suggest it is stronger in the form of attachment to an individual rather than to a specific space. In one case, a resident was shunned for his lack of membership in the affinity group. The director told us about Stanley, whose son was a high-ranking member, but who himself had never joined. Stanley was from a different part of the country and had a distinct regional accent. At Stonemont, Stanley became stigmatized by others. Several residents and staff commented on Stanley's differences from the other men. A resident shared his disapproval of Stanley's behavior noting, "Everybody knows Stanley and what he does," referring here to his flirtation with some of the women. It appears that Stanley has internalized this stigma, as evidenced by his apparent low self-esteem. He would not agree to a recorded interview. In field notes, an ethnographer described one of her interactions with him:

"I encountered Stanley by the door, in his usual seat ... I again asked him for an interview and he said once again, 'Why do you want to interview me?' And I again answered, 'Because I value your perspective and experiences.' 'I'm not worth it,' he said several times and followed this up with a very plain statement about his being 'a bum.' ... He seemed really sad and small this morning."

Not only did Stanley not belong to the affinity group, but he also did not follow its fixed gender roles and social norms. Instead of socializing primarily with men, Stanley flirted with women. The staff was aware of the situation. The Executive Director explained in her interview how his behavior is inappropriate:

"And he has some behaviors that are not always appropriate. So there have been complaints because he is not [a member of the affinity group] he doesn't understand how he is supposed to behave. ... Many of them tie it back to being [a member]. ... They aren't going to include them because ... you're not [a member] and you don't know what it's all about."

The stigma attached to Stanley as "the other" was so great that the men who once sat with him in the dining room all left his table one by one. They said they had nothing in common with him. Stanley's case shows how, in this affinity-based setting, individual differences can lead to stigmatizing behavior.

CONTRASTS BETWEEN TWO SITES

Although residents at Stonemont are grouped by care levels, the barriers to interaction between residents are not as evident as at The Riverside. Unlike the single link that connects the buildings at The Riverside, there are multiple intersections between care levels at Stonemont. These intersections reduce physical separations between residents of varying care levels. We suggest that the presence of shared spaces, or social ecotones, may diffuse stigmatizing behavior.

Whether driven by the way the spaces are designed or by social factors (e.g., corporate policy), Stonemont appears to be more socially integrated than The Riverside. The medical unit at Stonemont has its own activities calendar, but independent living and assisted living, including assisted living in the terrace of the new wing, share a calendar. At The Riverside there are three separate calendars for the three care levels, independent living, assisted living, and the DCU.

The stigma observed at Stonemont seemed directed more at individuals rather than at a particular place. Social cliques and exclusionary behaviors existed, as we have found in most of the settings we have studied, but these did not seem to have the focus on a place that was observed in The Riverside (Dobbs et al., 2008).

CONCLUSIONS

Lawton (1998) stated that "What has been referred to as 'external stimulation' has a more direct and immediate association with the environment than do the 'internal' aspects'" (p. 17). The external situation of increasing levels of care and dependence as manifested in the built environment is internalized in the anticipated loss of control that threatens the imagined future self. Fear and avoidance of that place and those people may become embedded in the culture of the setting.

Many factors can mitigate or aggravate stigma. Each setting we have studied has unique issues associated with collective living. Senior housing communities, by definition, group people who are experiencing or anticipating age-related loss of physical or cognitive abilities. Most residents expect to age-in place (i.e., die in the setting). Many residents share cohort memories and values of past times. Why, then, is there a profound and disturbing distancing from housemates who exhibit signs of decline?

When The Riverside was built, its founders envisioned a lovely setting where older adults could transition smoothly from one care level to the next. However, in its second decade, the fear and avoidance of the assisted living building by independent living residents negatively influences perceptions of residents who live in assisted living, and this fear prohibits social interactions. Friends who move from independent living to assisted living are often forgotten; they have moved on. The belief that the move into The Riverside's independent apartment would be the last move, from the perspective of the resident, has been proven false. A move to the "dark side," although still on the same campus, is possible and often traumatic.

Stonemont may not be as efficient as The Riverside, with its warren of hallways and mixed levels of care; however, the interaction that is promoted by the prevalence of social ecotones in shared spaces and shared activities appears to diffuse the stigma that is associated with age-related decline. Stigma does exist at Stonemont, but it appears to be more focused on individuals, particularly among the men, than on physically identified care levels, with the exception of the residual stigma attached to one floor of the health care wing and the "sleeping zones" in the medical unit. The social ecotones at Stonemont blend independent living and assisted living in ways that cannot happen at The Riverside. Further study is needed to understand how social ecotones in the built environment may promote relationships between groups that would not otherwise interact and in turn, mitigate stigma.

In all of the sites in which we have conducted fieldwork for the larger study, we have observed instances when stigmatizing behavior appeared to negatively affect the health of residents. We have seen residents hide evidence of falls, and family members go to great lengths to delay a loved-one's move to higher care levels. We have heard many voices in every site we've studied describe the hurtful effects of exclusion and shunning. This article described the stigmatizing behavior we observed in two unique sites and how the culture of the places reflects the built environment; how meaning can be attached to physical space.

As we prepare for the increasing number of older adults over the coming years, it is important to consider what we have learned about purpose-built senior housing and how space frames culture and culture reflects space. Understanding how stigma manifests in various physical environments may lead to changes that improve the lives of current and future residents in collective living settings.

REFERENCES

Becker, H. S. (1963). *Outsiders: Studies in the sociology of deviance.* New York, NY: The Free Press.

Carder, P. C. (2002). The social world of assisted living. *Journal of Aging Studies, 16,* 1–18.

Crocker, J., Major, B., & Steele, C. (1998). Social stigma. In S. Fiske, D. Gilbert, & G. Lindzey (Eds.), *Handbook of social psychology* (vol. 2, pp. 504–553). Boston, MA: McGraw-Hill.

Dobbs, D., Eckert, J. K., Rubinstein, R. L., Keimig, L., Clarke, L., Frankowski, A. C., et al (2008). Stigma and ageism in assisted living. *The Gerontologist, 48*, 517–526.

Doyle, P. J., de Medeiros, K., & Saunders, P. (2011). Nested social groups within the social environment of a dementia care assisted living. *Dementia, 12*, 1–17. doi:10.1177/1471301211421188.

Eckert, J. K., Carder, P., Morgan, L., Frankowski, A. C., & Roth, E. (2009). *Inside assisted living: The search for home.* Baltimore, MD: Johns Hopkins University Press.

Goffman, E. (1963). *Stigma: Notes on the management of spoiled identity.* New York, NY: Prentice Hall.

Lawton, M. P. (1998). Environment and aging: Theory revisited. In R. J. Scheidt & P. G. Windley (Eds.), *Environment and aging theory: A focus on housing* (pp. 1–31). Westport, CT: Greenwood Press.

Major, B., & O'Brien, L. (2005). The social psychology of stigma. *Annual Review of Psychology, 56*, 393–421.

Nakashima, M., Chapin, R. K., MacMillan, K., & Zimmerman, M. (2004). Decision making in long-term care: Approaches used by older adults and implications for social work practice. *Journal of Gerontological Social Work, 43*, 79–102.

Roth, E., & Eckert, J. K. (2011). The vernacular landscape of assisted living. *Journal of Aging Studies, 25*, 215–224.

Rubinstein, R. L. (1998). The phenomenology of housing for older people. In R. J. Scheidt & P. G. Windley (Eds.), *Environment and aging theory: A focus on housing* (pp. 89–110). Westport, CT: Greenwood Press.

The Role of the Social Environment on Physical and Mental Health of Older Adults

JULIE A. NORSTRAND

Graduate School of Social Work, Boston College, Chestnut Hill, Massachusetts, USA

ALLEN GLICKSMAN

Philadelphia Corporation for Aging, Philadelphia, Pennsylvania, USA

JAMES LUBBEN

Graduate School of Social Work, Boston College, Chestnut Hill, Massachusetts, USA

MORTON KLEBAN

Abramson Center for Jewish Life, North Wales, Pennsylvania, USA

Understanding the complex relationship between the environmental context and the well-being of older adults is paramount as aging in place is increasingly acknowledged as a policy goal. This study investigated how the social environment (measured by social capital) was related to both physical and mental health. A sample of 3,219 older adults (60 years and older) from Philadelphia, Pennsylvania, and 4 surrounding counties were obtained from the Philadelphia Health Management Corporation survey collected in 2006. Binary and ordinal logistic regressions of self-rated health and depression symptoms were regressed on sociodemographic and six social capital items. Participation in groups, sense of belonging, and neighbors willing to help were associated with self-rated health, whereas trust in neighbors and sense of belonging and neighbors willing to help were associated with depressive symptoms even when sociodemographic indicators were controlled. This study furthers our understanding of how social capital may relate to the physical and mental health of the elderly and illustrates the usefulness of this important concept in environmental gerontology.

INTRODUCTION

Aging-in-place is increasingly acknowledged as a crucial policy goal as the number of people reaching old age increases (Markwood, 2006; World Health Organization [WHO], 2007). There are increased efforts to ensure age-friendly or livable communities for all ages on a global basis (WHO, 2007). Environmental gerontology has "focused on the description, explanation, and modification or optimization of the relation between elderly persons and their socio-spatial surroundings" (Wahl & Weisman, 2003, p. 616). Considerable work within environmental gerontology has focused on the physical environment, although greater attention has been paid to social, organizational, and cultural environments more recently (Wahl & Weisman, 2003). The need for specific focus on social aspects of the environment are highlighted by a recent publication by the WHO, titled "Social Determinants Approaches to Public Health: From Concepts to Practice" (Blas, Sommerfield, & Kurup, 2011). In this report, they argue: "Although many public health programmes have achieved considerable success in reducing mortality and morbidity, they often fail to capitalize on interventions that address the social context and conditions in which people live" (Blass et al., 2011, p. 2). The critical role of the social environment is highlighted by Wahl and Oswald (2010), who stated that "the management of the relationship between interior and exterior worlds in later life is often reduced to the social environment" (p. 115). The authors do also emphasize the importance of examining the physical environment as well.

One approach to studying the social environment is through social capital, a concept that emphasizes social relationships between groups of people. Despite considerable research on theories including place attachment within environmental gerontology, social capital has received little specific mention. This is a critical point because social capital captures additional features of place not captured by sense of belonging, including norms and networks. The study of social capital continues to require attention; according to Walker and Hiller (2007), limited understanding of how social capital operates for specific subgroups, such as older adults, persists. Specifically, more research needs to be performed to examine the effect that social capital has on physical and mental health among older adults. In this study, older adults were considered to be individuals aged 60 years and older because gerontologists traditionally focus on individuals aged 60 years and older (WHO, n.d.).

Considerable inconsistency exists regarding the definition of social capital in the literature (Szreter & Woolcock, 2004). Because much of the health-related research has used Putnam's definition of social capital (Stephens, 2008), his definition was applied in this study: "features of social organization, such as trust, norms, and networks that can improve the efficiency of society by facilitating coordinated aims" (Putnam, Leonardi, & Nanetti,

1993, p. 167). Also, the dataset used for this study had items that reflected Putnam's core features of social capital. The reason for Putnam's significant impact on the social capital literature may be that he was able to show, through vast quantitative analyses, the influence of changing attitudes of trust, reciprocity, and civic engagement on the political and social life of Italy (Putnam, Leonardi, & Nanetti, 1993). Later, Putnam emphasized the important connection between social capital and health. For example, in 2000 he stated: "Of all the domains in which I have traced the consequences of social capital, in none is the importance of social connectedness so well established as in the case of health and well-being" (p. 326).

Today a substantial body of research has been performed exploring the relationship between social capital with physical and mental health among the general population. However, relatively little research has examined the relationship between social capital and health among older adults, as highlighted by Almedom's (2005) interdisciplinary review of social capital and mental health. Notable research has looked at single dimensions of social capital (such as trust, social networks, civic engagement, or religious attendance) in terms of health. It is the opinion of the authors that these studies do not adequately capture the multifaceted concept of social capital as defined in this study. As described above, Putnam (2000) conceptualized social capital along key dimensions, including trust, norms of reciprocity, and networks. This study has attempted to capture these key features of social capital.

The need for further examination of social capital among older adults is convincing because of the unique relationship between older adults and their neighborhood, described in greater detail below. Furthermore, social capital may be particularly important for this sector of the population due to their increased risk of social exclusion and potentially higher need for social support (de Souza & Grundy, 2007; Scharf, Phillipson, & Smith, 2003). Also, according to Pollack and Knesebeck (2004), "Social capital is one such factor that has been linked to health in the general population and may be of particular salience for the older adult" (p. 383).

Older adults may be considered to have a unique relationship to their neighborhood. This special relationship occurs for several reasons. First, retirement increases the time spent at home and social interactions shift over to family, neighbors, church, or community (Moen, Fields, Quick, & Hofmeister, 2000; Phillipson, Bernard, Phillips, & Ogg, 2001a, 2001b). Second, older people are more likely than younger people to suffer from chronic health problems, which ultimately reduce their mobility, so they are more likely to stay within their neighborhood (Thomese & Tilburg, 2000). This narrows not only their social interactions, but also their interaction with the surrounding physical environment (Glass & Balfour, 2004). Third, in many cases, older people have spent many years in their neighborhood and may be more emotionally invested in their neighborhoods than younger people (Oswald,

Jopp, Rott, & Wahl, 2011; Walker & Hiller, 2007). All of these examples emphasize the need for carefully examining the relationship between social capital and health among older adults.

Evidence of a significant relationship between social capital and health among older adults could have important policy implications. The overall goals of this study are to determine whether a relationship between social capital and health exists among older adults and to examine the nature of this relationship in terms of both physical and mental health. Self-rated health was used as a measure of physical health, and the number of depressive symptoms was used as a measure of mental health. The two research questions are:

1. Does social capital relate to physical and mental health among older adults?
2. How does the relationship between social capital and physical health versus social capital and mental health differ?

METHODS

Data Source

The sample was drawn from the Public Health Management Corporation's Community Health Data Base, a representative telephone survey conducted cross-sectionally every 2 years since 1994 with approximately 10,000 households in a five-county southeastern Pennsylvania region: Bucks, Chester, Delaware, Montgomery, and Philadelphia counties. Households were contacted using computerized Random Digit Dialing so that households with unpublished numbers and residents who had recently moved would be included in the sample. The response rate was 22%. When needed, interviews were conducted in Spanish. Also, if a randomly selected adult respondent was unable to be interviewed because of health impairments or language barriers, the interview was conducted with an adult proxy. All adult proxies were related to the selected respondent and lived in the same household at the time of the interview. The survey included an over-sample of individuals 60 years of age and older. A wide range of questions were asked regarding socioeconomic status, health behaviors, housing characteristics, physical and mental health, and domains of social capital. For this study, the 2006 data were analyzed.

Study Sample

Older adults (60 years and older) from a five-county Southeastern Pennsylvania region, formed the sample in this study. The sample size for this study was 3,219.

Measures

INDEPENDENT MEASURES

Social capital was measured by 6 items. The items were taken from the Social Capital Community Benchmark Survey (Kennedy School of Government, 2000). The questions were rephrased to be similar to other questions in the PHMC survey. No previous psychometric assessment has been performed on these questions. The 6 items were:

1. Participation in groups: "How many local groups or organizations in your neighborhood do you currently participate in such as social, political, religious, school-related, or athletic organizations?" Responses were recoded from 0-36 into 4 categories (0 = 0; 1 = 1; 2 = 2, 3 thru 36 = 3).
2. Neighbors willing to help: "Please rate how likely people in your neighborhood are willing to help their neighbors with routine activities such as picking up their trash cans, or helping to shovel snow. Would you say that most people in your neighborhood are always, often, sometimes, rarely, or never willing to help their neighbors?" This was recoded into four categories: always (4), often (3), sometimes (2), and rarely or never (1).
3. Sense of belonging: "Please tell me if you strongly agree (4), agree (3), disagree (2), or strongly disagree (1) with the following statement: I feel that I belong and am a part of my neighborhood."
4. Trust in neighbors: "Please tell me if you strongly agree (4), agree (3), disagree (2), or strongly disagree (1) with the following statement: Most people in my neighborhood can be trusted."
5. Talk to friends/relatives: "About how often do you talk with friends or relatives on the telephone?" Response categories included several times a day (6), once a day (5), a few times a week (4), once a week (3), less often than once a week (2), and never (1).
6. See friends/family: "About how often do you see friends or family members who do not live with you? Response categories included almost every day (6), a few times a week (5), once a week (4), a few times a month (3), once a month (2), less than once a month, and never (1).

COVARIATE MEASURES: SOCIODEMOGRAPHIC ITEMS

The items selected were those that the literature has suggested are correlates of physical and/or mental health status (Flores, Bauchner, Feinstein, & Nguyen, 1999; Franks, Gold, & Fiscella, 2003; Phillips, Hammock, & Blanton, 2005). These items included: age, which ranged from 60 to 99 years; sex; race, which was a dichotomized variable representing White and minority status (includes all non-White and all Hispanics of any race); poverty, which was dichotomized into at or below 200% of the poverty line (0) or not poor/above 200% level (1); and education, which was categorized into less than high school graduate (0–11 years), high school graduate (12 years), some college (13–15 years), college graduate (16 years), and post-college (more than 16 years). Poverty at 200% was selected for this study because it represents a more reasonable cut-off for poverty than 100% (Elder Economic Security Initiative, 2008).

DEPENDENT MEASURES

Dependent measures included were self-rated health (proxy for physical health) and number of depressive symptoms (proxy for mental health). Self-rated health was assessed using a single item where individuals were asked to rate their own health on a 4-point Likert scale: "Would you say (his/her) health, in general, is excellent, good, fair or poor?" (Moss, Hoffman, Mossey, & Rovine, 2007).

The number of depressive symptoms was measured using a 10-item version of the Center for Epidemiological Studies Depression Scale (CES-D) (Radloff, 1977). The 10-item version of the CES-D scale was generated from the 20-item original version by item–total correlations and elimination of redundant items (Anderson, Malmgren, Carter, & Patrick, 1994). Respondents were asked to respond either yes or no to "Please tell me if you felt this way much of the time in the past week" for a list of 10 statements about feelings (Table 1).

For this study, the 10-item version of the CES-D scale was dichotomized, with 0 representing 0-3 depressive symptoms and 1 representing 4 or more depressive symptoms. This cutoff was set because this is consistent with the proposed use of the CES-D as a screening instrument, which has been found to best detect major depression. Therefore, this split makes the most clinical sense (Irwin, Artin, & Oxman, 1999).

TABLE 1 Questions from 10-item version of CES-D

Please tell me if you felt this way much of the time in the past week:
1. I felt depressed.
2. I felt that everything I did was an effort.
3. My sleep was restless.
4. I was happy.
5. I felt lonely.
6. People were unfriendly.
7. I enjoyed life.
8. I felt sad.
9. I felt that people disliked me.
10. I could not get going.

Data Analysis

The statistical software package used was Stata version 11.0 (StataCorp, College Station, Tex).

Pearson Correlations

Pearson correlations were performed among the 6 social capital items, as well as the covariate measures and the dependent health measures, to better understand the relationships.

Binary and Ordinal Logistic Regressions

Due to varying degrees of non-normal distribution for many of the items, logistic regressions were performed because predictor variables do not have to be normally distributed (Tabachnick & Fidell, 2001). Furthermore, when dichotomizing the distribution of scores on number of depressive symptoms, giving an 88:12 split (0-3 symptoms vs. 4+ symptoms), the optimal statistical approach was binary regression.

Binary logistic regression was run with the dependent variable—number of depressive symptoms (a dichotomized item), which was regressed on predictors (age, sex, race, education, and poverty—and the 6 social capital items (participation in groups, trust in neighbors, sense of belonging, neighbors willing to help, talk to friends/relatives, and see friends/family).

For ordinal logistic regression, the dependent variable was self-rated health (an ordinal item), which was regressed on the same predictors.

RESULTS

Sociodemographics

The sample consisted of 3,219 older adults from a five-county Southeastern Pennsylvania region. The mean age was 71 years (SD = 8 years). The majority were women (68%), and a quarter were minorities. In terms of education, the largest proportion of older adults had completed a high school diploma (40%). The sociodemographic details of the sample appear in Table 2.

Health Characteristics

Health was represented by self-rated health (proxy for physical health) and the number of depressive symptoms (proxy for mental health). In this sample, approximately one-third (32%) of participants rated their health as fair

TABLE 2 Sociodemographic Characteristics of the Sample

Measure	Prevalence	N
Age, years, range (mean ± SD)	60–99 (71 ± 0)	3219
Sex (%)		
Male	32	1051
Female	68	2168
Race (%)		
White	75	2385
Minority	25	787
Poverty (%)	32	1015
Education (%)		
Less than HS (0–11 yrs)	15	488
HS graduate (12 yrs)	40	1268
Some college (13–15 yrs)	18	564
College graduate (16 yrs)	15	468
Post-college (16+ yrs)	13	408

or poor. The number of depressive symptoms existed on a continuum from 0 to 10, and the number of self-reported symptoms for this sample was low, with the majority (45%) reporting no symptoms. The health characteristics of the sample are shown in Table 3.

Social Capital Characteristics

Social capital items indicated that just over half (54%) of the older adults in this sample participated in groups. Neighbors were perceived as generally being willing to help because only 15% indicated that neighbors were rarely or never willing to help. Furthermore, the majority participants felt that they belonged to the neighborhood and that neighbors could be trusted. The majority indicated seeing friends and family almost every day (24%) or few times a week (39%). This was also the case for talking with friends and

TABLE 3 Health Characteristics of the Sample

Measure	Prevalence	N
Self-rated health (%)		
Poor	8	249
Fair	24	763
Good	48	1544
Excellent	20	648
Depressive symptoms (%)		
0	45	1316
1	22	658
2	13	384
3	8	231
4+	12	353

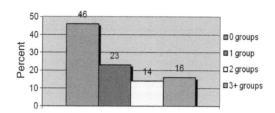

FIGURE 1 Participation in groups.

relatives, with participants indicating that they talked to friends and relatives several times a day (39%) or once a day (25%) (Figures 1–6).

Pearson Correlation

Pearson correlations were significant among all the social capital items ($r =$ .21–0.45, $p \leq .01$). Complete results can be obtained from the author on request.

Binary and Ordinal Logistic Regressions

SELF-RATED HEALTH

The fit of this model was statistically significant in terms of predicting self-rated health ($\chi^2 = 402.16$, $df = 11$, $p < .001$); however, the Pseudo R^2 was 0.066. Thus, the model explained 7% of the total variance for self-rated health. The outcome of the ordinal logistic regression indicated that participation in groups, sense of belonging, and neighbors willing to help were significantly associated with self-rated health. In other words, an increase in participation in groups was associated with a 15% increase in the odds of more positive self-rated health (odds ratio [OR] = 1.15); an increase in sense of belonging was associated with a 11% increase in the odds of more positive self-rated health; and a rise in willingness of neighbors to help was also associated with a 15% increase in odds of more positive self-rated health (OR = 1.15). In addition, sociodemographic measures (age, race, education, and poverty) were also significantly associated with self-rated health.

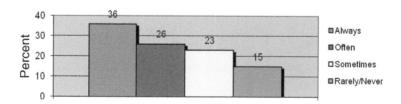

FIGURE 2 Neighbors willing to help.

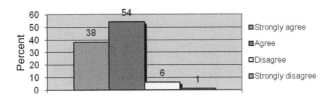

FIGURE 3 Belonging to neighborhood.

Specifically, incorporating age, being a minority, having a lower education level and being poor increased the likelihood of poorer self-rated health (Table 4).

NUMBER OF DEPRESSIVE SYMPTOMS

The fit of the overall model was statistically significant in terms of predicting number of depressive symptoms ($\chi^2 = 140.68$, $df = 11$, $p < .001$), and the Pseudo R^2 was 0.083; thus, the model explained 8% of the total variance for the number of depressive symptoms. The outcome of binary logistic regression indicated that trust in neighbors, sense of belonging, and neighbors willing to help were significantly associated with depressive symptoms. In other words, a decrease in trust in neighbors was associated with a 22% increase in odds of increased depressive symptomatology (OR = 0.78). A decrease in sense of belonging was associated with a 15% increase in odds of increased depressive symptomatology (OR = 0.85). Also, a decrease in willingness of neighbors to help was associated with a 19% increase in odds of increased depressive symptomatology (OR = 0.81). In addition, poverty was also significantly associated with the number of depressive symptoms. Specifically, being poor was associated with an increased likelihood of higher depressive symptomatology (Table 5).

DISCUSSION

The findings indicate that social capital, as measured in this study, may play a significant role in both self-rated health (proxy for physical health)

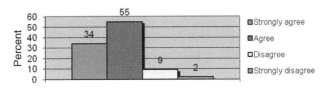

FIGURE 4 Trust in neighbors.

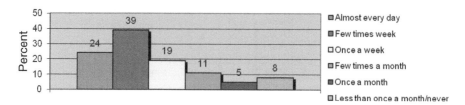

FIGURE 5 See friends/family.

and the number of depressive symptoms (proxy for mental health) of older adults. However, it is important not to overstate the role of social capital because both models explained only a small portion of the outcomes. Regression results showed that, even when taking into account well-known sociodemographic indicators, all social capital items (except for talking to friends and relatives and seeing friends and family) continued to be independently associated with either self-rated health or number of depressive symptoms. Specifically, participation in groups, sense of belonging, and neighbors willing to help were independently related to self-rated health, whereas trust in neighbors, sense of belonging, and neighbors willing to help were all significantly associated with number of depressive symptoms.

An important contribution of this study is that it furthers our understanding of the complex relationship between the social context and health of older adults. Calls continue for further theoretical development within environmental gerontology (Wahl & Oswald, 2010). Although social capital has been studied widely, especially among nonelderly populations, little attention has been paid to this concept within environmental gerontology. This study highlights the importance of social capital as a theoretical approach to examining the social environment. Specific focus on the influence of social capital on older adults makes intuitive sense when taking into account that the physical and social space of older adults decreases over time due to physical and cognitive limitations (Thomese & Tilburg, 2000).

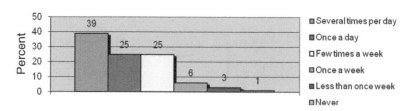

FIGURE 6 Talk to friends/relatives.

TABLE 4 Regression Coefficients and Odds Ratios for Self-Rated Health Among Older Adults

Outcome variable	Beta Coefficient	SE	OR	95% CI	P
Age, years	−0.03	0.00	0.97	(−0.04, −0.02)	***
Sex	0.15	0.08	1.16	(−0.01, 0.32)	
Education	0.25	0.04	1.28	(0.18, 0.32)	***
Race (minority)	−0.59	0.10	0.56	(−0.78, −0.39)	***
Poverty	0.60	0.10	1.82	(0.41, 0.79)	***
Participate	0.14	0.04	1.15	(0.06, 0.22)	***
Trust	0.06	0.04	1.06	(−0.03, 0.15)	
Belong	0.10	0.05	1.11	(0.01, 0.19)	*
Neighbor help	0.14	0.04	1.15	(0.05, 0.22)	**
Talk to friends abd relative	0.00	0.04	1.00	(−0.09, 0.08)	
See friends and family	0.08	0.04	1.08	(−0.00, 0.16)	

Number of obs = 2519
LR chi^2 (11) = 402.16
Prob > chi^2 = 0.0000
Log likelihood = −2825.00
Pseudo R^2 = 0.0664
*P < .05; **P < .01; ***P< .001.
Abbreviations: SE = standard error; OR = odds ratio; CI = confidence interval.

Implications for Research and Practice

This study focused on the role of the social context in terms of the health of older adults. Although it is fully acknowledged that the physical environment plays a critical role in the well-being of older individuals, the decision to focus solely on the social environment is done with the hope

TABLE 5 Regression Coefficients and Odds Ratios for Number of Depressive Symptoms Among Older Adults

Outcome Variable	Beta Coefficient	SE	OR	95% CI	P
Age, years	−0.01	0.01	0.99	(−0.02, 0.01)	
Sex	0.30	0.16	1.34	(−0.01, 0.60)	
Education	−0.12	0.07	0.89	(−0.25, 0.01)	
Race (minority)	−0.11	0.16	0.89	(−0.43, 0.20)	
Poverty	−0.88	0.15	0.42	(−1.18, −0.57)	***
Participate	−0.07	0.08	0.93	(−0.22, 0.08)	
Trust	−0.25	0.07	0.78	(−0.39, −0.10)	***
Belong	−0.16	0.07	0.85	(−0.31, −0.02)	*
Neighbor help	−0.21	0.07	0.81	(−0.36, −0.07)	**
Talk to friends and relative	−0.05	0.07	0.95	(−0.20, 0.09)	
See friends and family	−0.06	0.07	0.95	(−0.20, 0.88)	
Constant	−0.35	0.83		(−1.99, 1.28)	

Number of obs = 2397
LR chi^2 (11) = 140.68
Prob > chi^2 = 0.0000
Log likelihood = −769.27
Pseudo R^2 = 0.0838
*P < .05; **p < .01; *** P < .001.
Abbreviations: SE = standard error; OR = odds ratio; CI = confidence interval.

of furthering the theoretical framework of social capital, which to this day remains a controversial concept (Szreter & Woolcock, 2004); and thereby illustrating the usefulness of this important concept in environmental gerontology. Furthermore, the key role of the social context for frail elderly has been demonstrated in previous research. For example, cognitive and social dimensions were shown to be critical for elders with severe mobility impairment or blindness (Oswald & Wahl, 2005). Indeed, with age comes a decrease in mobility and agency, but an increase in a sense of belonging (Wahl & Oswald, 2010). Efforts to maximize the social dimension (i.e., sense of belonging) may be advantageous in that it can increase motivation for ensuring continued aging-in-place. This can be accomplished through changes to the physical dimension of the environment, such as with home modifications.

The findings of this study benefit research in that they may help guide the development of future measures of social capital. First, the significant role that the items sense of belonging to the neighborhood and belief that neighbors are willing to help may play for both the physical and mental health of older adults is a notable finding in this study. This is because when considering the academic research that has focused on the social predictors of health of older adults, has typically put greater emphasis on social networks. The findings in this study suggest that more attention may need to be paid to understanding how individuals perceive their neighbors. The role of neighbors (rather than family) in the lives of older adults requires greater focus. Litwin (2011) emphasized the importance of friends and neighbors in the lives of older people. Furthermore, due to decreased fertility rates, increased divorces rates, and low rates of remarriage, the availability of spouses or children to provide care for aging parents is expected to diminish in the near future (Karuza, 2007). Hence, reliance on neighbors will likely grow.

Another important consideration regarding developing measures of social capital is the importance of quantity versus quality of interactions with others. This study found that neither of the items relating to social networks (i.e., see friends and relatives and talk to friends and family) was significantly associated with either self-rated health or number of depressive symptoms. This is a surprising finding because considerable research has found significant associations between social network size and various health outcomes (Grundy & Sloggett, 2003). However, as Grundy and Sloggett (2003) pointed out, in some cases social networks have been found to have little or no effect. One point to consider is that previous research has underscored the fact that it is not the frequency of contact (as was measured in this study), but rather the level of support provided by the network that is the critical factor for both physical and mental health (Lubben et al., 2006; Lubben & Gironda, 2003a). Furthermore, social network type may also be an important factor to take into account (Fiori, Antonucci, & Cortina, 2006; Lubben et al., 2006).

It is hoped that the findings of this study will strengthen the policy dialogue on the role of social capital in terms of physical and mental health of older adults. This is a critical issue because we are entering a phase of unprecedented growth in the number of older adults living in our communities, of which many wish to age in place. Policy and programmatic interventions aimed at improving the well-being of older adults are encouraged to focus on ways of building social capital, such as increasing a sense of trust and belonging and encouraging neighbors to help. The willingness of neighbors to help could be a vital resource for older adults because these neighbors could provide transport to stores and medical appointments and attend to any immediate household needs, such as changing a light bulb. Fundamentally, interventions that encourage neighborly interactions could increase these key elements of social capital. Civic engagement and social clubs could be ways of increasing neighbor linkages. Furthermore, physical spaces, such as parks within urban settings, could be another approach to encouraging interactions between neighborhood residents (Litman, 2009).

According to the results of this study, the implications for increasing social capital among older adults are improvements in both self-rated health and the number of depressive symptoms. For example, improvements in depressive symptoms has been shown to diminish mortality, suicide, functional impairments, productivity losses, and general medical costs (Hong, Hasche, & Bowland, 2009). Thus, efforts to increase social capital could have extremely important positive effects for the older individual and society in general. Ultimately, professionals focused on community based interventions are encouraged to develop methods of screening for social capital and for developing clinical approaches that can maximize the social capital of older adults as they age.

It is hoped that this study may provide insight into ways of improving the measurement of social capital. In light of this, some important limitations of this study must be considered. Controversy remains about the definition and measurements of social capital. When selecting the items to reflect social capital, there was concern about how appropriate some of these items were for older adults. This was especially the case with the item participation in groups. It was not possible to determine what type of involvement, or commitment, membership in a group required. For example, participation in groups could reflect simply paying membership fees; if so, physical limitations would not affect the ability to participate in groups. Furthermore, the two social capital items—frequency of seeing friend and relatives and frequency of seeing friends and family—may be considered ambiguous in the sense they did not give a clear indication of the geographical location of these social relationships. For this study, it would have been helpful to determine which friends and relatives were located within the neighborhood of the elder. Such ambiguities clearly calls for more thought to be given to how social capital is measured when dealing with a specific subgroup of the population, such as older adults. Another important limitation of this study was the cross-sectional nature of the data. This means that it is not possible to determine the nature of the relationships between social capital and health; in other words, did low participation in groups result in poor physical health or did poor physical health limit the participation in groups? This limitation speaks to the need for longitudinal studies of social capital. Furthermore, as Wahl and Oswald (2010) have argued that "the real test will come only with controlled intervention research" (p. 120).

The overall findings of this study support the literature that has found a significant link between social capital and health. This study was unique in that it examined the effect of social capital on both physical and mental health among community dwelling older adults from southeastern Pennsylvania. Ultimately, this study reemphasizes the importance of social capital for older adults in our communities. This study highlighted key aspects (i.e., participation in groups, trust in neighbors, sense of belonging, and willingness of neighbors to help) of social capital that may be important for health of older adults. It is hoped that these findings may assist policymakers and the practice community in better serving populations aging-in-place. It is hoped that the findings of this study may also guide development of improved social capital measures. Through improvement of this concept, it is hoped that social capital may become incorporated into environmental gerontology. It is not until an accepted definition (and measurement) of the social environment is established for the elderly that environmental gerontology can better obtain its aim, which is "to describe, explain and modify/optimize the relationship between the ageing person and his/her physical-social environment" (Wahl & Oswald, 2010, p. 112).

REFERENCES

Almedom, A. M. (2005). Social capital and mental health: An interdisciplinary review of primary evidence. *Social Science & Medicine, 61*, 943–964.

Anderson, E. M., Malmgren, J. A., Carter, W. B., & Patrick, D. L. (1994). Screening for depression in well older adults: Evaluation of a short form of the CES-D. *American Journal of Preventative Medicine, 10*, 77–84.

Blas, E., Sommerfield, J., & Kurup, A. S. (2011). *Social determinants approaches to public health: from concept to practice.* Retrieved from http://whqlibdoc.who. int/publications/2011/9789241564137_eng.pdf

de Souza, E. M., & Grundy, E. (2007). Intergenerational interaction, social capital and health: Results from a randomized trial in Brazil. *Social Science & Medicine, 65*, 1397–1409.

Elder Economic Security Initiative. (2008). *The elder economic security standard™ index for Pennsylvania.* Retrieved from http://www.wowonline. org/pdf/WOW_PA_Index_FINAL.pdf

Fiori, K. L., Antonucci, T. C., & Cortina, K. S. (2006). Social network typologies and mental health among older adults: A replication. *Journal of Gerontology: Psychological Sciences, 61B,* 25–32.

Flores, G., Bauchner, H., Feinstein, A., & Nguyen, U. (1999). The impact of ethnicity, family, income and parental education on children's health and use of health services. *American Journal of Public Health, 89,* 1066–1071.

Franks, P., Gold, M. R., & Fiscella, K. (2003). Sociodemographics, self-rated health, and mortality in the US. *Social Science & Medicine, 56,* 2505–2514.

Glass, T., & Balfour J. (2003). Neighborhoods, aging, and functional limitations. In Kawachi, I., & Berkman, L. (Eds.). *Neighborhoods and health* (pp. 303–334). Oxford, United Kingdom: Oxford University Press.

Grundy, E., & Sloggett, A. (2003). Health inequalities in the older populations: the role of personal capital resources and socio-economic circumstances. *Social Science & Medicine, 56,* 935–947.

Hong, S. L., Hasche, L., & Bowland, S. (2009). Structural relationships between social activities and longitudinal trajectories of depression among older adults. *Gerontologist, 49*(1), 1–11.

Irwin, M., Artin, K. H., & Oxman, M. (1999). Criterion Validity of the 10-Item Center for Epidemiological Studies Depression Scale (CES-D). *Archives of Internal Medicine, 159,* 1701–1704.

Karuza, J. (2007). Social Support. In E. H. Duthie, P. R. Katz, & M. L. Malone (Eds.), *Practice of Geriatrics* (pp. 53–59). Philadelphia, PA: Saunders Elsevier.

Kennedy School of Government. (2000). *Social capital community benchmark survey.* Retrieved from http://www.cfsv.org/communitysurvey/docs/survey_instrument.pdf

Litman, T. (2009). *Community cohesion as a transport planning objective. Victoria Transport Policy Institute.* Retrieved from http://www.vtpi.org/cohesion.pdf

Litwin, H. (2011). Social network type and subjective well-being in a national sample of older Americans. *Gerontologist, 51,* 379–388.

Lubben, J., Blozik, E., Gillmann, G., Iliffe, S., von Renteln Kruse, W., Beck, J. C., & Stuck, A.E. (2006). Performance of an abbreviated version of the Lubben Social Network Scale among three european community-dwelling older adult populations. *Gerontologist, 46,* 503–513.

Lubben, J. E., & Gironda, M. W. (2003a). Centrality of social ties to the health and well-being of older adults. In B. Berkman & L. K. Harooytan (Eds.), *Social work and health care in an aging world* (pp. 319–350). New York, NY: Springer.

Markwood, S. (2006). The maturing of America: Getting communities on track for an aging population. Retrieved from http://www.n4a.org/pdf/MOAFinalReport.pdf

Moen, P., Fields, V., Quick, H. E., & Hofmeister, H. (2000). A life-course approach to retirement and social integration. In K. Pillmer, P. Moen, E. Wethington, & N. Glasgow (Eds.), *Social integration in the second half of life* (pp. 75–107). Baltimore, MD: Johns Hopkins University.

Moss, M. S., Hoffman, C. J., Mossey, J., & Rovine, M. (2007). Changes over 4 years in health, quality of life, mental health, and valuation of life. *Journal of Aging & Health, 19,* 1025–1044.

Oswald, F., & Wahl, H.-W. (2005). Dimensions of the meaning of home in later life. In G. D. Rowles & H. Chaudhury (Eds.), *Home and identity in later life: International perspectives* (pp. 21–46). New York, NY: Springer.

Oswald, F., Jopp, D., Rott, C., & Wahl, H.-W. (2011). Is aging in place a resource for or risk to life satisfaction? *Gerontologist, 51*, 238–250.

Phillips, L. J., Hammock, R. L., & Blanton, J. M. (2005). Predictors of self-rated health status among Texas residents. Prev Chronic Dis [serial online]. Retrieved from URL:http://www.cdc.gov/pcd/issues/2005/oct/04_0147.htm

Phillipson, C., Bernard, M., Phillips, J., & Ogg, J. (2001a). Household structure and social networks in later life. In C. Phillipson, M. Bernard, J. Phillips, J. Ogg (Eds.), *The family and community life of older people: Social networks and social support in three urban areas* (pp. 55–80). New York, NY: Routledge.

Phillipson, C., Bernard, M., Phillips, J., & Ogg, J. (2001b). The social world of older people: The experience of retirement and leisure. In C. Phillipson, M. Bernard, J. Phillips, J. Ogg, (Eds.), *The family and community life of older people: Social networks and social support in three urban areas* (pp. 229–248). New York, NY: Routledge.

Pollack, C. E., & Knesebeck, V. O. (2004). Social capital and health among the aged: comparisons between the United States and Germany. *Health and Place, 10*, 383–391.

Putnam, R. (2000). *Bowling alone: The collapse and revival of American community.* New York, NY: Simon and Schuster.

Putnam, R., Leonardi, R., & Nanetti, R. (1993). *Making democracy work: Civic traditions in modern Italy.* Princeton, NJ: Princeton University.

Radloff, L.S. (1977). The CES-D scale: A self report depression scale for research in the general population. *Applied Psychological Measurement, 1*(3), 385–401.

Scharf, T., Phillipson, C., & Smith, A. (2003). Older people's perceptions of the neighborhood: Evidence from socially deprived urban areas. *Sociological Research Online, 8*(4). Retrieved from http://www.socresonline.org.uk/8/4/scharf.html

Stephens, C. (2008). Social capital in its place: Using social theory to understand social capital and inequalities in health. *Social Science and Medicine, 66*, 1174–1184.

Szreter, S., & Woolcock, M. (2004). Health by association? Social capital, social theory, and the political economy of public health. *International Journal of Epidemiology, 33*, 1–18.

Tabachnick, B. G., & Fidell, L. S. (2001). *Using multivariate statistics* (4th ed.). Boston, MA: Allyn & Bacon.

Thomese, F., & Van Tilburg, T. (2000). Neighbouring networks and environmental dependency. Differential effects of neighborhood characteristics on the relative size and composition of neighbouring networks of older adults in the Netherlands. *Ageing and Society, 20*, 55–78.

Wahl, H.-W., & Oswald, F. (2010). Environmental perspectives on ageing. In D. Dannefer & C. Phillipson (Eds.), *The SAGE handbook of social gerontology* (pp. 111–124). London, United Kingdom: SAGE.

Wahl, H.-W., & Weisman, G. D. (2003). Environmental gerontology at the beginning of the new millennium: Reflections on its historical, empirical, and theoretical development. *Gerontologist, 43*, 616–627.

Walker, R. B., & Hiller, J. (2007). Places and health: A qualitative study to explore how older women living alone perceive the social and physical dimensions of their neighborhoods. *Social Science and Medicine, 65,* 1154–1165.

World Health Organization. (2007). *Global age friendly cities: A guide.* Retrieved from http://www.who.int/ageing/publications/Global_age_friendly_cities_Guide_English.pdf

World Health Organization. (n.d.). *Definition of an older or elderly person.* Retrieved from http://www.who.int/healthinfo/survey/ageingdefnolder/en/index.html

Last Words

RICK J. SCHEIDT and BENYAMIN SCHWARZ

Nearly three dozen researchers and scholars across disciplines of environmental gerontology have offered their views in this special issue of both current activities and future directions in several areas. The authors are all active, productive thinkers who are influential in shaping the current and future status of environmental gerontology. In this final article, we summarize the major suggestions emerging from the five content domains of the special issue and reflect on the future of the field.

PARADIGMS, THEORIES, AND CONTEXT: STOCK-TAKING AND NEW GROUND

Schwarz and Pastalan offer contrasting views about the scientific status of environmental gerontology. Both have their misgivings about "if and whether" environmental gerontology operates out of an appropriate "structural-theoretical" model or paradigm appropriately useful for a science of aging-behavior relations. Schwarz recommends adopting a context-driven perspective that is local in orientation, focusing on practical activity and practical knowledge derived from actual everyday applications. He urges us to apply the case study strategy to purposively selected precedents and exemplars connected to real-life problems.

Pastalan asserts that a radical "rewiring our way of thinking" and argues that conducting science within environmental gerontology is necessary. He believes that paradigm changes in other major fields of science affect not only those specific fields, but also have huge spin-off implications for other fields, including environment–behavior research. He advises environmental gerontologists to explore the new theoretical and empirical fruits emerging from paradigm changes that have occurred in major scientific fields, such as physics, medicine, and communication technology. Thus, cognitive neuroscience and activity pattern analysis of entire populations have rich implications for studying environmental transactions of elders at micro- and macro-levels. It is clear that our discussion of "world views" in environmental gerontology will continue. Discussion might begin with this question: Is the current malaise due to a fundamental failure of dominant paradigms within the field to produce an adequate science for understanding person–environment transactions or to a failure of researchers in the ecology of aging to adequately translate relevant science into terms useful for our more pragmatic disciplines? Perhaps both?

Golant offers an agenda for the future that has immediacy for both understanding and improving residential satisfaction of and by elders. Advancing the constructs of security and autonomy, the sweet spot of residential normalcy occurs when elders emotionally appraise their residence as falling within their personal comfort and mastery zones. This model can easily be translated into more precise theoretical and empirical terms (e.g., unpacking the psychological meaning of emotional experiences, assessing thresholds for comfort zones, refining relationships among components of the model, or linking the subjective appraisals to objective features of the residence). At a broader level, Golant predicts a future where larger numbers of elders will be able to live in their own residences by achieving the appropriate balance between comfort and mastery. Toward this end, he urges environmental gerontologists to be more aggressive in claiming this goal as their intellectual territory.

The agenda set by Geboy, Diaz Moore, and Smith is much in agreement. They also urge environmental gerontologists to redirect attention toward the residential environments of choice of older adults and away from the historical focus on institutions. Their own work illustrates their recommendation for future research in this arena—integrating existing theories in environmental gerontology with a focus on Third Age cohorts seeking a delicate balance on the comfort and mastery teeter-totter. Specifically, they believe that future research on current and emerging models of community-based living should be informed by the eclectic theoretical perspectives within environmental gerontology as well as by lateral areas such as lifespan human development. Interestingly, they advocate for a greater focus on place experience at the group level—beyond individualistic experience—to allow a consensual understanding that might inform improved environmental design.

METHODS AND MEASURES: ISSUES AND APPLICATIONS

Iwarsson's review of the work that she and her colleagues have done with The Housing Enabler illustrates the rewards that extend from excellent training and application of measurement development strategies in the ecology of aging. Based on Lawton and Nahemow's (1973) General Ecological Model, in addition to its historical significance as perhaps the first instrument to assess person–environment fit, it continues to generate data within a coherent strategy involving methodology development, outcome research, and solution-oriented projects. After nearly two decades of work attempting to implement findings from this and other methods into practice settings, she offers observations for researchers and practitioners who might team up to work together in the future.

Oswald and Kaspar share their continuing efforts to inform the construct validity of a measure derived from the multidimensional measure of perceived housing derived from the multinational European ENABLE-AGE study. In addition to the results that emerged from this study, a primary windfall of this effort was the development of an array of unique measures designed to assess both subjective and objective environmental features. Arguably, few researchers have modeled the conceptual and empirical process of concept and measurement development in environmental gerontology as Oswald and Kaspar attempted to do. They promise to continue practicing the less dramatic but essential cycle in environmental measurement, specifying constructs in nominal and operational terms, observing their empirical interactions, providing evidence for supportive validity and stability, and putting them into service in the field.

Using a Delphi technique, Kaup, Proffitt, and Abushousheh generated a practice-based research agenda for long-term care—Culture Change/Household Model—with practitioners and providers, researchers, designers and consultants, policy regulators, and vendors. Their effort is notable at two levels. First in its empirically generated, action-research approach for agenda setting, and second in using populations of experts whose views are rarely considered, much less compared, when establishing targets for future research. Their agenda targets five inductively derived goals for future research involving contributions of both researchers and practitioners, including the promotion of deep system change using socially relevant place types, developing benchmark measures to assess the progress achieved by particular implementation strategies, and how involvement of practitioners can advance research-generated knowledge in long-term care. This is an important treatise for environmental gerontologists interested in forming effective researcher–practitioner partnerships in other settings as well.

TRANSFORMING ENVIRONMENTS: HOME AND COMMUNITY CONTEXTS

Clark and Glicksman's report on the dynamic and exciting Age-friendly Philadelphia (AfP) initiative—one of about 300 existing in the nation—shows how partnerships between policy makers, planners, researchers, and indigenous organizations and agencies can transform the physical and social environments of entire communities to create neighborhood cohesion and to support independence of elderly residents. Their case study offers a roadmap for this particular effort, illustrating how practice initiatives may be established among researchers, planners, policymakers, and local organizations.

This project illustrates how researchers can "collaborate around aging issues," although many of the AfP initiatives are generically targeted to benefit citizens of all ages. One of the most challenging future tasks for these partnerships is evaluation, including operational criteria for progress, sorting out determinants of change, and considerations regarding whether diverse and context-bound initiatives have features of generalizable processes and lessons across environments that range in scale from the supra-personal to the personal.

Pynoos and his colleagues deal with a much more pointed target—fall prevention—but lay out in a similar way a detailed future agenda that involves direct and indirect partnerships between practitioners, policymakers, public health experts, aging services, housing specialists, and researchers. They present interesting recommendations for researchers and practitioners who inform their work with data. For instance, they suggest that programs serving older adults should have access to research results that are both widely disseminated and easy to understand. Among the many useful recommendations, they also suggest new sources of data collection about falls, such as EMT personnel as well as emergency room discharge data, and advocate development of measures that might be used to collect better data.

From the perspectives of an adult daughter and as one familiar with the language of aging in place, Tofle offers a close-up, personal account of the transition of her mother "from living independently, to hospital, to nursing home, to grave." Her phenomenological case study recounts her own transition as well, as she accompanies her mother on her journey to death, launched by a stark awareness that "I know this is the last time she will walk out of her own home." Her story is an eloquent reminder that environmental gerontologists must be aware of the fuller meanings of home and community context. In this instance, family members, terminally ill older relatives, and professionals who are total strangers do the hard work of creating physical, social, and psychological contexts that make "a good death" possible. Tofle's account reminds us that among the "terms of the person" in the ecological equation, the perceived or personal environment is more than a phrase. As seen through this case study, the motif of aging and dying, to use her terms, offers rich ground for the study of generational relationships, the meanings of housing transitions for both elderly individuals and their families, ethical conundrums involving short-term life extension, and how these partnerships may create places that support successful dying.

TRANSFORMING ENVIRONMENTS: CARE-BASED SETTINGS

Lemke offers a brief history of the evolution of nursing home care within the Department of Veterans Affairs (VA) from its post-Civil War birth as the

National Home to the 133 facilities now called community living centers. Clearly, when viewed from the long historical perspective, the extent and quality of care for elderly veterans has improved dramatically. VA long-term care has adopted the culture change model of resident-oriented care, and Lemke describes the tension within the VA system regarding this model of nursing care within the broader infrastructure of the VA medical centers. Those familiar with the culture change model are aware of the challenges that exist in the everyday attempts to balance resident autonomy with safety and security. Lemke's progress report on VA efforts to successfully install the model in its community living centers provides a documentation of change referenced against non-community living centers facilities. She moves beyond anecdotal examples of success and includes data drawn from measures designed to track change in several domains. She provides a case study of a community living center facility that has had award-winning success and describes a recently launched modular free-standing "small home" model (Green House home). In the VA assessment approach, structure and process measures are linked to desired and measured outcomes.

Culture change attempts to replace the depriving environmental conditions associated with the total institution or medical model of long-term care. However, at the community level the goal of environmental design is not to replace a faulty model with a better one, but rather to sustain a model of residential normalcy that simultaneously accommodates the functional losses experienced by older residents. Regnier and Danes share their views and their work in this regard. Regnier outlines features and advantages of "the northern European model" (and variants) as an option deserving of greater attention in the United States. In contrast to the prevalent U.S. model where "care institutions have separated themselves from the surrounding context and operate like mini-hospitals," Regnier discusses the advantages for older residents, many of whom have memory problems, of living in small group clusters containing 10 to 12 people connected to their neighborhoods through ad hoc service and care systems. "Choice is respected and you live in a more 'normal' environment with friends for which you have a reciprocal obligation to help and feel appreciated and valued. ... You make people feel as if they have control over living a satisfying lifestyle that is not that different than what they've had during the first 75 years of life." At another level, he discusses how small, novel changes in the social environments of culture change nursing homes can make powerful differences for residents on an everyday level.

Danes, who is from the Perkins Eastman Research Collaborative, illustrates lessons learned from the design of Woodside Place and adaptations to three other facilities for people with dementia. She notes the importance of taking into account the broader socio-historical and cohort-related forces that pose challenges to design for residents with dementia. These include advances in our knowledge of Alzheimer's disease, pressures to produce affordable long-term dementia care, higher levels of impairment of residents at entrance, alternative community-based residential care for elders with dementia and memory problems, and how cultural traditions affect the portability of Western models of dementia care to other settings. Danes offers a guide book of lessons gleaned from her post-occupancy evaluations conducted within Woodside Place and its successors. Given the increasing trend for provision of community-based care around the "aging-in-place" Zeitgeist, she demonstrates how specific features of the Woodside Place model has been useful for informing the design of dementia care units in two new community-based settings—a customized single-family house that would allow "a person with dementia to continue to live at home with a spouse or caregiver as opposed to moving into a care facility"—and a daycare facility with an apartment for a resident caretaker. Still in the planning stages, Danes notes that these projects "suggest prospectively what the next generation of dementia care facilities may offer."

INTO THE LIGHT: POPULATIONS AND TOPICS DESERVING MORE ATTENTION

Three other contributions to this special issue illustrate issues that should be on the to do lists of environmental gerontologists. Scheidt and Norris-Baker urge environmental gerontologists to set an agenda for future research that includes understudied older populations and contexts. They discuss the benefits of studying relatively ignored populations for applied science predominantly focused on an "environmental gerontology of the usual." They present a more detailed agenda for research on older male and female prisoners, as well as older residents of small, dying rural communities or "ghost towns." Other populations include aging adults with intellectual disabilities and developmental delays, migrating and migrant elders (including illegal immigrants), older Native Americans, and "avatar" elders who create and occupy social worlds in virtual environments.

Despite an active record of research in social gerontology on age stereotyping and negative implicit age-related attitudes (self-stigmatization), surprisingly little research exists within environmental gerontology on place-associated stigma, the individual and environmental dynamics that in its creation, and how it affects both the labeler and the targets—whether an individual or a setting. This may be an arena where place- or resident-associated stigma affects researchers and stigmatized populations, reducing the likelihood of attention from environmental gerontologists as well. We suspect this is one of the reasons why the field has seen so little research on older prisoners and, to some extent, on residents of dying communities. Hrybyk and collegues provide an in-depth ethnographic record of the dynamics of stigma operating within 2 (of 7) collective living environments for older adults—which they term "the dark side." Both settings, one purpose-built and the other an older affinity setting, contained independent living and assisted living residential levels. "Othering" occurred among independent living residents toward assisted living movers and, especially in the purpose-built setting, toward the assisted living space itself. These researchers provide anecdotal evidence of the harmful effects of stigmatizing behavior on the health of the residents. They urge further study of the ways that the built environment shapes the culture it contains and of the factors that can "mitigate or aggravate stigma" in order to improve the lives of residents of these settings.

Norstrand and her colleagues make a case for more considered research on an important but understudied aspect of the social environment—social capital. Their empirical data show relatively small effects of a multi-faceted measure of social capital on physical and mental health for a large 5-county sample of older Pennsylvanians. They urge future research on the construct, including improved measurement, prior to studying its impact on relevant and adequate empirical measures of physical and mental health. The authors also call for examination of the place of social capital in environment–aging theories. Inserting multi-faceted environmental indicators in quantitative algorithms or appreciating environmental conditions revealed in ethnographic research will provide fuller meaning for the construct. For example, viewing social capital as an expendable commodity is useful for understanding why older volunteers in economically threatened, underpopulated small towns often over-invest themselves in ways that lead to burnout.

THE BROADER HORIZON

Amalgamating the various approaches to environmental gerontology in this compendium is not an easy task. Still, a few themes emerge from the diverse contributions. From a theoretical perspective, the special issue echoes the major contrasts in the larger field of gerontology as expressed by Gans, Putney, Bengtson, and Silverstein (2009): (1) Should researchers in the field focus on large, overarching theories or should theorizing in environmental gerontology be limited to single aspects of environment–person relationships? (2) Faced with the growing uncertainty in the lives of older adults due to globalization, economic uncertainty, and the shifting welfare programs and old age policies, should the field emphasize predictability in the positivist approach or develop strategies to deal with the challenges of uncertainty? (3) Should the field focus on variability rather than universality? Is it feasible to claim universality in a field that is so firmly linked to specific settings and contexts?

Perhaps the most significant theme that emerges from the writings is the significance of cross-disciplinarity. Clearly, research on the person–environment transaction can considerably benefit from collaboration among researchers and practitioners from various disciplines. Several articles in the special issue illustrate that most, if not all, researchers in environmental gerontology have moved away from the uni-disciplinary model. Authors recognize the importance of cross-fertilization among disciplines in the search for explanations and theories in the study of environment and aging. One can anticipate that the trend will intensify in the future as disciplines will be forced to transgress their internal and external boundaries in search for research opportunities in the public open space and garner financial support. We believe that researchers in environmental gerontology have positioned themselves in the right place in anticipation for this dynamic future.

Simultaneously, a growing recognition exists among scholars in the field that applied research and knowledge production in the context of application are essential to the future of this discipline. These developments occur despite the challenging relationships between basic research and practice. The tension between theoretical knowledge and application in practice may still linger because the demand for practical solutions tends to surpass the capacities of basic science to deliver them. As Lawton (1990) observed in reference to the design of housing for the elderly: "[t]he researcher faces the dilemma of communicating unsatisfying small amounts of knowledge delivered from research that meets acceptable methodological standards or, on the other hand, going significantly beyond the data so as to provide concrete design assistance. Either way someone loses, the practitioner in frustration over the limited amount of guidance available from the academic, or the researcher in risking loss of integrity in going beyond the data" (p. 351). However, to successfully manage forces interested in knowledge in the context of application, as indicated in many of the articles, more scholars will have to move their research work to contexts of application. Furthermore, knowledge in context is rarely uni-disciplinary knowledge. Rather it is located in multi-disciplinary context, which justify the cross-disciplinary model described above. In addition, this type of knowledge is expected to work and is accepted as relevant in the context of application. That is, it is knowledge tested by practitioners who are in a position where the results of the practice determine if the knowledge is workable.

Alan Kay, the American computer scientist, noted that "the best way to predict the future is to invent it." We hope this special issues makes this contribution to environmental gerontology.

REFERENCES

Gans, D., Putney, N. M., Bengtson, V. L., & Silverstein, M. (2009). The future of theories of aging. In V. L. Bengtson, M. Silverstein, N. M. Putney, & D. Gans (Eds.), *Handbook of theories of aging* (2nd ed., pp. 723–737). New York, NY: Springer.

Lawton, M.P., & Nahemow, L. (1973). Ecology and the aging process. In C. Eisdorfer & M. P. Lawton (Eds.), *Psychology of adult development and aging* (pp. 619–674). Washington, DC: American Psychological Association.

Lawton, M. P. (1990). An environmental psychologist ages. In I. Altman & K. Christensen (Eds.), *Environment and behavior studies: Emergence of intellectual traditions* (pp. 339–363). New York, NY: Plenum Press.

Index